MUSCULOSKELETAL RADIOLOGY

MUSCULOSKELETAL RADIOLOGY

HARRY GRIFFITHS

University of Florida
Jacksonville, Florida, USA

informa

healthcare

New York London

Informa Healthcare USA, Inc.
52 Vanderbilt Avenue
New York, NY 10017

© 2008 by Informa Healthcare USA, Inc.
Informa Healthcare is an Informa business

No claim to original U.S. Government works
Printed in the United States of America on acid-free paper
10 9 8 7 6 5 4 3 2 1

International Standard Book Number-10: 0-8493-9390-6 (Hardcover)
International Standard Book Number-13: 978-0-8493-9390-7 (Hardcover)

Library of Congress Cataloging-in-Publication Data

Griffiths, Harry J.
   Musculoskeletal radiology / Harry Griffiths.
      p. ; cm.
   Includes bibliographical references and index.
   ISBN-13: 978-0-8493-9390-7 (hardcover : alk. paper)
   ISBN-10: 0-8493-9390-6 (hardcover : alk. paper) 1. Musculoskeletal
system—Imaging. 2. Musculoskeletal system—Diseases—Diagnosis. I.
Title.
   [DNLM: 1. Musculoskeletal Diseases—diagnosis. 2. Diagnostic
Imaging—methods. WE 141 G855m 2008]
   RC925.7.G74   2008
   616.7'07548—dc22
                                                      2008029126

For Corporate Sales and Reprint Permissions call 212-520-2700 or write to: Sales Department, 52 Vanderbilt Avenue, 16th floor, New York, NY 10017.

**Visit the Informa Web site at
www.informa.com**

**and the Informa Healthcare Web site at
www.informahealthcare.com**

This book is dedicated to all my fellows, residents and medical students from whom I have always learnt a lot and who have helped keep me young.

Preface

This book is based on over 35 years of being involved with academic musculoskeletal (MSK) radiology. The text incorporates much of my old "plain film" teaching collection with my extensive experience with CT, MRI, and other special procedures involving the MSK system. I have also been involved with orthopaedists from the start, and in fact while I was at the Peter Bent Brigham, Clem Sledge had me elected to the American Association of Orthopaedic Surgeons—at that time one of only four radiologists to be a member of that prestigious organization. Thus, I have an extensive knowledge of orthopaedic devices and their history over the past 35 years—hence the chapter on orthopedic hardware. In my present department, we perform over 100 bone and soft tissue biopsies every year as well as many arthrograms usually prior to MRIs and joint aspirations, some of which are performed under ultrasound guidance. My special academic interests will become obvious to the reader but include bone and soft-tissue tumors, rheumatology, and sports medicine. Yet in the old days, I did a lot of paediatric radiology and collected a huge number of the bone dysplasias, hence the fairly extensive coverage of these rare conditions, which are no longer on the American boards exam. With this in mind, the book is intended to be both inclusive and up-to-date.

On the one hand, some of my views are controversial and do not coincide with what is in the literature. This is not necessarily perversity on my behalf but extensive practical experience and knowledge of that particular topic. On the other hand, "new" conditions are described every day, although many can be found in the older literature under different names, the latest being ace tabular impingement syndrome, which is not in this book—yet. I hope you enjoy reading this book as much as I had fun putting a lifetime's experience into one volume.

The intended audience for this book includes radiologists and radiological residents, orthopaedists and orthopaedic residents, physical medicine physicians and physiatrists and their residents, as well as osteopathic doctors and their residents. Chiropractors who want an up-to-date and comprehensive MSK text should also be interested in reading this book.

ACKNOWLEDGMENTS

I cannot possibly thank all the people who have helped me over the years, but naming a few names is appropriate. I was taught by all the giants in the field including Ronald Murray, Frank Doyle, John Kirkpatrick, Bill Martell, Bob Wilkinson, and Harold

Jacobson. Over the years, I have relied on the friendship and support of Don Resnick, Harry Genant, Lee Rogers, Murali Sundaram, Murray Dalinka, and too many others to name individually in the United States. In the United Kingdom, Ian Beggs, Iain McCall, Jake Davidson, and Ian Watt have usually managed to keep me honest! My particular group of "cronies" also need to be mentioned by name—Henry Jones, Ann Brower, and Stanley Bohrer, with whom I enjoyed many good ISS meetings, not to mention excellent food and wine. The book began in Minneapolis where Clemmer Wait who was my secretary at that time and remains a good friend did all the original typing. When I eventually moved down to Florida and started work on the book again, Jim Perin did all the work of putting the text and illustrations together for the publisher—a computer-based task that I would be totally incapable of undertaking! I would particularly like to thank the production team at Informa Healthcare, both Joseph Stubenrauch and Naman Mahisauria, who were very considerate and helpful.

Finally, I would like to convey my special thanks to Jim Perin, M.D., Lori Deitte, M.D., and Clemmer Wait, M.S. for the extraordinary help in completing this publication.

Harry Griffiths

Contents

1

Trauma

TRAUMA

Although many people have attempted to classify fractures, I believe that this is unnecessary, except perhaps in the ankle, where the mechanism of the injury is important for us to understand the fracture pattern. Elsewhere, we should simply describe the fracture. For example, is it transverse, vertical, spiral, or oblique? Is it comminuted or not (so-called simple)? Does it involve the joint, i.e., is it intra-articular? The question of it being compound (i.e., connects to the outside world) or not is usually a clinical and not a radiological one. If it is comminuted, we should describe any large, triangular fragments, which are known as butterfly fragments. In fact, most fractures are comminuted and are either oblique or spiral. Most fractures near the ends of long bones are intra-articular and thus more difficult to manage and treat. But that does not mean that you do not have to specifically look for that finding.

There are some basic rules: First, always take the proximal body part as being in the correct anatomical position, and refer the position and angulation of the distal body part to the proximal part, i.e., describe fractures of the foot with relation to the ankle and the proximal tibia to the distal femur or knee joint. Secondly, there is a concept of a "ring of bone" where, if one bone of a pair or one part of a ring gets fractured, then the other either fractures or subluxes. The pelvis is also a ring of bone, so always look for more than one fracture. The classical example of the former is the radius and ulna and the tibia and fibula.

These will all be discussed in the appropriate subsections later in the chapter.

If there is a dislocation, look for concomitant fractures and describe the distal dislocated bone with respect to its anatomic relationship to the proximal undislocated side of the joint. For example, in anterior dislocations of the shoulder, the humeral head lies anterior to the glenoid. And, in anterior dislocations of the tibiotalar joint, the foot lies anterior to the distal tibia.

Other types of fractures occur, particularly in children, where we can see greenstick and torus fractures as well as fractures of the growth plate (Salter fractures). Once again, all of these will be discussed later in this chapter. Athletes get what are known as avulsion fractures where, for instance, the olecranon is avulsed off the proximal ulna by the pull of the triceps tendon, or the ischial tuberosity is avulsed off the ischium by the pull of the hamstring muscles. Salter fractures are classified depending on where the fracture line runs.

Type I	Through the growth plate (GP). These can often be difficult to see radiologically (S).
Type II	Through the GP with an extension through the metaphysis (A).
Type III	Through the epiphysis (L).
Type IV	Fracture through both the metaphysis and epiphysis (T).
Type V	Severe injury through the GP so that the child needs to go to the emergency room (ER).

So what does SALTER spell ??? This is an easy way to remember the classification.

Stress and insufficiency fractures also need to be considered in athletes for the former and in patients with osteopenia for the latter. Pseudofractures can be seen in rickets and hyperparathyroidism, mainly secondary to renal failure. Incremental fractures are seen in those metabolic diseases that cause bowing of long bones, such as Paget's disease and fibrous dysplasia. Pathological fractures are seen in association with any form of weakness in the bone, typically in association with metastases, primary bone tumors, and infections.

The complications of fractures also need to be considered. The acute complications include pneumothorax seen with rib fractures, arterial damage in comminuted proximal tibial fractures, or urethral damage in fractures around the symphysis pubis. Late complications include nonunion, avascular necrosis and infections. Each of these complications needs to be looked for as the fracture is healing.

Finally, although many of these findings can be seen on plain films, sometimes it is necessary to use computed tomography (CT) scanning or radionuclide bone scans to confirm the presence of a fracture or the configuration of fracture fragments. For example, CT scanning is essential in all complex pelvic fractures and in most shoulder girdle fractures. Bone scanning is useful in suspected sacral fractures as well as in stress fractures, although magnetic resonance imaging (MRI) is just as sensitive, but more specific.

A brief description of fracture healing is also useful so that the radiologist will know what to expect. Classically, there are three phases of healing: the inflammatory phase (usually 1–3 weeks), the reparative phase (3–8 weeks), and the remodeling phase (8 weeks onward). Healing obviously takes longer in older people than in the young, longer in large bones than in small ones, and longer in major fractures than in minor ones. Radiologically, the first signs of healing are the resorption of bone around the fracture site (i.e., increasing lucency and bone resorption). This is then followed by new bone formation, both periosteal and endosteal.

Once remodeling has started, the healing process can be clearly followed by radiographs. The late complications such as infection, nonunion, and avascular necrosis become obvious over time, but must be considered, particularly in association with specific fractures, i.e., nonunion of the tibia, avascular necrosis of the proximal pole of the scaphoid, and avascular necrosis of the femoral head in transcervical fractures of the femoral neck. Following fractures of weight-bearing bones, disuse osteoporosis is inevitable, becoming obvious by four weeks and usually reaching a peak by three months. Disuse osteoporosis is more unusual in fractures of the upper extremity, although it can be seen in elderly patients with distal radial fractures. A fairly common complication of fractures must also be looked for, and that is what appears to be delayed disuse osteoporosis. This is a specific syndrome known as Sudek's atrophy or, more correctly now, as *reflex sympathetic dystrophy*,

which starts at three months and reaches a peak at about one year. This will be discussed later. Finally, the management of fractures with internal fixation will be briefly discussed in chapter 7.

Nonunion of a fracture can be a difficult diagnosis to make, since one of the stages of healing is fibrous union. So, how can a radiologist make a competent, confident diagnosis of nonunion: only if both ends of the fractured bone develop sclerotic margins and especially if motion can be seen through the fracture site. Most radiologists will use the term "delayed union" rather than nonunion if they are not completely sure of the diagnosis. More recently, MRI has been used to determine if solid fibrous tissue has occurred across the fracture site or not, and this might be the way to go in the future.

SHOULDER

The Shoulder Girdle

The shoulder girdle consists of three bones and two joints: the scapula, the clavicle, and the proximal humerus, as well as the glenohumeral and acromioclavicular joints. Most fractures of the clavicle occur either in the midshaft or the distal end, mainly because the coracoclavicular ligament is fan shaped and is rather strong, so the fractures occur at either side of this (Fig. 1A, B).

There is an old orthopedic aphorism that states that fractures of the clavicle will reunite if they are in the same room. However, this is not entirely true, and occasionally one can see a nonunion, probably as a result of a soft-tissue interposition.

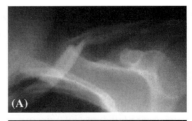

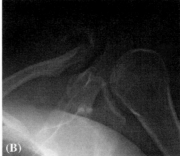

Figure 1 (**A**) There is a midshaft fracture of the clavicle with some angulation. (**B**) There is a fracture of the distal clavicle with evidence of motion.

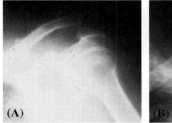 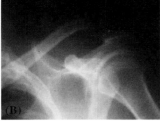

Figure 2 (**A**) There is a grade III acromioclavicular joint separation (*arrow*). (**B**) There is a grade III acromioclavicular joint separation.

There are three grades of separation of the acromioclavicular joint: grade I, with a 50% overlap; grade II, no overlap, but no upward displacement; and grade III, with at least 1 cm of upward displacement of the distal clavicle (Fig. 2A, B).

Grade III implies that there are complete tears of the collateral ligaments of the joint, as well as a tear of the coracoclavicular ligament. In grade I injuries, it is customary to x-ray both sides on the same film (the other, normal, side for comparison) and to take a film with and without the patient carrying a 10-lb weight in each hand, which exaggerates any acromioclavicular separation that may be present.

The Sternoclavicular Joint and Proximal Clavicle

The sternoclavicular joint is rarely involved in trauma unless a direct blow is sustained. However, resorption of the sternoclavicular joint occurs in renal bone disease and osteolysis of the proximal clavicle as well as septic arthritis of the sternoclavicular joint can be seen in diabetics, drug users, and in patients with in-dwelling catheters. Involvement of the sternoclavicular joint with new bone formation is an integral part of the SAPHO (Synovitis, Acne, Palmarplantar Pustolosis, Hyperostosis, Osteitis) syndrome, which will be dealt with later. However, occasionally, posterior dislocation of the sternoclavicular joint does occur and is frequently difficult to diagnose on plain film. Nowadays, CT scanning is probably the best way to determine if a fracture or a dislocation has occurred.

Fractures of the Scapula

Fractures of the scapula are not as rare as once thought. They usually occur as a result of a direct blow, either to the blade of the scapula from behind or to one of its component parts such as the coracoid process or the acromion (Fig. 3A, B).

In patients with severe trauma, scapular fractures are frequently missed for days, if not weeks, mainly because the musculature surrounding the bone is inclined to hold the fracture fragments in close apposition. The diagnosis can be confirmed by special views, including the scapula

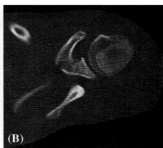 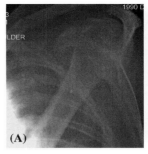

Figure 3 Fracture of the base of the glenoid and acromion. (**A**) Scapula "Y" view. (**B**) CT scan. *Abbreviation*: CT, computed tomography.

"Y" view. Once again, CT scanning can be useful in confirming any fracture that may be suspected.

Scapular fractures represent 1% of all fractures involving the skeleton. Ten percent of these involve the glenoid, of which 10% are displaced. Ninety percent of scapular fractures are associated with other injuries: ipsilateral rib fractures in 50%, humeral fractures in 35%, lung injury and/ or pneumothorax in 25%, and clavicle fractures in 25%.

There are a number of classifications of glenoid fractures. One of the accepted ones is by Ideberg, which had four different types. Recently, Heggland has modified this classification to describe six different types of glenoid fracture:

1. Type I—(a) anterior glenoid rim avulsion fracture associated with an anterior shoulder dislocation. These are common and actually represent what we know as a Bankart lesion (Fig. 4). (b) posterior glenoid rim avulsion fracture.
2. Type II—transverse fracture through the glenoid fossa with downward displacement of the glenohumeral joint.
3. Type III—transverse fracture of the glenoid fossa with cephalad oblique extension through the neck of the scapula (Fig. 5A, B).

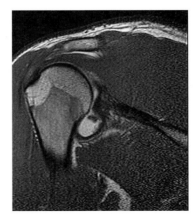

Figure 4 Bankart lesion. On this paracoronal slice from an MR image, a separated fracture fragment can be seen off the distal part of the glenoid. This is typical of a Bankart lesion. *Abbreviation*: MR, magnetic resonance.

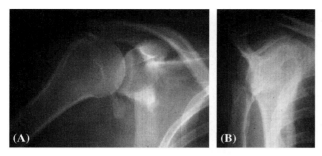

Figure 5 (A, B) Tranverse glenoid fracture.

4. Type IV—transverse fracture of the glenoid fossa continuing through the neck and the body of the scapula.
5. Type V—combined fractures.
6. Type VI—severely comminuted fractures.

Fractures of the Proximal Humerus

The proximal humerus is much more vulnerable, and fractures of the humeral neck are common in the elderly. These are usually seen in patients with profound osteopenia who fall on their outstretched hand. The fracture involves the thinned metaphyseal trabecular bone and impacts with a buckle often seen on the inner surface of the humerus. True fractures of the humeral head are seen as a result of direct trauma, and, some years ago, Neer proposed a classification on the basis of number of parts (or fragments) (Fig. 6).

However, this has recently been invalidated by the orthopedic community, so there is little need for radiologists to learn this classification. Eighty percent of fractures involving the proximal humerus are either undisplaced or only minimally displaced. Fractures may be of the surgical neck (transverse metaphyseal), anatomic neck (oblique through the remnant of the growth plate), greater tuberosity, or lesser tuberosity (Figs. 7 and 8).

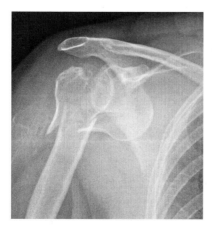

Figure 6 Comminuted humeral head fracture.

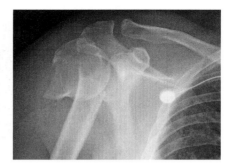

Figure 7 Surgical neck fracture of the proximal humerus in an overweight 65-year-old lady who fell on her shoulder. Note the overlapping of the fracture fragments as well as the rotation of the proximal fragment.

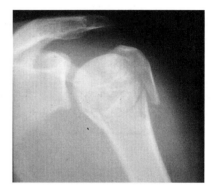

Figure 8 Greater tuberosity fracture. There is a vertical, linear fracture of the greater tuberosity with some upward displacement. Note that the fracture is basically held in place by an intact deltoid muscle.

At least two of these may occur at the same time, and any of them can also be associated with subluxation or actual dislocation of the glenohumeral joint. On the other hand, isolated fractures of the greater tuberosity are not uncommon and may be difficult to see because of the pressure of the deltoid muscle surrounding the proximal humerus that keeps them in place. Isolated fractures of the lesser tuberosity are rare and are also difficult to diagnose unless the anatomy is carefully studied. In young people, most humeral fractures heal well without complications. Badly comminuted fractures of the humeral head are often difficult to repair and so the head will be replaced with an endoprosthesis.

Shoulder Dislocations

Dislocations of the glenohumeral joint are quite common, particularly anterior dislocations, which account for 90% of all shoulder dislocations. The humeral head is pulled medially and downward and thus is easy to diagnose both clinically and radiologically (Fig. 9A, B, C, D).

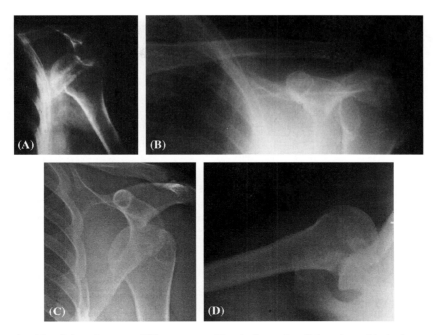

Figure 9 (**A**) Anterior shoulder dislocation, two different cases. Classical anterior dislocation with the humeral head being displaced medially and inferiorly below the glenoid. Note the large Hill-Sachs deformity. (**B**) and (**C**) A second patient once again showing the classical anterior displacement of the humeral head below the glenoid. (**D**) Axial view, which shows that the humeral head lying anterior to the glenoid.

On the whole, a single anterior dislocation does little damage apart from stretching the capsule and bruising. However, recurrent dislocation leads to flattening on the posterolateral surface of the humeral head (known as a Hill-Sachs deformity) and to irregularity of the inferior glenoid surface, as well as loss of the inferior glenoid labrum (a Bankart lesion) (Fig. 4).

Hill-Sachs deformity was first described in 1940 and usually occurs as a result of recurrent dislocations where significant defects occur in at least 60% of patients. In a patient with a first-time dislocation, significant Hill-Sachs deformities are rare. They occur because the upper posterior surface of the humeral head impacts against the anterior inferior surface of the glenoid labrum. This will ultimately cause damage to the glenoid and lead to a so-called *Bankart lesion*. Most Bankart lesions cannot be seen on plain film since they are entirely cartilaginous, although the majority of Hill-Sachs lesions are bony and thus obvious. Recurrent dislocations are common in young people, with a stated incidence of 80% in patients younger than 20 years, but only 10% in those older than 40 years. Following initial plain film evaluation, MRI is now the investigative procedure of choice to demonstrate the anatomy following recurrent shoulder dislocations.

Posterior shoulder dislocations are quite difficult to diagnose; in fact, about 60% are missed on the initial set of radiographs (Fig. 10A, B, C, D).

But, if one remembers, we should be able to see a space between the articular surface of the humeral head and the articular surface of the glenoid fossa because of the presence of articular cartilage; if a radiograph apparently shows overlapping of the glenoid and the humeral head, it is likely that a posterior dislocation is present. This can be confirmed by a number of views, including a scapula Y view, a Grashey view, or an axillary view, which will show the humeral head to lie posteriorly. There are few complications of posterior dislocation of the shoulder, apart from stretching the joint capsule and bruising, although occasionally the force of the dislocation may cause damage to the glenoid labrum.

There is one rare dislocation of the glenohumeral joint caused by major axial trauma to the arm, such as is seen in a patient who falls off a ladder or a roof head downward with the arm outstretched. This inferior dislocation occurs in less than 1% of all shoulder dislocations and is known as *luxatio erecta* (Fig. 11A, B).

Unlike either anterior or posterior dislocations, luxatio erecta is associated with severe damage to the brachial plexus and to the axillary vessels.

HUMERAL SHAFT FRACTURES

These may be transverse, oblique, or spiral, and simple or comminuted (Fig. 12).

In the upper humerus, the upper fragment is usually pulled inward by the pectoral muscles, whereas the distal fragment is pulled outward by the triceps muscle.

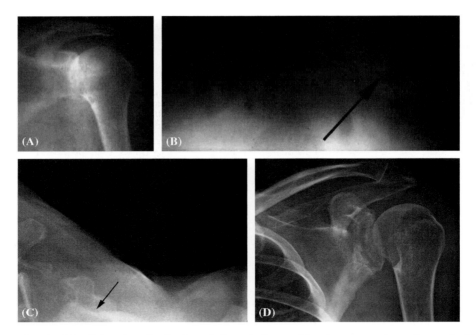

Figure 10 (**A**) Posterior shoulder dislocation. On the frontal view, the humeral head appears to be well seated, although it appears to be overlying the glenoid. (**B**) Axial view nicely shows that the humeral head lies behind the glenoid fossa. (**C**) Axial view in a different patient nicely shows that the humeral head lies behind the glenoid fossa. (**D**) Posterior shoulder dislocation. Frontal view, the humeral head appears to be well seated, although it appears to be overlying the glenoid.

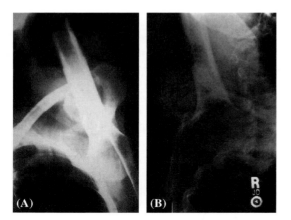

Figure 11 Luxatio erecta. (**A**) Note that the humeral head lies below the glenoid and between the blade of the scapula and the rib cage. (**B**) This oblique view confirms the diagnosis.

ELBOW

Most of the fractures that adults sustain around the elbow joint are in the proximal radius and ulna, whereas most of the fractures that one sees in children are in the distal humerus. Whatever the type of fracture, if it is intra-articular, then an effusion should be easily apparent on a good lateral flexed view. The anterior fat pad can often be seen in normal people as a vertical fat stripe in front of the distal humerus. The posterior fat pad is virtually never seen in people without effusions. When an effusion is present,

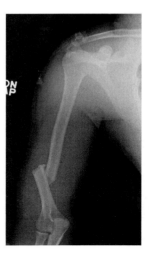

Figure 12 Transverse fracture of the distal humeral shaft with typical overlap and angulation of the two fracture fragments caused by the pull of the respective muscles, with the upper humerus being pulled inward and the lower humerus being pulled outward.

the anterior fat pad is pushed upward and outward and resembles the sail of a sailing ship (*the "sail" sign*) and the posterior fat pad is pushed outward and somewhat upward to appear more like a reversed comma (Fig. 13A, B).

However, if the joint capsule becomes torn, it is possible to have an intra-articular fracture involving the elbow joint without an obvious effusion, and although this is rare, it occurs frequently enough for one to be cautious.

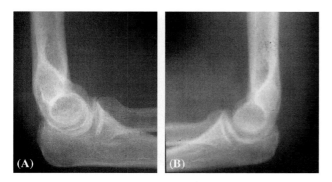

Figure 13 (**A** and **B**) Both of these patients have elbow effusions with a large sail sign anteriorly and a visible fat pad posteriorly. *Source*: From Ref. 1.

Fractures of the distal humerus in adults may be horizontal (in which case they are rarely intra-articular), T shaped, Y shaped, or unicondylar (Fig. 14).

None of these are particularly common, and most of these are obvious radiographically. On the other hand, supracondylar fractures in children are very common and can be particularly difficult to diagnose. In very young children, it is well worth remembering that if one drops a vertical line down the anterior cortex of the humerus on

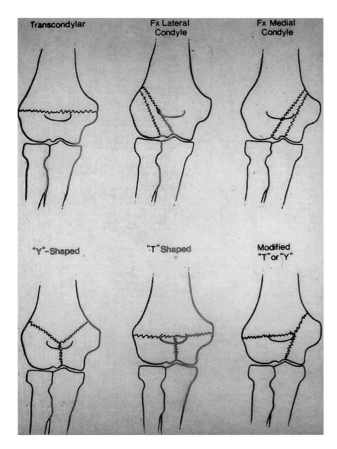

Figure 14 Fractures of the distal humerus. *Source*: Courtesy of Lee Rogers, MD.

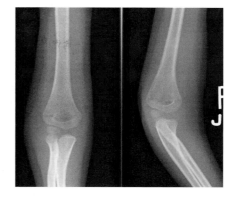

Figure 15 Supracondylar fracture of the elbow. This is the typical transverse supracondylar fracture of the elbow seen in children with posterior displacement of the distal fragments on the proximal ones.

the lateral view, this should bisect the condyles or, to be exact, go through the middle third of the capitellum. This line can be used at any age, but is most useful in children younger than four years. A second line (the radiocapitellar line) should run up the shaft of the radius and bisect the capitellum on every view (Fig. 15).

For a fuller understanding of distal humeral fractures in children, knowledge of the age of appearance of the various ossification centers is useful, and many people use a mnemonic CRITO: capitellum, one year; internal (medial) epicondyle, seven years; trochlear, 10 years; and external (lateral or outer) epicondyle, 11 years. In other words, concerning the distal humerus, 1-7-10-11 done in the form of an "X" (Fig. 16).

Supracondylar fractures in children represent over 60% of fractures about the elbow. If an effusion is present and the two lines are drawn, most of them are easy to see. If necessary, one can always x-ray the other side for comparison. Supracondylar fractures in children may also be horizontal, Y shaped, or T shaped. The most common site of injury in the distal humerus is the medial epicondyle, which is the site of attachment of the ulnar collateral ligaments. Avulsion injuries are common and may be difficult to diagnose. Most importantly, the medial epicondyle can get pulled off and drawn into the joint where it gets trapped. Surprisingly, this is difficult to diagnose in children younger than 12 years, because one can mistake the avulsed fragment as a trochlear growth center; however, this does not appear until the age of 10 years. One final pediatric injury that is also characteristic is the so-called *nursemaid's elbow,* which is seen in children aged two to five years and is caused by the radial head slipping out from under the annular ligament and getting trapped in the joint, leading to pain (Fig. 17A, B).

This is usually diagnosed by the technician who has noticed that the child's arm is rotated and flexed. In fact, in attempting to straighten the arm to take the film, the

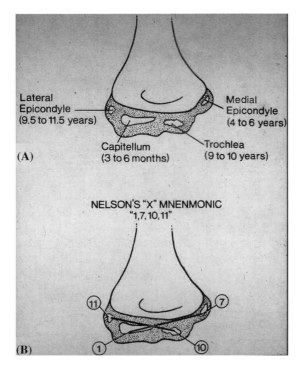

Figure 16 Ossification centers of the distal humerus. *Source*: From Ref. 1.

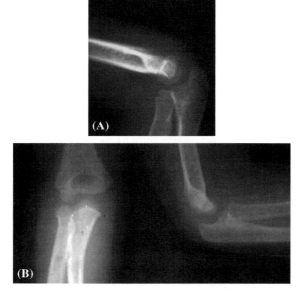

Figure 17 Nursemaid's elbow. (**A**) On the initial lateral film, the radius does not line up with the capitellum—it lies above it. (**B**) The radio-capitellar joint has been relocated.

technician will often relocate the elbow joint. Radiographically, the radiocapitellar line will be intact on the lateral view, but the two bones will not line up on the anteroposterior (AP) view.

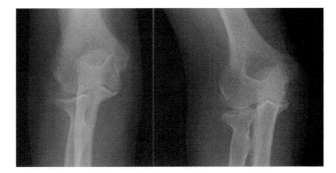

Figure 18 Radial head fracture. This is a segmental fracture of the radial head following a fall on the elbow.

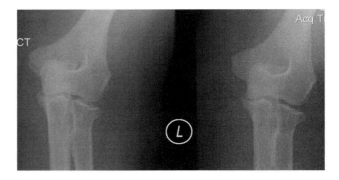

Figure 19 Radial head fracture. This is a segmental fracture of the radial head, following a fall on the elbow in a different patient.

Fractures of the radial head account for approximately 60% of all elbow fractures in adults. Many of these are virtually undisplaced and may be very difficult to see, although the patient will have an effusion (Fig. 13). Special views such as the notch view and the internal oblique view can help in the diagnosis, although sometimes one has to wait 10 to 14 days and to re-x-ray the patient to confirm the fracture. Fractures of the radial head may be simple or comminuted, vertical or horizontal (through the neck), or incremental (like a piece of pie) (Figs. 18 and 19).

They may be impacted, or the radial head may be fragmented. Most heal without complication, although sometimes it is necessary to remove the entire radial head if the fracture is very comminuted and to replace it with a prosthesis.

Fractures of the proximal ulna are also common (over 20% of injuries to the adult elbow). They are often of the avulsion type of fracture, with the force of the triceps tendon pulling the avulsed fragment upward. Some are only minimally displaced, but most of them need to be internally fixed with tension wiring and screws. Fractures of the coronoid process can also occur, but are usually without much consequence if isolated. Fractures of the radial head and proximal ulna are rare in children.

Dislocations of the elbow are not uncommon (the shoulder is the commonest site of dislocation in the body, interphalangeal dislocations are the second most common, and the elbow is the third most common site of dislocations). Ninety percent of elbow dislocations are posterior or posterolateral, i.e., the radius and ulna end up posterior to the distal humerus. Obviously, significant soft-tissue damage ensues. Very rarely, the interosseous ligament may be split so that a divergent dislocation of the radius (going outward) and the ulna (going inward) occurs. The collateral ligaments both tear or avulse, and the median nerve may become entrapped, particularly following reduction. Most elbow dislocations are associated with fractures: fractures of the medial epicondyle, separation of the medial epicondyle, radial head fractures, or coronoid process fractures.

Before we finish this segment, one other fracture/dislocation involves the elbow joint, and that is the *Monteggia fracture/dislocation,* where the radial head dislocates and the upper shaft or metaphyseal region of the proximal ulna sustains a fracture, which is usually oblique (Fig. 20A, B).

The most common direction for the radial head to go is anterior (65%) and the next most common is posterolaterally (20%). Although the fracture of the ulna is usually obvious, a surprisingly large number of radial head dislocations get missed. Remember to draw the radiocapitellar line—a line running up the midshaft of the radius has to bisect the capitellum in all views. Monteggia fracture/dislocations can be seen in all ages and, although initially described in children where the ulnar fracture may be a greenstick-type fracture, Monteggia injuries are actually more common in adults.

One interesting complication of elbow fractures, which will be dealt with in more detail later in this chapter, is myositis ossificans, which frequently occurs not only in the anterior musculature (brachialis muscle particularly) but also in the capsule and surrounding joints.

RADIUS AND ULNA SHAFT FRACTURES

Most fractures of the radial and ulnar shaft are straightforward and usually horizontal or oblique in alignment, although frequently occurring at different levels. Segmental fractures are also not uncommon. However, it is possible to get a solitary fracture of the ulna, the so-called *nightstick fracture,* where the patient sustains a direct blow to the midshaft of the bone when the arm is lifted over the head to ward off a blow from a nightstick (Fig. 21).

Children will get *greenstick fractures* in the midshaft of the radius often, apparently, solitary, but subluxation of the distal radial-ulna joint or a bowing deformity of the ulna can also be seen (Fig. 22).

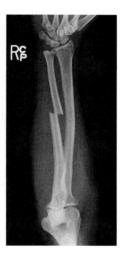

Figure 21 Nightstick fracture. This is a result of a direct blow to the midshaft of the ulna with a transverse fracture. The radius is intact.

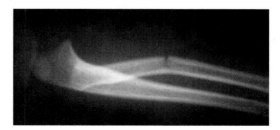

Figure 22 Greenstick fracture. This is the typical "greenstick" fracture of the proximal ulna seen in a young child who fell off a swing.

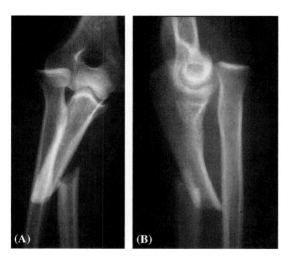

(A) (B)

Figure 20 Monteggia Fracture/dislocation (**A**) AP view and (**B**) Lateral view. The Monteggia fracture dislocation is a fracture of the proximal shaft of the ulna and a dislocation of the proximal radio-humeral joint as is well seen on these two films.

An impacted metaphyseal fracture of the ulna also needs to be searched for.

FRACTURES OF THE WRIST

The best known and also the commonest fracture of the distal radius and ulna is the *Colles fracture,* which was first described in 1814 in Dublin by Abraham Colles when he described a fracture that occurred in a colleague who fell on his outstretched hand (Figs. 23A, B and 24).

By definition, a Colles fracture is a comminuted, basically horizontal fracture of the distal radius, with dorsal angulation, frequently, but not necessarily, associated with a fracture of the ulnar styloid (only in 60%). Obviously, Colles did not describe this part of the fracture since he did not have the advantage of X rays to guide him! Colles's original clinical description stands today, and the phrase "dinner-fork deformity" has been applied to the dorsal displacement and swelling that one sees clinically. Colles fractures are typically seen in elderly patients, particularly women older than 60 years who

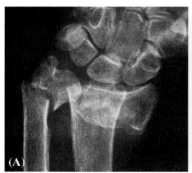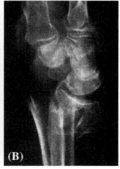

Figure 23 (**A**) Colles fracture of the distal radius and ulna with transverse fractures of both bones. The fractures have marked dorsal angulation well seen on the lateral view. (**B**) The fractures show marked dorsal angulation well seen on the lateral view.

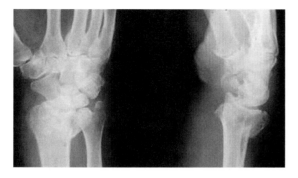

Figure 24 Colles fracture. Not quite so severe a fracture, although with marked distortion of the distal radius and ulna as well as dorsal angulation.

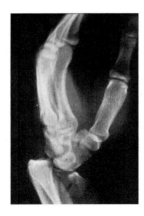

Figure 25 Smith's fracture. This is the typical appearance of a reversed Colles or a Smith's fracture with the wrist or hand lying in a volar position relative to the distal radius and ulna.

fall on their outstretched hand. They are quite often associated with fractures of the proximal humerus (10%) and hip fractures (8%). On the lateral view, the normal volar angulation of the distal radius is about 12% to 15%; in Colles fractures, this often becomes a dorsal angulation of 20° or more. Most Colles fractures that occur in either severely osteoporotic patients or in the extremely elderly will also impact, and it is this foreshortening and dorsal angulation that causes the most problems with attempts to reduce the fracture. However, external fixators or other traction systems are used in many of these patients with good results.

A "reversed" Colles fracture with volar angulation is much less common and is known as a *Smith's fracture* (Fig. 25).

On the AP view, Colles and Smith's fractures can appear identical, so the lateral view is important to differentiate them, dorsal angulation in a Colles fracture and volar angulation in a Smith's fracture.

There are many more types of distal radial fracture, and most of them have eponyms.

Classical *Barton's fractures* are of the posterior aspect of the outer radial rim of the distal radius and are usually associated with dislocations of the carpus, particularly lunate and perilunate, as well as avulsion fractures of the ulnar styloid (Fig. 26).

The so-called *reversed Barton's fracture* is a similar fracture of the anterior rim, which is actually twice as common as the originally described posterior rim fracture. It is obvious that there is some overlap between these fractures and Colles fractures (the classical Barton's fracture) and Smith's fractures (the reverse Barton's fracture). However, Barton's fractures are only of the rim and only involve up to 50% of the articular surface. Typically Colles and Smith's fractures do not involve the radiocarpal joint, and Barton's fractures are frequently associated with radiocarpal or carpal dislocations.

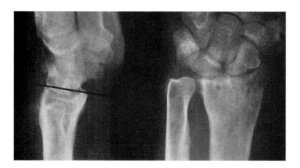

Figure 26 Barton's fracture. This is a fracture of the outer radial rim of the distal radius, which can often be difficult to see on plain films.

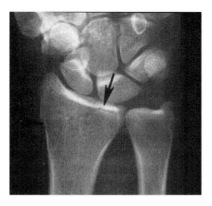

Figure 27 Chauffeur's fracture. This is an oblique fracture of the radial styloid, again this is often difficult to see on a plain film.

Fractures of the radial styloid are usually avulsion fractures, with the radial collateral ligament pulling off a fragment of bone. These are also known as *chauffeur's fractures* (or Hutchinson's fractures) and may be complete or incomplete and can be very difficult to see because they may be only minimally displaced (Fig. 27).

The original term for these fractures is due to the fact that chauffeurs used to crank up car engines to start them, and, if they inadvertently let go of the handle, it reversed direction and clipped them smartly on the back of the wrist, thus causing the fracture.

Obviously, there are many variations of all these types of fractures, as well as more simple transverse and vertical fractures of the distal radius. Radiologically, it is important to determine the degree of displacement as well as to determine whether the fracture extends into the joint or not. Fractures of the ulnar styloid occur in association with many of these other fractures, and although appear to be relatively insignificant, can lead to ulnar instability if not corrected.

Dislocations of the wrist are largely carpal, although separations, subluxation, or even dislocation of the distal radio-ulnar joint may be seen in association with radial or

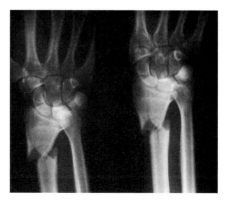

Figure 28 Galleazzi fracture/dislocation. This follows a fall on the outstretched hand with a fracture of the distal radius and a dislocation of the distal radioulnar joint.

ulnar shaft fractures as part of the *Galleazzi fracture/ dislocation* and are obviously seen in association with Colles and Smith's fractures (Fig. 28).

Surprisingly, dislocations of the radio-ulnar joint are difficult to diagnose because, on the true lateral view of the wrist in a normal person, the distal ulna appears to project far posterior to the distal radius, and it is easy to misdiagnose this dislocation. In that case, go and examine the patient!

Fractures of the distal radius and ulna in children are usually fairly easy to diagnose; buckle or impaction fractures occur classically in the distal radius in children younger than six years. If they are complete or circumferential, they are called *torus fractures* (a torus being the ring around the base of a Greek column) (Fig. 29).

However, partial buckle fractures are much more common and may be associated with a bowing deformity of

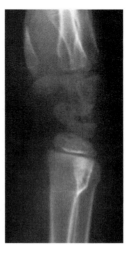

Figure 29 Torus fracture. This is the typical buckle fracture usually seen in children aged four to six years, following a fall on the outstretched hand.

the distal ulna. In older children, transverse fractures of the distal radius occur classically 2 to 4 cm proximal to the distal growth plate. Greenstick fractures of the distal radius are relatively uncommon, although older children can get Colles fractures and other fractures similar to those seen in adults (Fig. 22).

Salter fractures of the distal radius associated with ulnar styloid fractures are considered the adolescent equivalent of the Colles fracture. Salter II fractures are the most common epiphyseal fractures seen in children aged between 10 and 14 years, whereas Salter I fractures are seen more often in children aged between 8 and 10 years and are usually difficult to diagnose.

FRACTURES OF THE CARPAL BONES

Fractures of individual carpal bones without other injury to the wrist are quite rare except for scaphoid fractures, which actually account for approximately 70% of all solitary carpal injuries. Since triquetral fractures account for 10% to 15% of solitary carpal injuries, this only leaves approximately 10% of solitary injuries involving the other six carpal bones. If one excludes scaphoid and triquetral fractures, the probable order of involvement of the other carpal bones are hamate, trapezium, lunate, capitate, and pisiform. The scaphoid is quite vulnerable since it lies between a rock and a hard place, i.e., when a patient falls on the outstretched arm, they land usually on the radial aspect of the palm, and thus the scaphoid is compressed between the ground and the distal radius, which in this instance is carrying all the weight of the body. Most scaphoid fractures are seen in patients aged between 15 and 40 years, and 70% of them are transverse or horizontal fractures of the waist of the bone (Fig. 30).

The word, scaphoid, or navicular, refers to the boatlike shape of the bone, which makes the waist the most vulnerable part. However, any part of the bone may fracture, and avulsion fractures of the scaphoid tuberosity

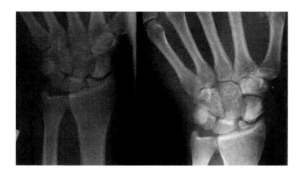

Figure 30 Scaphoid fracture. There is a transverse fracture of the scaphoid with separation of the two fragments. This example is a subacute fracture.

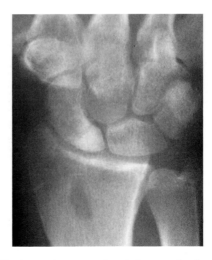

Figure 31 Avascular necrosis of the proximal pole of the scaphoid. Note that the proximal pole of the scaphoid is sclerotic, which is a typical sign of avascular necrosis.

account for 10% of scaphoid fractures. These are caused by avulsion of the radial collateral ligament, which inserts on the tuberosity on its way up to the trapezium and the base of the thumb.

The two well-known complications of scaphoid fractures are avascular necrosis and nonunion. Since the blood supply comes in mainly from the radial collateral ligament and enters the distal pole of the bone, the more proximal the fracture, the greater the risk of avascular necrosis, i.e., fractures of the proximal pole are associated with a 90% incidence of avascular necrosis, fractures of the waist of the scaphoid with a 30% incidence, and fractures of the distal pole with a 0% to 5% incidence of avascular necrosis (Fig. 31).

Avascular necrosis may occur even if the fracture unites satisfactorily, and it often takes three to six months to manifest itself radiologically, which it does by gradually increasing density of the proximal pole when compared with the other parts of the bone. But one must be aware that in the immediate posttraumatic period, the proximal pole of the scaphoid may appear relatively dense in comparison with the surrounding bone because of disuse of the other bones, particularly if the wrist is immobilized.

The second complication of scaphoid fractures is non-union or delayed union of the fracture, and this occurs particularly in those fractures of the waist that are widely separated. Nonunion occurs in approximately 30% of fractures of the waist of the bone and in approximately 50% of fractures involving the proximal pole. On the whole, it is wisest for the radiologist to refer to the appearance of wide separation of the fragments as delayed union until sclerotic margins develop along the edges, which implies that motion is occurring through the

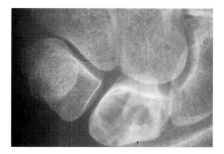

Figure 32 Kienboch's disease. Note the increased sclerosis and cyst formation within the lunate.

fracture site and, hence, nonunion. If either early avascular necrosis or nonunion is suspected, MRI is very helpful in the former, and thin-slice CT with reconstructions is useful in the latter.

The lunate is the second most common bone to sustain trauma, and, classically, this results in avascular necrosis rather than a fracture. Avascular necrosis of the lunate is known as *Kienboch's disease*. This is discussed in more detail elsewhere (Fig. 32).

The reason that triquetral fractures are the third commonest fracture in the carpus is that the dorsal radiocarpal ligaments have a strong attachment to the dorsal aspect of the triquetrum. Thus, if one falls backwards on a closed fist, a large amount of pressure is placed on these ligaments, and so triquetral avulsion fractures are not uncommon. They can usually only be seen on the lateral view of the wrist, so it is important to look carefully at the posterior aspect of the carpal bones on this view (Fig. 33A, B).

It is believed that fractures of the hook of the hamate are the next most common fracture of a solitary carpal bone. These occur frequently in racket sports or in golf,

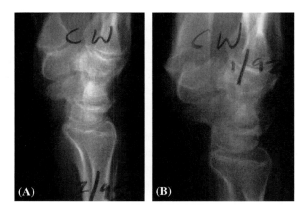

Figure 33 (A) Triquetral fracture in a lateral view of the wrist, a discrete fracture off the posterior aspect of the triquetrum can be seen. It was only present on this view (*arrow*). (B) Triquetral fracture. For comparison is a normal X ray of the same wrist taken three years before.

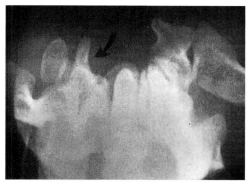

Figure 34 Hook of the hamate fracture. There is a transverse fracture of the hook of the hamate in this patient who was an avid golfer.

where the players lose control of their rackets or their clubs and the force is transmitted through the region of the carpal tunnel to the hook of the hamate (Fig. 34).

These fractures are also easy to miss on a straight AP or lateral film of the wrist, although a double ring sign has been described. If a fracture of the hook of the hamate is suspected, I recommend a carpal tunnel view or a CT scan to confirm it.

Individual solitary fractures of the other carpal bones occur usually as a result of a direct blow.

CARPAL DISLOCATIONS

On the other hand, complex fracture dislocations of the carpus are much more common, so this is probably a good place to discuss carpal dislocations (Fig. 35).

Up to recently, these were all considered to be individual injuries, but it is now thought that they actually represent a spectrum of trauma, depending upon differing amounts of stress to the wrist. *Lunate dislocations* (where the lunate dislocates volarly and separates both from the distal radius and the capitate) occur as a result of relatively minor trauma (Figs. 36 and 37).

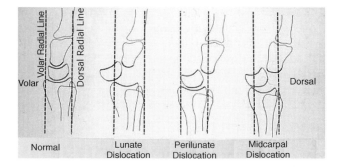

Figure 35 Line drawing to show the three different types of lunate and carpal dislocations. *Source*: From Ref. 1.

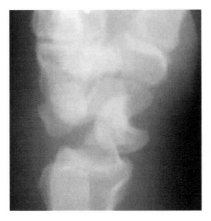

Figure 36 Lunate dislocation. On the lateral view, the lunate can be clearly seen lying anterior to a line drawn through the radius and the capitate. The remainder of the carpal bones have stayed with the capitate, and thus this is a solitary lunate dislocation.

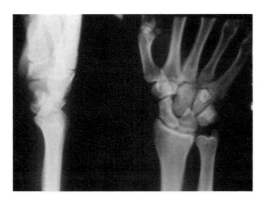

Figure 37 Another patient with a lunate dislocation, which is clearly seen on the lateral view. On the frontal view, the triangular shape of the lunate can be seen, which is a typical appearance of a dislocation of the lunate.

Perilunate dislocations occur when the lunate maintains its normal anatomic relationship with the radius, but the rest of the carpus dislocates posteriorly away from it, i.e., the scaphoid, capitate, and triquetrium, the metacarpals and the rest of the hand (Fig. 38A, B).

Next, *trans-scaphoid perilunate fracture/dislocations* occur as a result of even more stress placed on the wrist, and, since these are usually associated with dislocations of the triquetral hamate joint, they can also be known as midcarpal fracture/dislocations.

FRACTURE AND DISLOCATION OF THE METACARPALS

Fractures of the metacarpals represent approximately 20% to 25% of all hand injuries, with fractures of the fifth

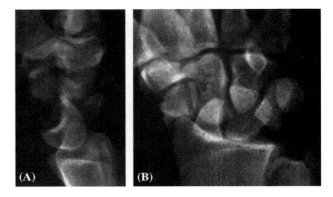

Figure 38 Perilunate dislocation. (**A**) On the lateral view, the lunate can be seen sitting in the fossa of the distal radius with the remainder of the carpus dislocated and lying posteriorly. (**B**) On the AP view, there is marked distortion of the carpus because of the perilunate dislocation.

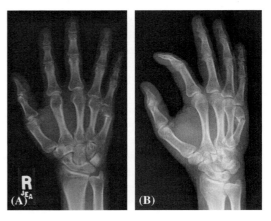

Figure 39 (**A**) A Boxer's fracture. Note the dorsally angulated fracture of the neck of the fifth metacarpal (*arrow*). (**B**) A Boxer's fracture in a different patient.

metacarpal being the most common (35%), followed by fractures of the first metacarpal (25%). Fractures of the second through fourth metacarpal are oftentimes transverse or oblique fractures of the midshaft of the bone. However, the best-known metacarpal fracture is that of the neck of the fifth metacarpal and is known as a *"Boxer's" fracture* (Fig. 39).

It should of course be called the non–Boxer's fracture since real boxers use their second and third knuckles to deliver the punches. Spiral fractures of the metacarpal shaft also result in rotation and shortening of the length of the bone. Often oblique views provide the most information.

Fractures of the base of the first metacarpal can be surprisingly difficult to see on routine AP and lateral views of the hand, and several specific oblique views of the first metacarpal with true AP and lateral views of the first ray may be necessary (Fig. 40A, B, C).

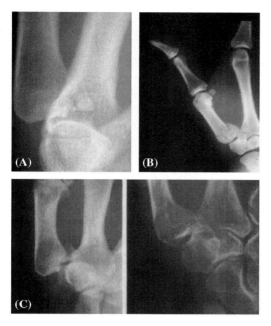

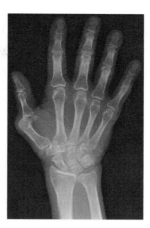

Figure 41 Gamekeeper's thumb. This implies a ligamentous injury to the collateral ligament of the first metacarpophalangeal joint. This can be seen as a subluxation of the joint and occasionally has a small avulsion fracture.

Figure 40 (**A**) Bennett's fracture. Fracture of a single condyle on the base of the first metacarpal. This usually involves the ulnar condyle and is known as a Bennett's fracture. (**B** and **C**) Rolando fracture. This is a fracture of both the radial and the ulnar condyles of the base of the first metacarpal.

Eighty percent of first metacarpal fractures involve the base of the metacarpal. They may be intra-articular (45%) or extra-articular (35%). The remainder are mixed. Bennett described the fracture dislocation of the first carpometacarpal bones in 1881. It was only when X rays became available that a full description of this injury became possible. A *Bennetts' fracture* is, by definition, an oblique fracture of the ulnar aspect of the base of the first metacarpal associated with subluxation or dislocation of the first metacarpal on the trapezium. The fracture fragment is held in place, whereas the abductor pollicus longus pulls the remainder of the bone outward. Bennett's fractures need to be internally fixed, and they represent 35% of metacarpal fractures.

Rolando fractures are less common (10% of metacarpal fractures) and are a comminuted intra-articular fracture of both the condyles of the base of the first metacarpal. This fracture may be Y shaped or T shaped, but can be extremely comminuted, in which case closed reduction and casting are used.

"*Gamekeeper's thumb*" is a term classically used for a tear of the first ulnar or radial metacarpo-phalangeal collateral ligament (Fig. 41).

It can be associated with an avulsion fracture of the ulnar aspect of the base of the proximal phalanx of the thumb. The term is derived from the fact that, in days of yore, gamekeepers used to throttle rabbits by holding the head and hyperextending and twisting the neck to kill them. This put a large amount of stress on the ulnar collateral ligament. Gamekeeper's thumb can be seen today as a result of many sports injuries, but particularly in skiers who keep their thumbs on top of their ski poles and are prone to injury when they fall. If there is no fracture visible radiologically, stress views will confirm the diagnosis. Otherwise, the avulsion fracture gives it away. If the avulsed fragment is large enough, it is pinned back into position. If there is only a ligamentous tear, casting is the usual method of treatment.

In children, metacarpal fractures are usually of the Salter 2 type, particularly at the base of the thumb. Otherwise, one can see transverse, spiral, and oblique fractures of the metacarpal shaft. Torus fractures of the neck of the fifth metacarpal childhood equivalent of Boxer's fractures.

Subluxations and dislocations of the first carpometacarpal joint are more complex and difficult to classify. Most of us have some motion at this joint, so it is often necessary to compare the two sides to see if there is any real subluxation on the side that hurts. Subluxation of the first carpo-metacarpal joint is prelude to early degenerative arthritis, and is well known to lead to early arthritis. Similar to any other joint, the early changes of degenerative arthritis include squaring off of the joint margins, subchondral sclerosis, early joint space narrowing, and osteophyte formation. However, if one reviews hand X rays of patients older than 60 years, a high percentage show these changes in this joint, and so I believe that degenerative arthritis of the first carpometacarpal joint is an almost inevitable accompaniment of aging.

On the other hand, fracture dislocation of the bases of the fourth and fifth metacarpals are a condition primarily seen in young people (Fig. 42A, B, C).

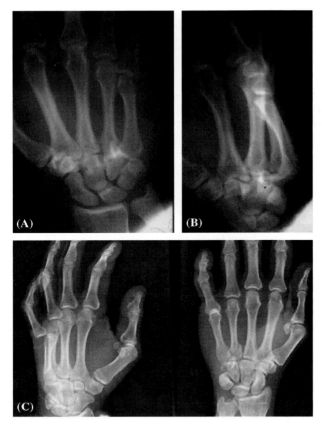

Figure 42 (**A** and **B**) Fracture at the base of the fourth and fifth metacarpals seen in this skateboard rider who crashed. The fracture at the base of the fourth metacarpal appears to be a simple fracture. There is also a dislocation of the fifth carpometacarpal joint. (**C**) Another patient with a fracture of the base of the fourth and fifth metacarpals and dislocation of the fifth carpometacarpal joint.

Lee Rogers (1), in his book, says that they are extraordinarily rare, but he did not practice in Minnesota, where rollerblading was invented. We were seeing these injuries increasingly in people who fall on their outstretched hand off rollerblades or skateboards, and they appear to occur if the person tries to save their wrist and rolls their fist up and falls rolling onto the dorsum of the wrist with all the force, thus causing a fracture/dislocation through the capitate and hamate or the bases of the fourth and fifth metacarpals.

FRACTURE AND DISLOCATIONS OF THE PHALANGES

Phalangeal fractures are usually due to direct blows and are often of little consequence unless they are intra-articular or condylar and the fragments are markedly separated. Fractures of the distal phalanx represent 50% and occur most frequently in the thumb and little finger. Fractures of the middle phalanx only account for 10%, and

fractures of the proximal phalanx, which also occur most commonly in the thumb and index finger, account for 40%.

They are often multiple (10%), particularly following a crush injury or motor vehicle accident. It is also important to remind you that pathological fractures occurring through an enchondroma are not uncommon and need to be looked for carefully if there is no real history of significant trauma.

Collateral ligament injuries to the interphalangeal joints are also not uncommon. They are often not accompanied by any visible fracture, and so radial and ulnar stress views are useful to show if there is any instability in the joint. Collateral ligament injuries to the interphalangeal joint of the thumb are particularly common, and particularly seen in conjunction with a gamekeeper's thumb–type injury.

Mallet finger (otherwise known as baseball finger) occurs as a result of avulsion of the extensor tendon off its insertion into dorsal aspect of the base of the digital phalanx (Fig. 43).

The injury maybe purely soft tissue without a fracture, or a fragment of bone may be avulsed with it, which then results in a characteristic flexed angulation through the distal interphalangeal joint, which is thought to resemble a mallet and needs to be attended to since the deformity will otherwise become permanent.

Volar plate fractures can occur at any level in the fingers but are more common, as well as being characteristic, at the proximal interphalangeal joint where the volar plate is larger (Fig. 44).

These are due to avulsion of the flexor digitorum tendon, the superficial part of which inserts into the

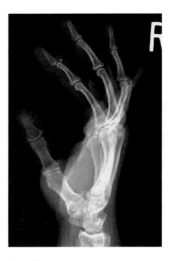

Figure 43 Mallet finger. This is the typical softball injury, with avulsion of the dorsal condyle at the base of the distal phalanx, usually of the index, middle, or ring finger. As a result of this, there is obviously a lack of flexion of the DIP joint. *Abbreviation*: DIP, distal interphalangeal joint.

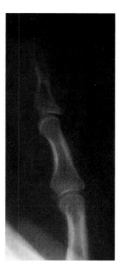

Figure 44 Volar plate fracture. These are not uncommon. They occur as an avulsion off the proximal end of the middle phalanx of one of the fingers, usually the long or index finger.

volar aspect of the middle phalanx, and the deep part of which (flexor digitorum profundis) inserts into the volar aspect of the proximal end of the distal phalanx. These are the results of a hyperflexion injury, such as being hit on the finger by a baseball or cricket ball. Once again, the avulsed fragment may be large or small, or nonexistent.

Boutonniere deformities are not uncommon in rheumatoid arthritis, and its variants, however, also may follow trauma with flexion at the proximal interphalangeal joint and extension at the distal interphalangeal joint as a result of rupture of the middle slip of the extension mechanism (Fig. 45).

The proximal interphalangeal (PIP) joint flexes, protruding through the gap and between the lateral slips of the deep tendon, which, in turn, pull the distal phalanx into extension.

Dislocations of the interphalangeal joints are not uncommon and are usually the result of hyperextension,

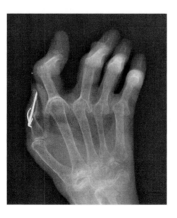

Figure 45 Boutonniere deformities occurring in a patient with severe rheumatoid arthritis.

with the affected phalanx being displaced posteriorly. They are often associated with volar plate injuries. Anterior dislocations are rare (Fig. 43C).

In children, fractures of the proximal phalanx represent over 50% of phalangeal fractures and are mainly of the Salter-Harris type II. However, fractures of any part of the phalanx may occur as a result of direct trauma; oblique, transverse, and spiral fractures of the shaft occur in 30% of phalangeal injuries. In younger children, greenstick and torus fractures of the phalanges may also be seen, particularly at the base of the proximal phalanges. Often AP and lateral views fail to show the fracture, and oblique views are necessary to confirm it.

HIP AND PELVIS

Pelvic Fractures

Introduction

In a simplistic explanation of pelvic fractures, there are those that are stable and those that are unstable. The pelvis consists of two arches of bone: one is the *weight-bearing arch* (the spine to the sacrum to the sacroiliac joints to the iliac wings to the acetabulae to the femurs), and the other is the *stabilizing arch* (one acetabulum to the sacrum to the other acetabulum and through the symphysis). If both of these get damaged, then the fracture is unstable, but, if only the stabilizing arch gets disrupted, the fracture is usually stable. Also, since the pelvis is a ring of bone, if there is a fracture or separation in one part of the ring, then there is usually a second fracture or separation elsewhere in the ring. Usually, a sacroiliac separation will accompany a separation of the symphysis; a fracture of the rami will accompany a fracture of the sacrum.

At first glance, pelvic fractures seem to be relatively straightforward; one looks at the various bones to see if they are intact, as well as see the sacrum, sacroiliac joints, symphysis pubis, and rami. However, the shape of the pelvis and the presence of the acetabulum and hip joint rather complicate things. Obviously, the way that pelvic fractures are worked up today is that an AP plain film is taken, and this is followed by a CT scan, often with sagittal and coronal reconstructions. However, it still remains important to fully evaluate the anterior and posterior walls of the acetabulum, as well as the acetabular columns. So 45° oblique Judet views are very useful. A right anterior oblique (RAO) view of the left hip will show the anterior wall and column of that hip, whereas a left anterior oblique (LAO) of the left hip will show the posterior column. Obviously, an RAO view not only shows the anterior column on the left but also the posterior column on the right. Similarly, an LAO view will show the anterior column on the right and the posterior column on the left.

Classifications

A very simple approach to pelvic fractures would be to classify them on the mechanism of injury:

1. AP compression fractures
    a. straddle (10%)
    b. open book
2. Lateral compression fractures
    a. ipsilateral AP and lateral compression
    b. contralateral (bucket handle)
    c. ramal and posterior fractures
3. Vertical shear fractures
    a. Malgaigne fractures (15%)

I have come across no less than seven classifications of pelvic fractures, but will only discuss two. The Bucholz classification is based on stability and has three types: type I, ramal fractures which are stable; type II, AP compression fractures or dislocations, where the anterior fracture or dislocation is unstable, but the posterior fracture/dislocation is stable; and type III, where both the anterior and posterior fractures are unstable. However, this classification excludes a number of other fractures and dislocations, particularly the vertical shear fracture or Malgaigne fracture, as well as the lateral compression fracture.

The Young/Burgess (2) classification concerns lateral compression fractures, and also has three categories: Type I, where the lateral force is projected predominantly posteriorly, causing a crush fracture of the sacrum or sacroiliac joint, and a coronal or horizontal fracture of the rami without any major ligamentous damage. Type II, where there is a crush fracture of the sacrum and a coronal fracture of the ramus. Significant posterior ligamentous injury also occurs involving the posterior aspect of the ipsilateral sacroiliac joint. Type III, where the lateral force is so severe that the internal force on the ipsilateral side is transferred to the contralateral side, causing posterior ligamentous injury on the ipsilateral side with involvement of the sacroiliac joint, as well as ligamentous injury on the contralateral side. Ramal fractures also occur, and a crush injury of the ipsilateral side of the sacrum can also be seen (Fig. 46A, B).

Stable Fractures

Ramal Fractures

Now let us return to the simplest classification. Stable fractures account for 66% of all pelvic fractures, and are either simple breaks in the pelvic rim or avulsion fractures and are usually the result of moderate trauma. Ramal fractures account for 50% of pelvic fractures, and these are usually stable (Fig. 47).

Duverney's fracture is a unilateral isolated fracture of one side of the iliac wing (7%); isolated sacral fractures

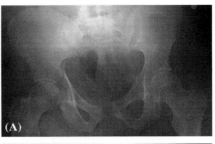
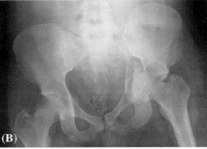

Figure 46 (**A**) These both represent lateral compression fractures of the pelvis. This pelvic film shows four ramal fractures as well as separation of the left sacroiliac joint. (**B**) Lateral compression fracture showing that the left hemipelvis has been compressed medially with separation of the left sacroiliac joint. There is also a linear fracture of the acetabulum as well as fractures of both the left pubic and ischial ramus.

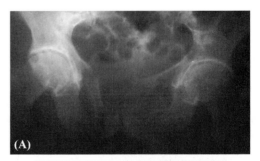
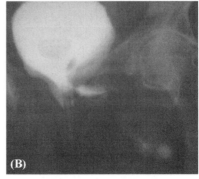

Figure 47 (**A**) Ramal fracture. This is a typical straddle fracture with fractures and distortion of all four rami. The symphysis pubis has been shifted downward. (**B**) Rupture of the bladder base in the same patient. Note the contrast leaking around the bladder base and into the soft tissues.

account for 5%, and avulsion fractures account for 2%. Thus, the commonest fracture is a ramal fracture, which may be bilateral or unilateral. In the ischium, ramal fractures are usually vertical and involve the medial margin of the obturator foramen, and they may appear either as a lucent line or may be impacted, in which case they are seen to be sclerotic. Ischial fractures may be associated with fractures within the acetabulum, like a transverse or T-shaped fracture, and a CT scan is required to exclude these. They also may be associated with mild disruption of the sacro-iliac joint. On the other hand, pubic ramus fractures maybe medial, in which case they are usually obvious, or more lateral, on the lateral margin of the obturator foramen, in which case they are more difficult to see. Fractures of both rami are quite common and can be only slightly or minimally displaced. However, if the patient has a "straddle" fracture with wide displacement, it is important to look for associated fractures of the posterior wing and of the sacrum or separation of the sacroiliac joint.

Single Fractures

Single fractures of various pelvic bones can also be seen, particularly of the sacrum and the coccyx, as well as avulsion fractures of either the anterior superior iliac spine (hurdlers and jumpers), or anterior inferior iliac spine (often in runners) (Fig. 48A, B).

Avulsion fractures of the inferior aspect of the ischial apophysis are often seen in young, adolescent baseball players who, while they are sliding into third base, get stopped suddenly, and the hamstring muscles pull off the ischial ramus. If this is recurrent, there can be considerable buildup of bone on the inferior surface of the ischial

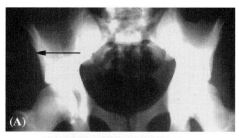

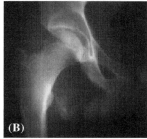

Figure 48 (**A**) Avulsion of the anterior superior iliac spine. (**B**) Avulsion of the hamstrings off the tibial tubercle in a different patient.

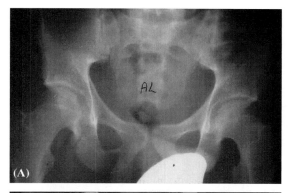

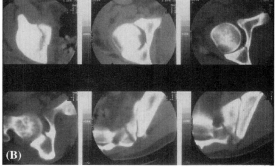

Figure 49 Sacral fracture. (**A**) Plain film. The sacral fracture is difficult to see on this film. (**B**) However, it becomes obvious on the CT scan. *Abbreviation*: CT, computed tomography.

ramus. If it is acute and there is a major separation of apophysis from the underlying bone, the apophysis needs to be replaced surgically.

Iliac Wing Fractures

Isolated fractures of the iliac wing can be large or small, and they are usually vertical (Duverney fractures) and are usually due to direct lateral compression. The fracture fragments become widely displaced because of all the muscular attachments.

Sacral Fractures

Sacral fractures are also not uncommon, either in combination with other injuries or as a solitary fracture due to a fall landing directly on the sacrum. They are often difficult to diagnose on plain films, although, if one follows the "eyebrows" of the sacral ala, they can often be identified (Fig. 49A, B).

The sacral eyebrows are usually smooth, curved, intact, and symmetric. CT scans and bone scans are often necessary to confirm sacral fractures (Fig. 50A, B, C).

Sacral fractures are usually horizontal and located below the level of the fourth sacral ala and are often the result of a direct fall on the backside or being hit by a steamroller. On a lateral radiograph, it is often easy to see them since the distal fragment is usually displaced forward.

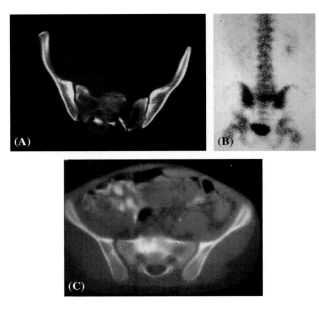

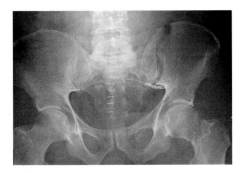

Figure 50 (**A**) A CT scan of a different patient shows a fracture of the left sacral ala. (**B**) This is confirmed by a bone scan, which shows a "Honda" sign. (**C**) An MRI in a different patient showing a sacral fracture on the right. *Abbreviation*: CT, computed tomography.

Coccygeal Fractures

Coccygeal fractures are usually transverse, and the inferior fragment is pushed inward. A good lateral radiograph or a coned-down view will show these. They may be painful, but not of any real clinical significance.

Unstable Fractures

Malgaigne Fractures

On the other hand, unstable fractures (33% of all pelvic fractures) are those in which there is disruption of the ring in two or more places and are usually the result of severe trauma, either a motor vehicle accident or a major fall. They are frequently associated with visceral and urinary tract injuries and often have more severe hemorrhages. Malgaigne fractures are vertical shear fractures and account for 14% of pelvic fractures (Fig. 51).

Straddle fractures, which are unstable fractures involving both pubic and both ischial rami, account for 10%; diastasis of both the sacroiliac joint and symphysis account for 5%, and an unclassifiable mix of comminuted, unstable fractures account for the rest.

Double Vertical Fractures

Malgaigne fractures were first described in 1850, well before the advent of radiographs, and they are usually on one side of the pelvis and are basically a vertical shear

Figure 51 Malgaigne fracture. This is typically a vertical fracture involving one half of the pelvis, including the left iliac bone, the left sacroiliac joint, and the left pubic and ischial rami.

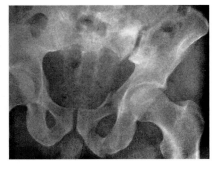

Figure 52 Malgaigne fracture. This is another typical example with separation of the left sacroiliac joint and shift of the left hemipelvis downward. There are also ramal fractures of the rami.

fracture. They separate a large fragment, which contains the hip joint, from the remainder of the pelvis, and the fracture is usually anterior in the rami, but posterior with displacement or dislocation of the sacroiliac joint. If a Malgaigne fracture is a single, vertical fracture, it is inherently stable, but this is actually rare, and most are unstable (Fig. 52).

Double vertical fractures and fracture dislocations are extremely unstable and, again, usually involve the same side of the pelvis, with a fracture of the sacrum and concomitant fracture of the pubic and ischial rami. However, they can be seen on opposite sides of the pelvis, and then this is known as a "bucket handle" fracture. These are severe injuries and usually occur as a result of a major motor vehicle accident. They are usually associated with other injuries, particularly other fractures of the extremities, head injuries, as well as damage to the thoracic and abdominal viscera. The iliac wing is usually displaced superiorly and posteriorly, and rotated externally, i.e., it becomes flattened out or rotated internally.

A basic rule for the radiologist is, if you see anterior arch fractures, you must look for fractures or separations in the posterior arch, i.e., the sacrum, the sacroiliac joint,

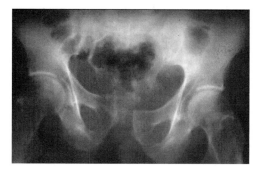

Figure 53 The typical separation of the right sacroiliac joint and symphysis pubis can be seen in this patient. Straight AP view. *Abbreviation*: AP, anteroposterior.

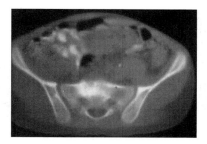

Figure 54 Insufficiency fracture of the sacrum shows the typical sclerotic line just on the right of the midline.

and the iliac crest. They are also commonly associated with fractures of the L5 transverse processes.

Iliac fractures are usually obvious and occur just lateral to the sacroiliac joint. The sacroiliac joint diastasis is usually obvious, but, if necessary, measure side to side and compare. Sacral fractures, which often occur in these complex injuries, are less obvious and frequently only show up on the CT scan. However, on the plain radiograph, if you follow the eyebrows, once again, you should be able to see the fracture on a plain film (Fig. 53).

Dislocations

Dislocations are similar to the unstable double fractures of the pelvis, except that here there is no actual fracture, just separation of the sacroiliac joint and the symphysis (Fig. 53). This situation is frequently associated with severe visceral and vascular injury and needs to be reduced and fixed. Presently, large cannulated compression screws through the sacroiliac joint are used, as well as a plate across the symphysis.

Straddle Fractures

Double vertical arch fractures, or straddle fractures, involve all four rami and are usually vertical, with the central fragment displaced superiorly. There is a substantial incidence of urethral (male patients) and bladder (female patients) injuries, accounting for some 20% of these patients (Fig. 47B).

Complex Fractures

This remaining 4% are very difficult to classify. This subcategory also includes what I still like to call the central fracture dislocation of the hip, where the femoral head is driven through the medial wall of the acetabulum,

usually in a posterior direction, but occasionally in an anterior or superior direction, depending on the force of injury.

Complications of Pelvic Fractures

Pelvic fractures are associated with many complications, including death, severe bleeding, and other injuries. Although arterial damage is relatively uncommon, venous damage is quite frequent. Damage to the ureters and sciatic nerve are rare. But urethral damage in men and tears of the bladder base in women are also relatively common (Fig. 54).

Overall, 10% to 20% of patients with severe pelvic injuries die, the majority die from exsanguination (70%), and 30% from sepsis as a result of a pelvic hematoma that gets infected. Open fractures of the pelvis are also fairly common and can often communicate directly with the vagina and rectum and are often associated with deep skin lacerations. One late complication of pelvic fractures is retroperitoneal abscess, which can be seen as late as three months after injury and in which the mortality is 50%.

Stress and Insufficiency Fractures

Stress fractures occur in patients who have normal bone mineral, but who experience abnormal stress, such as military recruits and long-distance runners. On the other hand, insufficiency fractures occur in patients with low bone mineral, but who are exposed to normal stress. Insufficiency fractures are frequently seen either in elderly patients with primary osteoporosis or in patients who are on long-term steroids and develop secondary osteoporosis (Fig. 54).

Classically, in the elderly, insufficiency fractures occur in the sacrum and are often difficult to diagnose on plain films and even on CT scans. However, a bone scan will show a characteristic "Honda" sign (or a half-Honda sign if only one side is involved). Insufficiency fractures can

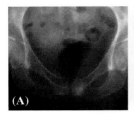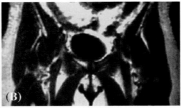

Figure 55 Insufficiency fractures of the pelvis. (**A**) Initial film shows the typical findings of an insufficiency fracture in the left parasymphyseal region, with a vertical sclerotic line running parallel to the symphysis through both the pubic and ischial rami. (**B**) MRI scan of the same patient confirms these findings: coronal slice. *Abbreviation*: MRI, magnetic resonance imaging.

also be seen in the rami, where they are often vertical in orientation. Another situation where vertical ramal fractures occur (particularly the ischial ramus) is when the mechanism of the hip joint is altered, usually following a total hip replacement. These ramal fractures classically occur one to two years after the implant and are a potent cause of chronic hip pain in these patients.

Parasymphyseal Fractures

These are quite common in the elderly and are really localized insufficiency fractures (Fig. 55A, B). They are usually somewhat sclerotic in appearance and are quite difficult to diagnose since they have a somewhat mixed, patchy lytic and sclerotic appearance. The differential diagnosis will include such things as metastases and chondrosarcomas; however, an MRI will confirm that they are, in fact, simple insufficiency fractures.

Pelvic Fractures in Children

Many pelvic fractures in children occur as a result of a pedestrian or motor vehicle accident. In fact, the incidence in several reported series is over 60%. The distribution of fractures in children is similar to that in adults, with about 40% of the fractures being unstable. The majority of these are Malgaigne-type fractures, with double vertical fractures of both the anterior and posterior arches. However, children only rarely fracture their sacrum, but more often disrupt the sacroiliac joint. Fractures of the acetabulum are also relatively rare in children, occurring in only about 3% or 4%. Fractures will also occur through the triradiate cartilage, and traumatic separation of the proximal femoral epiphysis can also be seen as a result of a motor vehicle accident. Children are more likely to get avulsion injuries than adults. Once again, the anterior superior iliac spine, which is the origin of the sartorius muscle, can be

avulsed in patients who are hurdlers, sprinters, long jumpers, and gymnasts. The anterior inferior iliac spine, which is the origin of the rectus femoris, can also be involved in these sports. Ischial tuberosity avulsions are certainly quite common and usually easy to recognize, since they can be compared to the opposite sides (Fig. 55A and B). In fact, it is possible to avulse almost any muscle origin in the pelvis, and avulsion injuries to the adductor tubercle adjacent to the symphysis pubis have also been described in young athletes. These are usually confirmed using MRI.

HIP

Fractures of the Upper Femur

Femoral neck fractures are the second most common fracture following fractures of the distal radius, and are seen predominantly in elderly female patients with osteoporosis. However, femoral neck fractures also can occur in younger people as a result of major trauma, often associated with pelvic fractures. There are various subdivisions of femoral neck fractures, but a simple one is to divide those that are *intercapsular* (63%) (subcapital, transcervical, and basicervical) and those which are intertrochanteric (37%) and, hence, *extracapsular*.

Subcapital fractures occur just under the femoral head at the upper portion of the femoral neck and account for 33% to 50% of all femoral neck fractures (Fig. 56A, B). They may be impacted and be either complete or incomplete or displaced, with the leg foreshortened and rotated internally. Subcapital fractures have a 3:1 female to male ratio and are associated with 6% to 8% fractures of either the distal radius or the proximal humerus. They are also associated with a 33% incidence of avascular necrosis and are usually managed by implanting a femoral endoprosthesis.

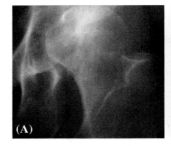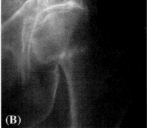

Figure 56 Early, discrete subcapital femoral neck fracture. (**A**) On this initial film, there is a suggestion of a break in the cortex just above the femoral calcar. (**B**) On a repeat film taken 10 days later with the patient non-weight bearing, a sclerotic healing subcapital fracture can be easily seen.

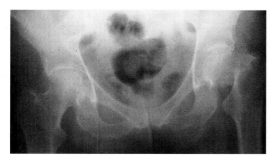

Figure 57 This is the typical transcervical fracture with marked angulation of the femoral head and neck on the inter-trochanteric region.

Transcervical fractures are rarer, and *basicervical fractures* are uncommon, accounting for only 10% of all femoral neck fractures (Fig. 57).

These are associated with a 20% incidence of avascular necrosis and are usually fixed by internal pinning, although femoral endoprostheses may also be used.

Intertrochanteric fractures account for 15% of femoral fractures in the elderly, but represent 50% of femoral neck fractures in younger patients without osteoporosis and have an equal sex incidence (Fig. 58).

Intertrochanteric fractures usually parallel the inter-trochanteric ridge and are most often comminuted, with

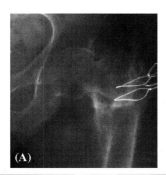

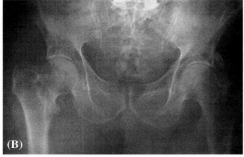

Figure 58 Intertrochanteric fractures (I/T). **(A)** This patient has an old I/T fracture which has now refractured and angled into a varus position. **(B)** A more recent I/T fracture in a different patient showing their typical oblique orientation.

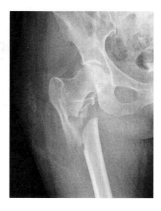

Figure 59 A comminuted subtrochanteric fracture.

separation of the lesser trochanter, greater trochanter, or both. If they are two part (i.e., a solitary fracture—25%) or three part with separation of the lesser trochanter (30%), they are stable, although the lesser trochanter will get pulled upward by the ilio-psoas muscle. If they are three part, involving the greater trochanter, or four part, they are unstable (45%) and are frequently displaced, with the fragments becoming separated with varus deformity of the hip. These are usually fixed by compression pin and plate.

Finally, *subtrochanteric fractures* account for 5% of femoral neck fractures in the elderly, but 20% of femoral neck fractures in younger patients (Fig. 59).

By definition, they occur within 3 in of the lesser trochanter, involving the proximal femoral shaft, and are all unstable. They are seen in association with osteoporosis in the elderly, with major trauma in the young, and also as pathological fractures in association with Paget's disease, fibrous dysplasia, and metastatic disease. They have a low incidence of avascular necrosis and are usually managed by a sliding compression pin and plate.

Osteochondral impaction fractures of the femoral head have been classified into three types and are known as Pipkin fractures (Fig. 60A, B).

These usually occur as an isolated injury as a result of a direct blow to the femoral head, although they have also been associated with posterior hip dislocations. Type I is a segmental linear fracture of the femoral head below the fovea and is the most common. These are difficult to see on plain films and usually require a CT scan (Fig. 60C).

Type II are through the fovea and type III, which are rare and comminuted and involve the whole of the femoral head.

Avulsion fractures of the proximal femur occur in young athletes and principally involve the lesser trochanter, which becomes avulsed in runners, hurdlers, and baseball players. Once avulsed, the lesser trochanter is drawn up proximally by the pull of the ilio-psoas muscle.

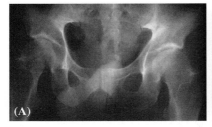
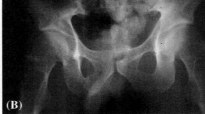
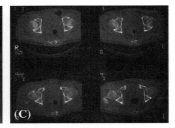

Figure 60 Type I Pipkin fracture. (**A**) On the initial film, no abnormality can be seen. (**B**) A film taken five days later; there is a suggestion of a linear fracture of the right femoral head. (**C**) This is confirmed by the CT scan, which shows a linear segmental fracture of the inner surface of the femoral head. This has very little displacement, which is why it is difficult to see on the plain films. *Abbreviation*: CT, computed tomography.

Dislocations of the Hip

Hip dislocations account for only 5% of all dislocations in the body, and, thus, they are quite rare: 90% are posterior and only 10% anterior, if one excludes the central fracture/dislocations, which have been discussed under section "Pelvic Fractures."

Posterior dislocations account for 90% of hip dislocations and occur when the knee hits the dashboard, while the hip is flexed and the femoral head gets driven posteriorly and superiorly between the iliac bone and the gluteal muscles (Fig. 61A, B).

They are often difficult to reduce, but, if allowed to remain out of the socket for over 24 hours, there is a 100% incidence of avascular necrosis, whereas if reduced within four hours, the incidence of avascular necrosis is virtually zero. Reducing them may result in an osteochondral

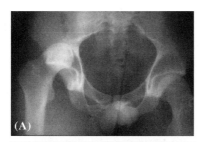
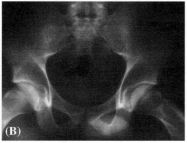

Figure 61 Posterior dislocation of the right hip. (**A**) On the initial film, the right femoral head can be seen lying above and posterior to the right acetabulum. (**B**) Following reduction, normal alignment has been achieved. No fracture can be seen.

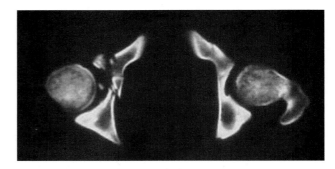

Figure 62 Postreduction of a posterior dislocation showing multiple bony fragments within the joint on CT scan. *Abbreviation*: CT, computed tomography.

fracture of the inferior medial aspect of the femoral head (Pipkin fracture). Sciatic nerve damage, either transient or permanent, is another complication of posterior hip dislocation and is seen in 10% of patients. Posterior hip dislocations are also associated with femoral neck fractures and/or femoral shaft fractures in 45%. On reducing them, either bone or cartilaginous fragments may get caught between the acetabulum and the femoral head, impeding their full reduction. CT scanning will often show the presence of the fragment that the surgeon may then remove arthroscopically (Fig. 62).

Anterior hip dislocations are uncommon (10%), and the femoral head slides anteriorly and inferiorly into the obturator notch in most patients (90%), although occasionally the head will go anteriorly and superiorly (10%), where it is associated with an anterior column acetabular fracture (Fig. 63).

Anterior hip dislocations occur with abduction and external rotation and may be associated with fractures of the acetabulum and elsewhere (20–25% of cases). They are rarely associated with femoral head fractures. The incidence of avascular necrosis will also depend on the length of time the femoral head is out of the acetabulum, but is lower than that seen with posterior dislocations. The overall incidence of avascular necrosis is 20% in anterior hip dislocations (Fig. 64).

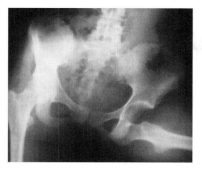

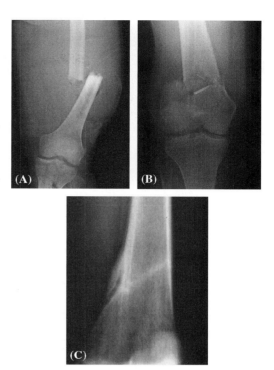

Figure 63 This is a typical anterior dislocation of the hip, with the femoral head lying in the obturator and the leg markedly abducted.

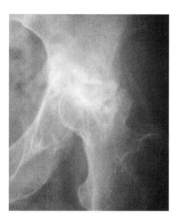

Figure 64 This patient sustained a posterior dislocation of the hip 10 years before this film and now has grade V avascular necrosis of the left femoral head with severe degenerative arthritis.

A recent paper looked at 50 patients with isolated hip dislocations. Four percent developed avascular necrosis; heterotopic ossification occurred in 8%, early osteoarthritis in 15%, and moderate osteoarthritis in 10%. This paper also noted an increasing complication rate when the patient had other injuries.

Injuries to the femoral head and neck in children are rare. Occasionally Salter I-type injuries can occur through the growth plate, but these are usually seen in association with pelvic fractures. Traumatic slipped capital femoral epiphyses are also rare, as are fractures of the femoral neck and intertrochanteric fractures. However, dislocations of the hip, particularly posteriorly, can be seen in children younger than 12 years.

Fractures of the Femoral Shaft

Usually the shaft is divided into three equal parts, starting 3 in below the level of the lesser trochanter down to the supracondylar region above the knees. Fractures of the midshaft are the most common, and they are often

Figure 65 Femoral shaft fracture in three different patients. (**A**) Typical midshaft fracture. (**B**) Comminuted supracondylar fracture. (**C**) This is a typical insufficiency fracture of the distal femur with an oblique healing fracture seen in the distal metaphyseal region.

transverse with only minimal comminution, or oblique, and comminuted with a butterfly fragment often breaking off on their medial aspect (Fig. 65A, B, C).

In 85%, the proximal fragment gets abducted by the pull of the glutei. The most important thing to remember about femoral shaft fractures is that 20% of patients have an associated injury in the same limb, so X-ray down from the pelvis and hip to the knee, and then down to the ankle, checking the complete length of both the femur and the tibia and fibula on the same side.

KNEE

Distal Femur/Proximal Tibia and Fibula

Injuries to the distal femur and proximal tibia are common, and most of them also involve the menisci and ligaments of the knee. To some extent, the knee is probably the most commonly injured area in the body, but many of these injuries are to the soft tissues alone, and are covered by the section on MRI of the Knee in chapter 8. However, many patients develop knee effusions after an injury. Effusions are best diagnosed above the patella, where the small, triangular fat pad above the patella itself becomes separated from the larger, rounded fat pad in

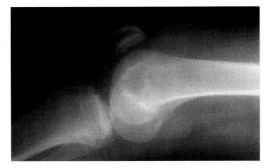

Figure 66 Knee effusion. Note the ovoid gray area lying above the patella, with the anterior femoral fat pad below it in a small prepatella fat pad above it. This is a typical appearance of a large effusion.

front of the femur, as fluid fills the suprapatellar pouch (Fig. 66).

You cannot diagnose knee effusions in the region of Hoffa's fat pad (lying deep to the patellar tendon and between the distal femur and proximal tibia). On the other hand, prepatellar bursitis as well as bursitis in the various bursae around the patellar mechanism can be diagnosed on a good lateral film of the knee. It is also difficult to diagnose a knee effusion posteriorly because the two gastrocnemius muscles produce a large, soft-tissue impression posteriorly. If the cortex is also damaged following an intra articular fracture, then a lipohemarthrosis can occur, and this is best demonstrated on a crosstable, lateral view of the knee, where the fat from the bone marrow layers out above the blood as a horizontal shadow in the suprapatellar pouch (Fig. 67A, B).

Nearly all fractures of the distal femur in young people are intra-articular, and, although there is no formal classification of them, they resemble the fractures seen in the distal humerus-transverse, such as supracondylar fractures (which mainly occur in elderly, osteoporotic patients), Y-and T-shaped intracondylar fractures, sagittal and coronal fractures, fractures of a single condyle, which are usually oblique, and coronal oblique fractures, which also largely occur in elderly, osteopenic patients (Fig. 68).

On the other hand, there is a classification of proximal tibial fractures, although I cannot recall anyone using it; 25% are depression fractures, 25% are vertical, or sagittal, split fractures, 25% are a combination of the two, and 25% are other fractures (Fig. 69).

Many proximal tibial fractures are associated with fractures of the head or neck of the fibula, or with dislocation of the proximal tibiofibular joint. Fractures of the proximal fibula may also occur separately, usually as a result of a direct blow, and these can be associated with damage to the common peroneal nerve. Fractures of the proximal fibula are also seen as part of the Maissoneuve fracture complex, where there are fractures of the posterior

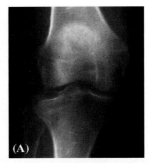

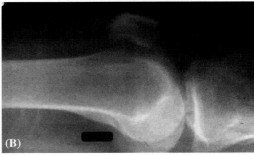

Figure 67 (A) There is a depressed fracture of the lateral tibial plateau with some comminution. AP view. (B) Crosstable lateral view to show the lipohemoarthrosis. *Abbreviation*: AP, anteroposterior.

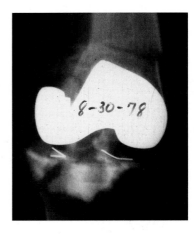

Figure 68 Elderly osteoporotic supracondylar fracture.

malleolus, a tear of the interosseous membrane, and a fracture of the fibular neck (Fig. 70A, B, C).

Associated soft-tissue injuries are common with tibial fractures and may involve the menisci, collateral ligaments, cruciate ligaments, or any combination of the three (see section on MRI of the Knee in chapter 8).

Other types of fractures may be seen in and around the knee, including stress fractures in military recruits and insufficiency fractures in the elderly or osteopenic, although these are more common in the upper third of the tibia than in the femur. Avulsion fractures of the tibial

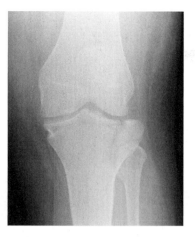

Figure 69 Vertical fracture lateral tibial plateau.

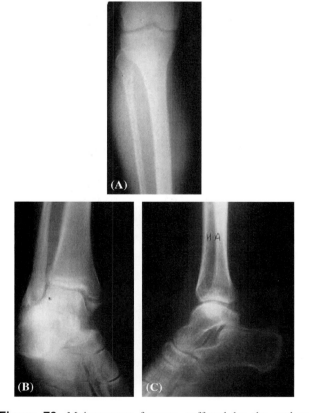

Figure 70 Maissoneuve fracture suffered by the author. (**A**) Fracture of fibular neck. (**B**) Fracture of the medial malleolus. (**C**) Fracture of posterior malleolus.

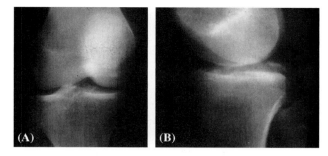

Figure 71 (**A**) Avulsion fracture of the tibial spine: AP view. This is inherently an avulsion fracture of the insertion of the anterior cruciate ligament. This can be seen with careful scrutiny of the plain films. (**B**) Avulsion fracture of the tibial spine: lateral view. This is inherently an avulsion fracture of the insertion of the anterior cruciate ligament. This can be seen with careful scrutiny of the plain films. *Abbreviation*: AP, anteroposterior.

spines are also quite common, occurring following a twisting injury such as in skiing injuries or falls off a bike (Fig. 71A, B).

These are, of course, really cruciate ligament injuries, with the anterior cruciate ligament inserting into the anterior tibial spine and the posterior cruciate ligament inserting far posteriorly behind the posterior tibial spine. Avulsion fractures may be virtually undisplaced (when you will need MRI to confirm them), hinged, completely detached and pulled proximally, or even inverted.

Dislocations of the knee are usually disastrous, since they are often associated with severe soft-tissue injury such as cruciate ligament tears, collateral ligament tears, and complete disruption of the posterolateral corner of the knee, as well as meniscal injuries. It takes considerable force to dislocate a knee, and arterial injury (usually to the popliteal artery) is seen in 30%, and peroneal nerve damage occurs in 15%. The most common knee dislocation is an *anterior dislocation* where the femur moves forward on the tibia.

This occurs as a result of acute hyperextension and produces tears of the posterior cruciate ligament and posterior capsule. *Posterior dislocations,* where the femur goes backward on the tibia are more serious and are associated with anterior cruciate ligament tears, arterial damage, as well as damage to the patellar mechanism (Fig. 72).

Isolated dislocations of the proximal tibiofibular joint can occur as a result of falls or twisting injuries, and are seen in jumpers and parachutists although they are most commonly seen in association with spiral fractures of the distal tibia (Fig. 73A, B).

Once again, damage to the common peroneal nerve is seen quite commonly in association with these injuries. The most common separation is anterolaterally, but the proximal tibiofibular joint may also dislocate posteromedially as a result of a direct blow. Remember that, if you see a superior dislocation, this is usually associated with a fracture distally at the ankle. Once again, let me stress that, if you see what appears to be an isolated fracture of the proximal fibula or an isolated dislocation of the proximal tibiofibular joint, you must x-ray the entire tibia and fibula from the knee down to and including the ankle (ring-of-bone concept).

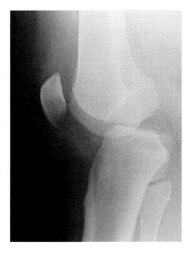

Figure 72   Posterior dislocation of the knee with the tibia lying markedly posterior to the femur. This injury is often associated with a tear of the patella tendon as well as tears of the cruciate ligaments.

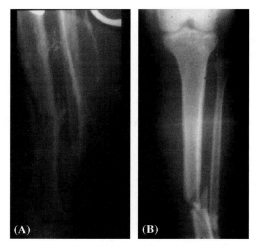

Figure 73   (**A**) Fractures of the midshaft of the tibia and fibula with arterial damage. (**B**) Another example with separation of the proximal tibiofibular joint and fractures of the distal tibia and fibula.

Patellar fractures occur in isolation or as a result of a direct blow or in association with other fractures or dislocations around the knee (Fig. 74A, B).

Sixty percent of them are transverse, 15% vertical, and 25% are comminuted or stellate. Avulsion fractures of the insertion of the quadriceps tendon into the superior pole and of the patella tendon off the inferior pole also occur and can be easily confirmed by the use of MRI. Osteochondral fractures of the undersurface of the patella can be seen following a direct blow to the patella, forcing it backward onto the trochlear notch of the femur. These are usually seen with either arthrography

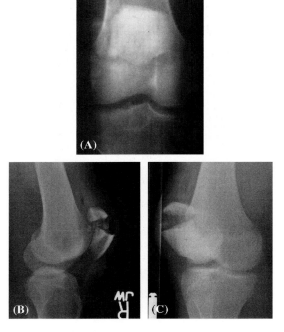

Figure 74   Patellar fractures in two different patients. (**A**) Vertical. This would be difficult to see on a lateral view. (**B**) Lateral view. Horizontal fracture. (**C**) Oblique view. Horizontal fracture.

or MRI. A congenital anomaly of the superior lateral pole of the patella, where the various growth centers fail to fuse, is commonly seen and is known as a bipartite patella (Fig. 75).

It is most often seen in the upper outer quadrant, but 5% can be seen elsewhere; 60% are bilateral. It is usually easy to distinguish between a fracture and a bipartite patella on clinical grounds alone; the latter does not hurt

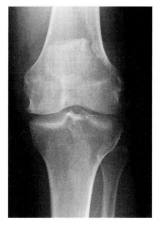

Figure 75   Bipartite patella. Note the separation of the upper/outer/lateral portion of the patella from the main bone. This is the typical appearance of a bipartite patella and is usually bilateral.

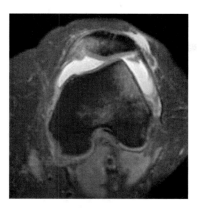

Figure 76 Results of patella dislocation. Axial MR scan. This shows the bone bruising on the lateral femoral condyle and the medial aspect of the patella, where there is also a patella retinacular tear. *Abbreviation*: MR, magnetic resonance.

and is usually bilateral, whereas a true fracture is painful and unilateral. However, occasionally it can be difficult to distinguish the two, and MRI is helpful. Sometimes bipartite patellae are almost undisplaced and, thus, invisible, which makes the diagnosis even more difficult to make.

Dislocations of the patella are quite common, usually lateral, and occur when the knee is flexed and in valgus (Fig. 76).

They may be transient or become locked in position, and this often depends on the shape of the undersurface of the patella. The relative angulation and size of the medial and lateral patellar condyles has been classified into five subgroups where type I is normal and type V is basically flat, which would obviously lead to recurrent patellar dislocation.

Many of the fractures around the knee can be seen in children; however, epiphyseal injuries also occur, although they are rare, accounting for only 1% of all epiphyseal injuries in the body. Seventy percent of distal femoral fractures are of the Salter II type, Salter III fractures (unicondylar) account for 15%, and Salter IV fractures for 10%. In the proximal tibia, the epiphyseal injuries are either Salter I or Salter II. In younger children, spiral fractures of the tibia associated with a bowing fracture of the fibula may occur, and, in fact, a "toddlers" fracture is a minimally displaced tibial fracture with or without a fibular fracture seen in under two-year olds.

FOOT AND ANKLE

Fractures of the Ankle

There are several different classifications of ankle fractures, but only two are widely used today; these are the Weber classification (3), which is probably too simple,

and the Lauge-Hansen (4) classification, which is probably too complex. On top of these classifications come various other fractures or types of fractures, all of which have eponyms. In fact, there is a complete chapter on ankle eponyms in Kelikian's (5) excellent book on the ankle. But first let us deal with the normal anatomy.

The ankle has been described as a "mortise" joint, with the lateral malleolus, medial malleolus, and posterior malleolus holding the talus in place. Between the tibia and fibula is an intraosseous membrane that holds the two bones roughly parallel and ends in a syndesmosis just above the ankle joint. This should be no greater than 4-mm wide and is best seen on a 15° oblique AP view of the ankle called a mortise view. The joint space between the three malleoli and the talus should be approximately equidistant, measuring from 2 to 3 mm in the average normal patient. Thus, the talus has articulating surfaces on its sides, as well as a curved superior surface that has two "domes" with a slight depression centrally on the AP view.

Finally, remember that the tibia and fibula act as a ring of bone, so that a fracture of the distal tibia may be accompanied by a fracture of the proximal fibula. Thus, full-length views of the tibia and fibula, as well as localized X rays of the ankle itself, should make up a complete ankle series in your practice.

Before we get into the specific classifications, the ankle and foot have acquired a number of directional terms that are not used elsewhere in the body:

Plantar flexion: flexion down toward the plantar surface.
Dorsi flexion: flexion up away from the plantar surface.
Inversion: inward rotation.
Eversion: outward rotation.
External rotation: lateral movement of the foot in relationship to the long axis of the leg.
Internal rotation: medial movement of the foot in relation to the long axis of the leg.
Abduction: inward displacement of the foot in relation to the tibia.
Adduction: outward displacement of the foot in relation to the tibia.
Supination: a combination of internal rotation and adduction.
Pronation: a combination of external rotation and abduction.

Having got this out of the way, let us consider the first and most simplistic classification of ankle fractures: the *Weber classification*.

Weber A fracture: the fibula is fractured below the ankle mortise.
Weber B fracture: the fibula is fractured at the level of the ankle mortise.
Weber C fracture: the fracture is above the ankle mortise and usually some 4 to 6 cm above the mortise itself.

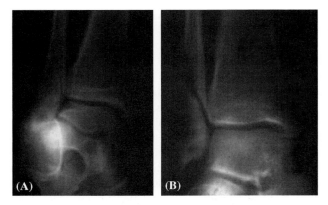

Figure 77 Weber type B fracture. (**A** and **B**) The classical Weber type B is a fracture that ends at the same level as the ankle mortise and apparently enters into it.

The type A fracture is an avulsion fracture of the distal fibula at or below the joint level with an associated fracture of the medial malleolus, which is usually oblique.

The Weber type B fracture is a spiral fibular fracture entering at the level of the ankle mortise with partial disruption of the tibiofibular ligament, as well as an avulsion fracture off the medial malleolus, which is usually horizontal. Alternatively, the medial malleolus may be intact, and there may be a rupture of the deltoid ligament (Fig. 77A, B).

The Weber type C injury is a high, usually oblique, fibular fracture with rupture of the tibiofibular ligament, as well as the interosseous membrane up to the level of the fracture. This is associated with an avulsion fracture of the medial malleolus, which is, once again, horizontal, or the medial malleolus may be intact and the deltoid ligament may rupture instead.

To go from one extreme to the other, the Lauge-Hansen classification (4) was also first described in 1972 and has five major subgroups, with many subtypes in each group, which add up to a total of 24 different types of ankle fracture in all. The major subgroups are

1. supination external rotation injury.
2. supination adduction rotation injury.
3. pronation external rotation injury.
4. pronation abduction injury.
5. pronation dorsiflexion injury.

The first word refers to the position of the foot at the time of the injury, and the second word to the direction that the talus goes as a result of the injury.

Supination External Rotation Injury

Stage 1 is rupture of the inferior anterior tibiofibular ligament. Stage 2 is stage 1 as well as an oblique spiral fracture of the lateral malleolus. Stage 3 is stage 2 as well

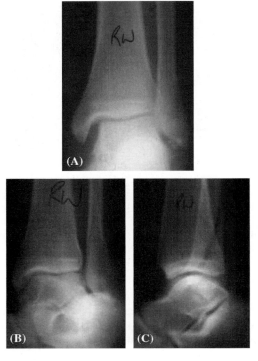

Figure 78 (**A**, **B**, **C**) Supination adduction injury. This is a typical supination adduction fracture with a spiral fracture of the distal fibula and separation of the syndesmosis as well as a tear of the deltoid ligament, leading to widening of the medial aspect of the ankle mortise.

as a fracture of the posterior lip of the tibia. Stage 4 is stage 3 as well as a transverse or oblique fracture of the medial malleolus or tear of the deltoid ligament. Thus, there are four stages, but five different outcomes in supination external rotation injuries.

Supination Adduction Rotation Injuries

Supination adduction injuries are somewhat more straightforward in that there are only two stages, but four outcomes. In stage 1, there is a transverse fracture of the lateral malleolus or a tear of the lateral collateral ligament. Stage 2 is with the addition of a vertical or oblique fracture of the medial malleolus. Thus, a supination adduction injury can be a classical bimalleolor fracture with a horizontal fracture of the distal fibula at the level of the ankle mortise and a vertical fracture of the medial malleolus (Fig. 78A, B, C).

Pronation External Rotation Injuries

These have four stages and, once again, eight different types of injury, depending on whether a fracture occurs or there is a tear of the ligaments (Fig. 79A, B).

Stage 1 is a transverse fracture of the medial malleolus or a tear of the deltoid ligament. Stage 2 is with the

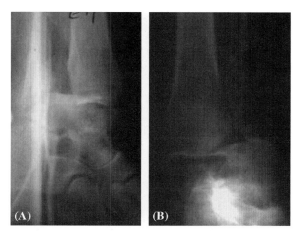

Figure 79 (**A** and **B**) Pronation external rotation injury. In this injury there is complete separation of the fibula from the tibia with fractures of the medial malleolus as well as the posterior malleolus and the distal fibula.

addition of a tear of the inferior anterior tibiofibular and intraosseous ligaments. Stage 3 is with the addition of a tear of the intraosseous membrane to the level of the spiral fracture of the fibula, 7 or 8 cm up the fibula, or a more proximal fracture at the tip of the lateral malleolus. Stage 4 is all of the above with the addition of an avulsion fracture off the posterior lip of the tibia at the attachment to the posterior inferior and inferior transverse tibiofibular ligament. This is a true *trimalleolar fracture*. Thus, pronation external rotation injuries are classically with a transverse fracture of the medial malleolus at the level of the ankle mortise and a high fracture of the fibula and a tear of the syndesmosis. There are eight subtypes of this injury.

Pronation Abduction Injuries

There are only three stages of this injury, but six subtypes, depending on if a fracture occurs or if ligamentous damage ensues. Stage 1 is a transverse fracture of the medial malleolus or a tear of the deltoid ligament. Stage 2 is with the addition of a rupture of the anterior and posterior inferior tibiotalar ligaments and the inferior transverse tibiofibular ligament, with a fracture of the posterior lip of the tibia. In this situation, the syndesmosis and intraosseous ligament will remain intact. Stage 3 is all of the above, with the addition of an oblique supramalleolar fracture of the fibula (Fig. 80A, B, C, D).

Pronation Dorsiflexion Injuries

These have four stages and only four subtypes. Stage 1 is a fracture of the medial malleolus. Stage 2 is with the addition of an avulsion off the anterior lip of the tibia. Stage 3 is with a fracture of the supramalleolar portion of

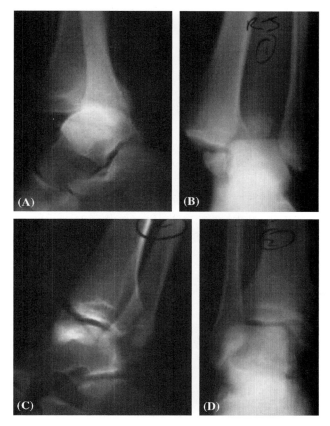

Figure 80 (**A**, **B**, **C**, **D**) Pronation abduction injury. This is an extreme example of a typical pronation abduction injury with fractures of all three malleoli as well as separation of the distal fibula and tibia syndesmosis.

the fibula, and stage 4 is with the addition of a transverse fracture of the dorsal part of the tibia at the level of the proximal margin of the large tibial fragment (Fig. 81).

Pronation dorsiflexion injuries are typically seen in patients who get their foot caught under the pedal of the car or fall forward with their foot fixed in a sagittal position.

Unfortunately, we have not finished with fractures about the ankle. There are a number of other fractures that have not been fully included by either classification, and perhaps the logical way to assess these is alphabetically.

Dupuytrens Fracture

This is a spiral fracture of the fibula associated with an ankle fracture, usually of the posterior tibial margin. This fracture occurs as a result of pronation and external rotation (Fig. 82A, B).

Maissoneuve Fracture

This fracture is one that the author has personal experience with (Fig. 70). This is a fracture of the posterior

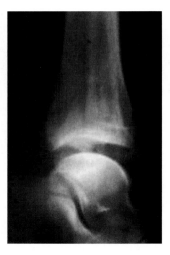

Figure 81 Pronation dorsiflexion injury. This lateral view shows a discrete fracture of the posterior malleolus as well as a fracture of the distal fibula.

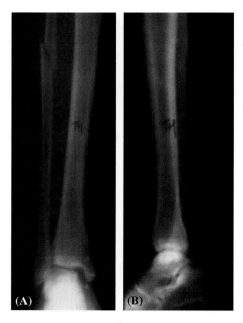

Figure 82 (**A**, **B**) Dupuytrens fracture with a spiral fracture of the proximal fibula and a discrete minimally displaced fracture of the posterior malleolus.

fibula associated with an ankle fracture in external rotation. The fracture of the fibula is often at the neck of the fibula, where it is remarkably pain free (see earlier).

Pilon Fractures

In 1911, Destot likened the tibiotalar joint to a pestle and mortar. The term "Pilon fracture" is used to describe four subgroups or subtypes of distal tibial fracture, all involving the tibial plafond, which is the anterior lip of the fibula (Fig. 83A, B).

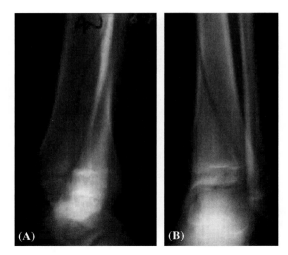

Figure 83 (**A**, **B**) Pilon fracture. There is a long spiral fracture of the distal tibia extending at least 10 cm up the tibial shaft.

Pilon fractures may or may not be accompanied by a fibular fracture. The difference between the various subtypes is the degree of involvement of the tibial articular surface: in an "explosion" fracture, it is pulverized, and in the supra-articular fracture, it is split. Pilon fractures occur as a result of axial compression in falls from altitudes, and the tibia fractures because the body of the talus is relatively stronger than the tibial vault. The difference between a fracture of the posterior malleolus and the Pilon fracture is the height and length of the tibial fragment; in Pilon fractures, the segment has to be at least 8-cm high.

Posterior Marginal Fractures, or Posterior Malleolar Fractures

These occur in association with many of the external rotation injuries described in the Lauge-Hansen classification. They are also an integral part of the Maissoneuve fracture, where the talus is forced against the posterior margin in forced plantar flexion. Anterior marginal, or anterior lip fractures, do not have to be as high or as long. The difference between a Tillaux fracture and an anterior marginal fracture is difficult to assess, but, on the whole, anterior marginal fractures are a result of a direct axial compression force, and Tillaux fractures are a result of an internal rotational force in a younger patient (Fig. 84).

Explosion fractures are what the word implies and are due to high-velocity accidents, where the talus is driven into the tibial vault and "explodes," the distal tibia shattering the tibial vault with severe comminution. These are typically seen as a result of a motor vehicle accident, where the driver of the vehicle has his foot on the brake pedal as he or she hits the back of a stationary truck at 70 m.p.h. Supra-articular fractures are a more minor version of explosion fractures, with only a horizontal component or two across the distal tibial metaphysis. In many supra-articular fractures, the tibial vault remains intact.

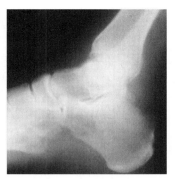

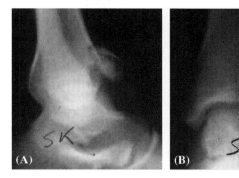

Figure 84 Posterior marginal fracture. On the lateral view, there is discrete separation of the posterior malleolus.

The term "Pilon fracture" does not refer to a pylon, but to a pestle. Most Pilon fractures are caused by high-velocity injuries, and the term refers to a comminuted fracture of the distal tibia, which often involves the tibial plafond. The overlap between Pilon fractures and other fractures of the distal tibia can be confusing. Posterior marginal fractures are the most common and are not treated surgically unless they involve more than 25% of the weight-bearing surface of the distal tibia. They are also more commonly associated with fibula fractures, as is the case with a Maissoneuve fracture.

Tillaux Fracture

This is an avulsion fracture of the anterior tibial tubercle, usually as a result of external rotation of the foot. In a child, it is equivalent to a Salter III fracture of the lateral half of the epiphysis. It may be in two or three planes. In

Figure 85 Tillaux fracture. These images show a typical avulsion fracture of the anterior tibial tubercle. (**A**) Lateral view. (**B**) AP view. *Abbreviation*: AP, anteroposterior.

adults, it is classically seen in association with pronation external rotation injuries (Fig. 85A, B).

Finally, let us discuss ankle fractures in children. Possibly the classical fracture in young children is a Salter II fracture of the distal tibia. However, they also get spiral fractures of the distal fibula, Tillaux fractures, and Pilon fractures, which have already been described. Greenstick fractures and torus fractures of both distal tibia and fibula will also occur, and, obviously, children can also get malleolar fractures, just as adults. However, children also get another fracture called the triplane fracture (Fig. 86A, B).

From its name, triplane is a fracture in three planes: a fracture of the lateral half of the tibial epiphysis (sagittal plane), with a posterior triangular metaphyseal fragment (angulated plane), and a fracture through the growth plate (horizontal plane). These occur only in the distal tibia, and the children are usually aged between 12 and 15 years.

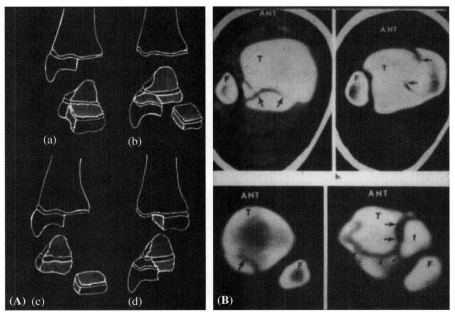

Figure 86 Triplane fracture. (**A**) Drawing. (**B**) CT scan showing both the transverse and the vertical planes of this complex fracture seen mainly in children. *Abbreviation*: CT, computed tomography. *Source*: From Ref. 1.

The majority of triplane fractures are actually only two-part injuries, and the three planes are really quite rare. The best way to evaluate the triplane fracture is a CT scan with sagittal and coronal reconstruction.

Talar Fractures

Not surprisingly, there are several classifications of talar fractures, many of which are associated with dislocations, either of the tibiotalar joint (ankle joint) or the subtalar joint. A simple classification would be

- fractures of the body of the talus
- fractures of the neck or waist of talus
- fractures of the head of the talus
- fractures of the posterior process (os trigonum)
- fractures of the anterior-superior process
- osteochondral fractures

It is estimated that at least 40% of all talar fractures are associated with dislocations, and fractures of the neck and body are associated with a much higher incidence of dislocation, perhaps as high as 70%.

Fractures of the talar body may be simple, in which case they are often oblique or vertical and mainly minimally displaced and are usually closed fractures (Fig. 87).

However, many talar body fractures are comminuted and open and associated with other fractures and dislocations.

Similarly, *fractures of the talar neck* may be vertical and minimally displaced, in which case there are few sequelae, or they may be open and associated with a fracture/dislocation, in which case the body of the talus usually swings around either 90° or 180° degrees, thus

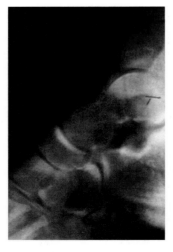

Figure 87 Fracture of the body of the talus. Note the discrete vertical, linear fracture running through the body of the bone with only minimal displacement.

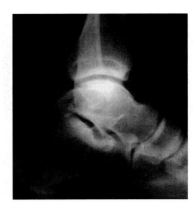

Figure 88 Fracture of posterior facet of the talus. (**A**) There is separation of the posterior facet of the talus in this young patient following an MVA. *Abbreviation*: MVA, motor vehicle accident.

producing a situation where the axis of the leg is coronal in position, and the foot is in the sagittal plane. In this case, the blood supply of the talus, which comes in posteriorly, is disrupted, and avascular necrosis occurs in virtually 100% of patients.

There is, in fact, a classification of fractures of the talar neck: type I virtually nondisplaced, vertical or oblique, and benign; type II displaced fracture, with subluxation or dislocation of the subtalar joint; and type III displaced fracture with dislocation of the body of the talus, both from above (the ankle joint) and below (the subtalar joint).

Fractures of the *head of the talus* are usually only minimally displaced and of little consequence. Fractures of the posterior process are controversial, with one side saying that they are developmental, with separation of a small posterior ossification center, and the other side saying that they are in fact true fractures (Fig. 88).

The situation is known as the *os trigonum syndrome* and will be dealt with in detail under MRI of the Ankle (see chap. 8). Fractures of the anterior superior process are invariably as a result of an avulsion-type injury seen in basketball players, for example, who excessively plantar flex their ankles.

This will ultimately produce a talar "beak," which is due to avulsion of the insertion of the anterior tibiotalar ligament, but may also be seen in tarsal coalitions, possibly for the same reason. Discrete avulsion fractures from the insertion of the various ankle ligaments into the talus are common, particularly on the medial side from the insertion of the deltoid ligament. These are frequently missed by the radiologist, but can be well seen low down on the mortise view, both medially (deltoid ligament) and laterally (anterior tibiofibular, fibulotalar, and posterior tibiofibular ligaments), if looked for carefully.

Osteochondral fractures are also quite common, even if one excludes osteochondritis dissecans of the talar dome, which is discussed elsewhere. Osteochondral

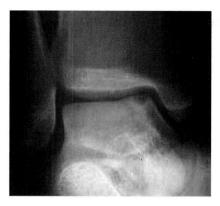

Figure 89 Osteochondral fracture following acute trauma and an inversion injury.

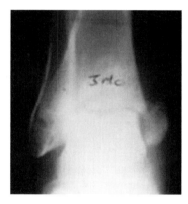

Figure 90 Premature degenerative arthritis of the ankle joint in a patient following a fracture of the waist of the talus.

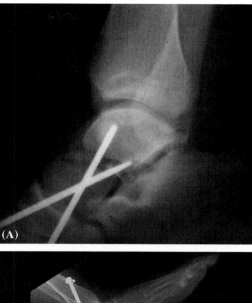

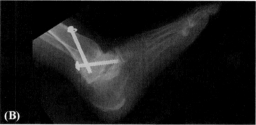

Figure 91 (**A**) Avascular necrosis of the talus. Single lateral ankle film showing markedly increased density of the head of the talus secondary to avascular necrosis one year after a non-union of a fracture of the waist of the talus. (**B**) Successful arthrodesis of the tibia-talar joint. Note the 2 cannulated screws running across the fused tibio-talar joint as well as the severe secondary degenerative changes in the subtalar joints.

fractures occur as a result of trauma and may be medial or lateral; these usually occur in active adults aged 20 to 40 years and have serious consequences only if a bony fragment is broken off into the joint (Fig. 89).

The two complications of talar fractures have already been alluded to: premature degenerative changes in either the tibiotalar joint or, more commonly, in the subtalar joint, and avascular necrosis (Fig. 90).

The patients' symptoms and radiographic appearance will confirm the diagnosis of degenerative arthritis, although occasionally CT scanning with sagittal reconstruction may be needed to fully evaluate subtalar arthritis. Avascular necrosis of the talus is easy to diagnose in its later stages, but can be quite difficult to diagnose early on. On the plain films, one of the earliest radiological signs of avascular necrosis of the talus is the presence of a subchondral lucency similar to that seen in the femoral head in early avascular necrosis and known as the "crescent" sign. In the talus, this subchondral lucency usually runs under only one of the talar domes, and cannot usually be seen until six to nine months after injury. This

is in comparison to a similar finding in disuse osteoporosis, although this is usually more generalized, with subchondral lucencies everywhere, including the tibial plafond as well as the lateral and medial borders of the talus, and occurs at four to eight weeks rather than six months. However, an MRI would now be able to confirm the diagnosis of early avascular necrosis with low signal on T1W and fat-sat T1W images with or without gadolinium. As the avascular necrosis progresses, the talus becomes increasingly dense and starts fragmenting and collapsing, at which stage arthrodesis is the best method of management (Fig. 91A, B).

Calcaneal Fractures

There are also a number of classifications of fractures of the calcaneus, which I have modified somewhat to include insufficiency fractures. Although there can be many different types of calcaneal fractures, the important ones are the compression fractures, which involve the subtalar joints and cause loss of *Boehler's angle*. On the lateral

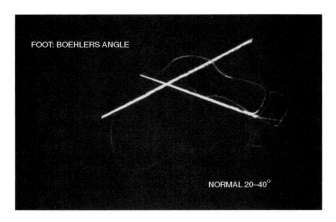

Figure 92 Boehler's angle. Drawing.

X ray, if one draws a line across the top of the anterior part of the calcaneus from the anterior process to the highest point on the bone and a second line from this point to the highest point posteriorly adjacent to the insertion of the Achilles tendon, they should cross at about 35°, with an anatomic range of 25° to 40°. This is referred to as Boehler's angle and, when below 20°, implies a calcaneal compression fracture (Fig. 92).

My modified classification of calcaneal fractures is as follows:

- Type I—fractures of the tuberosity, sustentaculum tali, and anterior process
- Type II—beak fractures of the insertion of the Achilles tendon
- Type III—insufficiency fractures
- Type IV—oblique fractures not involving the subtalar joints
- Type V—oblique fractures involving the subtalar joints
- Type VI—compression fractures

Fractures of the anterior process occur as a result of an inversion abduction injury when the anterior part of the calcaneus gets caught between the talus and the cuboid (Fig. 93).

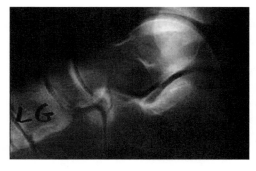

Figure 93 Fracture of the anterior process of the calcaneus.

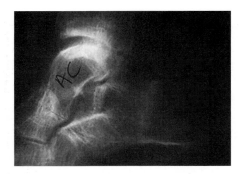

Figure 94 Insufficiency fracture of the calcaneus in a young male patient with poliomyelitis. Note the discrete sclerotic line running across the calcaneus.

These are often missed but are best seen on the lateral view. Similarly, fractures of the sustentaculum tali occur as a result of an inversion supination injury. Neither of these fractures appear to have any sequelae, although they may be the cause of chronic pain in the hind foot. Beak fractures off the posterior aspect of the calcaneus occur as a result of avulsion of the insertion of the Achilles tendon, but are rare, although, if they do occur, they are easy to diagnose, both clinically and radiologically. More often, patients will tear the tendon itself, and this is dealt with under MRI of the Ankle (see chap. 8). Insufficiency fractures usually have a characteristic curvilinear appearance parallel to the posterior aspect of the calcaneus and are seen in osteoporotic patients on high doses of steroids as well as in diabetic patients (Fig. 94).

In fact, diabetic patients sustain a number of different calcaneal fractures, and this will be discussed separately below.

The next three subtypes of calcaneal fractures are the clinically important fractures. The oblique nondisplaced fractures may be difficult to see on a simple lateral and AP view, but oblique views, and, more particularly, angled views such as the Harris view, which is a 45° anterior craniocaudad view taken along the longitudinal axis of the calcaneus, are very useful (Fig. 95A, B).

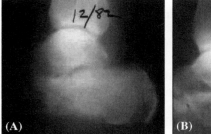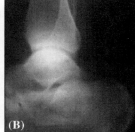

Figure 95 Oblique "nondisplaced" fracture of the calcaneus. (**A**) The initial film was read as normal. (**B**) Subsequent films taken one month later show the fracture and loss of Boehler's angle.

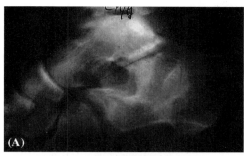

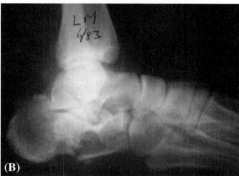

Figure 96 (**A**) Example of a compression fracture of the calcaneus with loss of Boehler's angle. (**B**) Another example of a severe compression fracture in a different patient who jumped from a bridge, where the talus has basically been pushed down through the calcaneus.

If the diagnosis is still unclear, CT scans with sagittal reconstructions are also very helpful to the surgeon. Oblique fractures involving the subtalar joints are usually obvious on the lateral view, with either partial or complete loss of Boehler's angle.

To reduce the incidence of subtalar arthritis, it is necessary to reconstitute this angle, hence, sagittal and coronal reconstructions are useful for the surgeon to identify the bony fragments and, often like a jigsaw puzzle, to reconstitute the bone. If the fracture is simple, then reverse traction with a calcaneal pin may be sufficient to reduce the fracture, but, more usually, it requires open reduction with several malleable plates and compression screws. Finally, compression fractures are the most serious fractures involving the calcaneus (Fig. 96A, B).

They are usually sustained by a fall from a considerable height. Usually obvious on the AP, and particularly the lateral view with loss of Boehler's angle, the most important part the radiologist can play is to identify the fragments, and, once again, CT scans with reconstruction are the technique of choice. Obviously, many of these patients will end up with premature arthritis in their subtalar joints, often necessitating arthrodesis. This, in turn, can also lead to premature degenerative arthritis in the ankle joint.

Fractures of the Other Tarsal Bones

Although rare, one can see isolated fractures of the cuboid, navicular, and cuneiforms. In isolation, the cuboid fractures usually occur as a result of a direct blow such as dropping a wardrobe on the outside of the foot (Fig. 97).

Isolated fractures of the cuneiforms are also very rare and mainly occur as a result of direct trauma. However, fractures of either the cuboid and the cuneiforms often accompany other fracture dislocations of the foot when they are not seen in isolation. On the other hand, longitudinal stress fractures through the body of the navicular are not uncommon in high-performance athletes as an isolated injury (Fig. 98A, B, C).

These are often difficult to diagnose off plain films, but either CT with reconstructions or MRI will make the diagnosis relatively easy. Avulsion fractures of the medial aspect of the navicular can occur as an occupational hazard in ballet dancers, but these are also usually easy to diagnose.

Fractures of the Metatarsals and Phalanges

Isolated fractures of any of the small bones of the foot can occur as a result of direct trauma, either by dropping an object on the foot or stubbing a toe, for example. However, there are two different types of metatarsal fractures that warrant separate discussion.

Jones fractures of the base of the fifth metatarsal occur as a result of an inversion injury, with the pull of the peroneus brevis tendon avulsing the proximal portion of the base of the fifth metatarsal (Fig. 99A, B, C).

First described by Sir Robert Jones in 1902 as a "transverse diaphyseal fracture approximately three-quarters of an inch from its base," this fracture needs to be differentiated from discrete avulsion fractures off the tip of the fifth metatarsal base caused by a pull of the plantar fascia, and also from an accessory apophysis, which often occurs in adolescent children (Fig. 99B, C).

Avulsion fractures occur within a few millimeters of the tip of the bone and an apophysis runs vertically and not horizontally. One of the reasons for this differentiation is that avulsion fractures heal rapidly and well, whereas the continuous pull of the peroneus brevis tendon leads to further distraction and nonhealing of a Jones fracture, which will often require internal fixation with a compression screw.

Stress fractures of the metatarsals are also not uncommon (Fig. 100).

Classically, these occur in athletes or military recruits and appear as transverse fractures of the neck of the second or third metatarsal. These are often impossible to see on the initial film, so that it is wise to recommend a follow-up film in 10 to 14 days if a stress fracture is suspected. However, stress fractures can occur at any age and in any

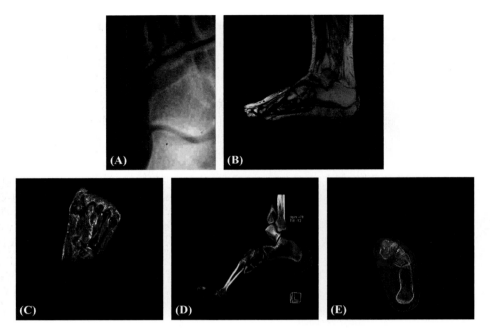

Figure 97 Fracture of the cuboid. (**A**) Plain film. Cuboid fractures are often difficult to see on plain films and easy to miss. This patient sustained this compression fracture one month previously. The sclerotic line infers that the fracture is subacute and healing. (**B**) Sagittal fat sat T1 MRI and (**C**) Coronal P.D. images show areas of abnormal signal in the cuboid typical of a healing fracture. (**D&E**) Sagittal and coronal CT scan reconstructions in the same patient confirmed the fracture. *Abbreviations*: MRI, magnetic resonance imaging; P.D., proton density.

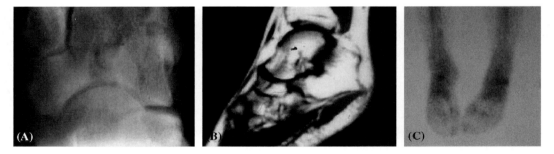

Figure 98 (**A**) Fracture tarsal/navicular. (**A**) Coned-down AP view of the navicular showing a typical vertical fracture. (**B**) MRI in a different patient showing clearly the fracture line of the navicular. (**C**) Bone scan showing high uptake in the region of the navicular—very sensitive but not as specific as the MRI. *Abbreviations*: AP, anteroposterior; MRI, magnetic resonance imaging.

patient, for instance, ballet dancers can get stress fractures of the base of the second metatarsal as a result of walking on their "points" too frequently. Older patients will get insufficiency fractures, often of the midshaft of the third and fourth metatarsals, and these are seen in patients either on high doses of steroids for one reason or another or in patients with advanced osteoporosis or osteomalacia. Similarly, patients with diabetes will get insufficiency fractures of their metatarsal shafts.

Dislocations of the Ankle Joint

Many of these have been discussed when we were going over fractures around the specific joints. *Isolated tibiotalar or ankle dislocations* are rare, although, the ankle joint will often sublux in association with bimalleolar and trimalleolar fractures (Fig. 101A, B).

In more major trauma, the talus may dislocate anteriorly, but usually goes posteriorly with respect to the

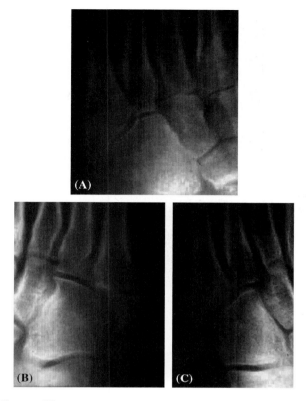

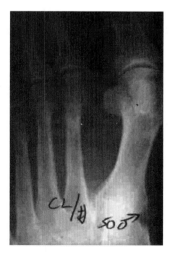

Figure 99 Fracture of the base of the fifth metatarsal. **(A)** Jones fracture. This is a typical Jones fracture approximately 2 cm distal to the proximal end of the bone. This occurs secondary to a pull by the peroneus brevis tendon. **(B)** Discrete fracture of the base of the fifth metatarsal. This is an avulsion fracture caused by a pull of the plantar fascia. **(C)** Normal epiphysis.

Figure 100 Stress fractures of the necks of the second and third metatarsals in a long-distance runner.

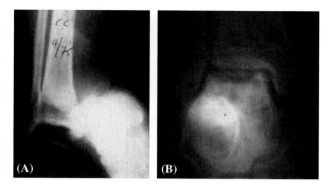

Figure 101 Tibiotalar dislocation. **(A)** Initial film showing complete separation of the tibiotalar joint. **(B)** AP film taken 10 years later, showing classical avascular necrosis of the talus. *Abbreviation*: AP, anteroposterior.

tibial plafond, and these subluxations are commonly associated with posterior malleolar fractures.

Subtalar dislocations are classified into three subtypes:

1. Type I—closed without associated injury
2. Type II—closed with associated injury

   a. soft-tissue damage, tendon or capsular tear (Fig. 102A, B)
   b. extra-articular fractures
   c. intra-articular fractures, particularly fractures of the talar neck or into the talonavicular joint or subtalar joint

3. Type III—open injuries with fractures of the body of the talus

As has been mentioned previously, all of these can be associated with premature degenerative arthritis in the subtalar joints, but type III injuries are also particularly associated with avascular necrosis of the talus (virtually 100% of patients).

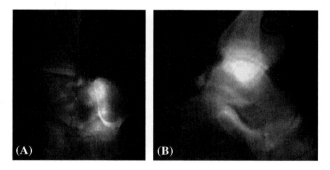

Figure 102 Subtalar dislocation. **(A)** AP view. Note that the talus stays in the ankle mortise, while the foot is dislocated laterally. This could be missed on this film. **(B)** Lateral view. Note that the talus stays in the ankle mortise and this may be missed on the lateral view. *Abbreviation*: AP, anteroposterior.

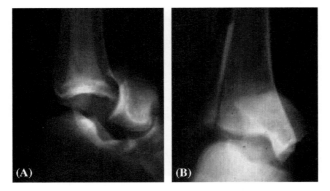

Figure 103 Talar dislocation. (**A**) Lateral view. In this situation the foot stays with the tibia and fibula, and the talus dislocates anteriorly and laterally. (**B**) AP view. In this situation the foot stays with the tibia and fibula, and the talus dislocates anteriorly and laterally. *Abbreviation*: AP, anteroposterior.

Isolated talar dislocations also occur, and are basically a combination of ankle dislocation and subtalar dislocation. They are also associated with a high incidence of both subtalar degenerative arthritis and avascular necrosis (Fig. 103A, B).

In the foot, *Chopart fracture dislocations* involve the joint between the hind foot and the midfoot, i.e., the talonavicular and calcaneocuboid joints (Fig. 104A, B).

These can be seen both as a result of direct trauma, such as a wheel running over your foot, or as a result of diabetes with a neuropathic element involved. Francois Chopart described an amputation between the hind foot and midfoot in 1791, and, thus, this has now become known as the Chopart joint. Most Chopart dislocations are associated with small avulsion fractures, particularly off the lowermost aspect of the talus and the uppermost aspect of the navicular since the navicular usually dislocates in a plantar direction. Similarly, since the cuboid is inclined to dislocate laterally on the calcaneus, small avulsion fractures can also be seen off the adjoining surfaces of these two bones.

Isolated subluxations of the calcaneocuboid joint are well described in the podiatric literature, but are largely dismissed by ours. However, one does occasionally see motion through this joint on stress views, which produces the patient's pain in people such as ballet dancers, acrobats, and gymnasts, for example.

Fracture/dislocations through the joint between the midfoot and forefoot are known as *Lisfranc fracture/dislocations* (Fig. 105A, B, C).

These are named after a French surgeon, Jacques Lisfranc, who lived from 1780 to 1847, and, in 1809, described an amputation through the base of the metatarsals in cavalry officers who sustained fracture dislocations at the midfoot/forefoot level as a result of falling off their

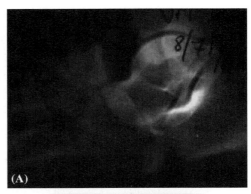

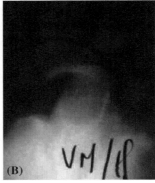

Figure 104 Chopart dislocation. There is a dislocation of the midfoot off the hind foot. (**A**) Lateral view showing the talarnavicular and calcaneus-cuboid dislocation, with the foot riding above the calcaneus and talus. (**B**) AP view showing that the forefoot has shifted medially on the hindfoot. *Abbreviation*: AP, anteroposterior.

horse with their boot firmly caught in the stirrup. Thus, the eponym "Lisfranc joint" has become applied to this joint. Neither the Chopart joint nor the Lisfranc joint lie particularly in any one plane. In the tarsometatarsal joint, the base of the second metatarsal interlocks between the first and third cuneiform as a "*keystone*" like in an archway. The first cuneiform is usually the largest and oblong in shape, the third cuneiform is somewhat smaller, and the second cuneiform is short and square. The base of the second metatarsal locks this joint into place. Lisfranc fracture dislocations are also sustained as a result of trauma, for instance, a foot caught under a pedal in a car, or being run over, or from a motorcycle accident when the cycle falls over with the driver's foot still under it, usually wearing a large boot. However, Lisfranc fracture dislocations are also frequently seen in diabetic patients with a neuropathic joint at the tarsometatarsal level.

There are several classifications of Lisfranc fracture dislocations, but the important decision to make is to decide if the fracture is "convergent" or "divergent." If the whole of the forefoot moves laterally on the midfoot, then it is considered to be convergent. If the first ray

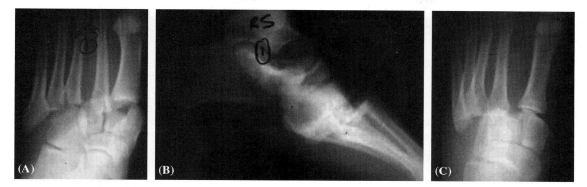

Figure 105 Lisfranc dislocation. (**A**) Showing the dislocation of the tarsometatarsal joint with lateral subluxation of all the metatarsals and a fracture of the base of the second. This is an example of the convergent type of Lisfranc. (**B**) Showing the dislocation of the tarsometatarsal joint with lateral subluxation of all the metatarsals and a fracture of the base of the second. This is an example of the convergent type of Lisfranc. (**C**) Lisfranc dislocation in a different patient illustrating the divergent type, with the first ray remaining basically in anatomic position.

remains in place and the second through fifth rays move lateral, then it is divergent. Alternatively, the first ray may be disrupted and sublux medially, whereas the second through fifth rays sublux laterally, producing a divergent Lisfranc fracture dislocation. Thus, to manage a Lisfranc fracture dislocation requires internal fixation of the second ray in a simple fracture dislocation and internal fixation of both the first and the fifth rays in a divergent type of injury.

Fractures of the Foot in Diabetic Patients

As has been mentioned elsewhere, there are five radiological components of "diabetic feet": medial wall vascular calcification; periosteal reaction around the metatarsal shafts; cellulitis, osteomyelitis, and septic joints; patchy osteopenia as well as generalized osteoporosis; and neuropathic or Charcot joints. Thus, patients with diabetes are a setup to get fractures and dislocations in their feet because of their loss of localized pain sensation and proprioception, as well as their increasing osteopenia. It would also appear that many discrete foot fractures in diabetic patients go unnoticed and undiagnosed and will evolve into neuropathic joints if left untreated. Diabetic patients can also get spontaneous dislocations, although these seem to be more prevalent at the talonavicular joint and at the tarsometatarsal joint. In a review of neuropathic joints in a group of diabetic patients, Forgacs[10] found that the majority were at the tarsometatarsal level (40%), 30% were in the tarsus, 15% were at the ankle, and 15% were in the interphalangeal joints, metatarsophalangeal joints, and elsewhere.

Finally, diabetic patients appear to get three distinct types of calcaneal fracture.

1. Avulsion fracture of their posterior tubercle as a result of an avulsion off the insertion of the Achilles tendon.

This is presumably because the bone is weaker than the tendon itself (Fig. 106A, B).
2. Curvilinear fractures in the posterior aspect of the calcaneus running approximately parallel to the posterior surface of the bone, but 2 to 3 cm inside. These have become known as "Iowa fractures" since they were first described in Iowa. These probably start as an insufficiency fracture, which is then made worse by the patient's neuropathy (Fig. 106C, D).
3. Compression-type fractures of the body of the calcaneus (Fig. 106E).

In each of these situations, the patient's loss of local pain sensation and lack of proprioception presumably lead to a late diagnosis and to a poor prognosis.

CERVICAL SPINE INJURIES

One of the most serious injuries that a person can sustain is to the cervical spine. Thus, it is essential to develop a system for looking at plain films of the spine, particularly the lateral view. Many patients who are involved in motor vehicle accidents will have a neck injury, either a fracture, a subluxation, a dislocation, or a whiplash-type injury. The patient will be admitted on a trauma board with their neck in a brace, and a cross-table lateral cervical spine film is taken routinely.

When I assess this film, I begin anteriorly and look at the width of the soft tissues (Fig. 107).

In the upper spine, in front of the arch of the atlas, this shadow may appear to be quite large, particularly in young people because of their tonsils. However, this retropharyngeal soft-tissue stripe narrows, so that in front of the body of C3, the anterior soft tissues should be no greater than 4 mm across. Where the esophagus begins at approximately C5, the soft tissues widen and

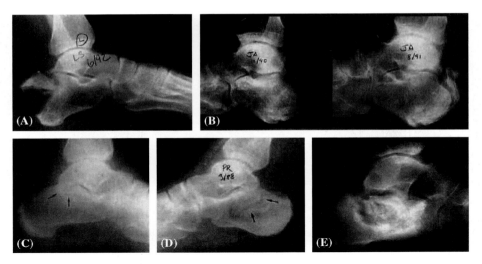

Figure 106 Diabetic calcaneal fracture. (**A**) Recent transverse fracture of the calcaneus "splitting" the bone in half. (**B**) Chronic avulsion type fracture posterior aspect of calcaneus. (**C and D**) Two examples of the "Iowa"-type fracture paralleling the subtalar joints. (**E**) Compression-type fracture in a severe diabetic patient.

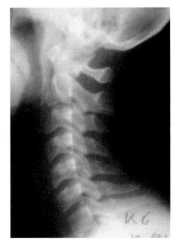

Figure 107 Normal lateral view of the cervical spine.

should measure no more than 12 mm. Crudely put, from C2 through C5 the soft tissues should measure half the width of a vertebral body, and from C5 downward, the soft tissues should be no greater than the whole width of a vertebral body. On many people, a discrete fat stripe can be seen 3 or 4 mm in front of the upper cervical vertebral bodies. This should run parallel to the anterior end plate of the bodies and should not be displaced forward. The next place to assess is the atlantoaxial joint, which should be parallel and no larger than 2-mm wide in adults. In children up to age nine years, the atlantoaxial space may be considerably wider, (the normally accepted width is up to 5 mm). From the age of 9 to 15 years or so, it may be wider than in adults (i.e., 3- to 4-mm wide), but, by 18 or 19 years of age, the atlantoaxial joint should become

normal and no greater than 2 mm. Below C2, the alignment of the anterior end plates (anterior vertebral line) should be in an even line with virtually no step-offs between vertebral bodies; i.e., no subluxation. Again, in young children whose cervical spines are more difficult to assess, frequent pseudosubluxations may be seen, but usually occur at each and every level in the cervical spine.

Next, go further back to the posterior aspects of the vertebral bodies from the dens down as low as you can see (usually C7 or T1). This is known as the posterior vertebral line. The posterior end plates should line up without any subluxation in adult patients.

Next, I look at the posterior aspect of the spine, particularly at the alignment of the spinous processes. The arch of C1 is very variable and often absent. In fact, over 5% of the population have congenital anomalies of C1. The spinous process of C2 is also quite variable, but, from C3 downward, the tips of the spinous processes should be in line and evenly spaced (Fig. 108).

I then look at the laminar line (or the spinal laminar line), which is, in fact, the vertical line seen on the anterior aspect of the spinous processes. Once again, this should be evenly spaced from the base of C2 downward. Finally, I look at the alignment of the facet joints and pillars, which can be difficult to assess. Basically, the lateral masses, or the "pillars," of each of the cervical vertebral bodies are rhomboid in shape on the lateral view and articulate through the facet joint with the pillar above and the pillar below at approximately 45° to the horizontal, and, of course, there is one pillar to each side. So, look at the alignment of both of the pillars, as well as both of the facet joints, which should overlap each other like shingles on a roof in a good lateral view. If all appears normal on the lateral view—do not relax, because at least 5% of cervical

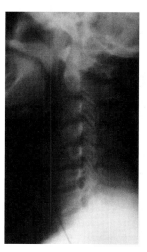

Figure 108 Normal lateral view of the cervical spine taken in a collar. Note that the spine is straight because of a collar.

fractures will still be missed on the single, cross-table, lateral view.

Take the patient out of the collar, and, if they are not complaining of neck pain, take an odontoid view and an AP view of the cervical spine. The odontoid view allows you to look for fractures of the arch and pillars of C1, as well as for displaced fractures of the odontoid (Fig. 109A, B).

Unfortunately, at least 30% of odontoid fractures are nondisplaced, so CT scanning is needed to "clear" the spine. On the AP view, look for the alignment of the vertebral bodies and disc spaces, look at the pillars and for the alignment of the facet joints, and look at the uncal joints, which are the small, laterally placed synovial joints between each vertebral body.

Almost all authorities on cervical spine injury, including Gehweiler et al. (6) and Daffner et al. (7), have published lists of the most important radiological signs to help diagnose cervical injury. I believe that their latest list is the easiest to use. The four most reliable signs are as follows:

- widening of the interspinous spaces
- widening of a facet joint
- widening of the retropharyngeal space
- displacement of the fat stripe

To which they add three other less reliable signs:

- loss of the normal lordosis
- kyphotic angulation
- tracheal deviation

If the spine on these preliminary views appears normally aligned without obvious fracture or displacement, and if the patient is conscious and has no neck symptoms, you have cleared the spine. However, if the patient is unconscious or semiconscious, or if you have seen something abnormal, then a CT scan is essential to clear the

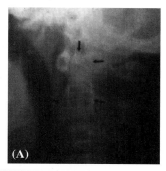

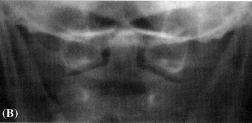

Figure 109 (**A** and **B**) Normal atlantoaxial joint. Note the space between the back of the dens and the arch of the atlas (predental space) is 2 mm. Note that the dens sits squarely within the atlas on the AP view, with equidistance between the pillars bilaterally. *Abbreviation*: AP, anteroposterior.

spine. The concept of clearing the spine is relatively new, but is particularly important in unconscious patients and with those who are severely traumatized elsewhere, so that the surgeons and orthopedists can get on with their jobs without worrying about the neck. In approximately 2% of patients in these circumstances, it is impossible to clear the spine for one reason or another, and then the patient is usually kept in a collar until such time that repeat films or a CT scan can be taken to clear the spine at a later date.

If all appears normal at this stage, flexion and extension views are performed. For these to be adequate, we need to see from the base of the skull down to C7, we need to be able to see the whole of each vertebral body, and there should be reasonable excursion of the spine. In other words, in full flexion, the spinous processes should be almost touching posteriorly, and there should be a smooth curve of the vertebral bodies anteriorly. In full extension, the chin should be on the chest, and posteriorly, the spinous processes should be splayed out evenly from C2 downward. The bodies should be curved in a uniform line anteriorly. Once again, on each of these views, go through your protocol: soft tissues, anterior vertebral line, posterior vertebral line, spinous processes, spinal laminar line, facet joints, and pillars. If all appears normal, then you have excluded the vast majority of significant cervical spine injuries, although, once again, you will have missed some 2% to 3% of fractures, most of which are considered minor, although some horizontal fractures of the base of the dens may still be missed.

There are various classifications of cervical spine injury. They are all based on a similar anatomic classification: flexion injuries, extension injuries, rotary injuries, and compression injuries. *Flexion injuries* account for approximately 60% of the total injuries and consist of hyperflexion sprain injuries, hyperflexion dislocations, with or without facet lock, which, in turn, may be bilateral or unilateral, comminuted fractures of the vertebral body (which are known as flexion teardrop fractures), burst fractures, and fracture dislocations. There are also a number of flexion injuries to the C1-C2 complex, which are dealt with below. Minor flexion injuries to the cervical spine include fractures of the spinous processes (clay-shoveler's fracture), wedge-compression fractures, laminar fractures, and isolated fractures of the transverse process, uncinate process, and articular pillar, most of which are only detected with CT scanning in any case.

Extension injuries to the cervical spine account for approximately 30% of the injuries and consist of the "hangman's" fracture of the arch of C2, hyperextension sprain, and two injuries to the dens: posterior fracture dislocation and posterior atlantoaxial dislocation. Minor extension injuries include minimally displaced horizontal fractures of the arch of the atlas, anterior inferior fractures of the vertebral body (extension teardrop fractures), spinous process fractures, and isolated fractures of the posterior arch of C1.

All *rotary injuries* where the patient experiences an abnormal rotational force are considered major, although they account for only 5% of injuries to the cervical spine. They can involve the atlantoaxial joint, where they produce either subluxation or dislocation, or they may involve the lower cervical spine and be associated with unilateral pillar fractures, unilateral facet lock, or other rotational hyperflexion and hyperextension injuries. These injuries are frequently associated with the death of the patient. Finally, axial compression fractures represent approximately 8% of all cervical spine injuries, and the major injuries include burst fractures of C1 (Jefferson fracture), as well as vertical and oblique fractures of C2, and major fractures of the occipital condyle. Minor axial compression injuries include lateral mass fractures.

Fractures and Dislocations of the C1-C2 Complex

The arch of C1 and the dens (the odontoid process), which constitutes C1 anatomically, and the body and arch of C2 produce a complex structure inherently, locking the skull to the upper cervical spine. There are articulating facets between the front of the dens and the arch of C1, and there is a transverse ligament crossing behind the dens and holding it in place. There are articulating facets between the base of the skull and the pillars of C1, between the

pillars of C1 and C2, and between the pillars of C2 and C3. Approximately 5% of the population have congenital anomalies of C1, including failure of fusion, failure of ossification, and fusion either with the base of the skull or with C2. These obviously complicate matters when we are trying to assess the cervical spine for injury.

Anderson and D'Alonso (8) classified these fractures into three types:

* Type I—a separation of the tip of the dens, now largely considered to be developmental and not a true fracture
* Type II—a transverse fracture of the base of the dens (~40%)
* Type III—a true fracture of the body of C2 (Figs. 110, 111A, B, and 112A, B, C)

Congenital and Developmental Abnormalities of the C1-C2 Complex

There are a number of syndromes associated with either an absent dens or atlantoaxial instability. The dens is absent in Morquio's syndrome, as well as in Down's syndrome and achondroplasia. Atlantoaxial instability and either hypoplasia or aplasia of the dens may be also seen in Down's syndrome. However, by far the commonest cause of atlantoaxial instability is rheumatoid arthritis, although it may also be seen following trauma, in ankylosing spondylitis, with calcium pyrophosphate disease, and following an infection.

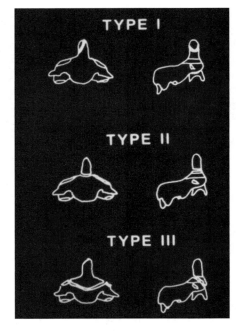

Figure 110 A diagram of the three types of D'Alonso dens fractures. *Source*: Courtesy of Lee Rogers, MD.

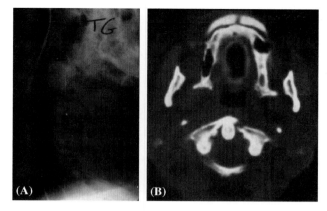

Figure 111 This is a chronic D'Alonso type II fracture at the base of the dens. (**A**) On the plain film the sclerosis can be seen showing that the dens is rocking on the body of C2. (**B**) A CT scan confirming the fractures of both the anterior arch and the posterior lamina. *Abbreviation*: CT, computed tomography.

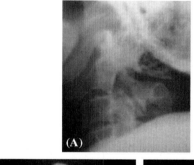

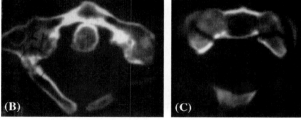

Figure 112 D'Alonso type III dens fracture. (**A**) Plain film appears to be relatively normal. (**B**) and (**C**) CT scans confirm the fractures of the posterior elements of the arch of the atlas and the body of C2. *Abbreviation*: CT, computed tomography.

In normal young people, the *predental space* (i.e., the gap between the posterior aspect of the axis and the anterior aspect of the dens) may angulate and have a "V" shape. In patients younger than 18 years, a V-shaped predental space is normal. In older patients, it usually occurs as a result of a partial tear of the transverse ligament holding the dens in place.

Finally, a brief mention of the os odontoideum needs to be made. This is a small unfused ossicle on the top of the dens. This may be due to a congenital failure of fusion between two growth centers, or it may be acquired as a result of a D'Alonso type I fracture.

Common Cervical Spine Fractures

At this stage of the discussion, I felt that an alphabetical listing of the most common cervical spine fractures and their eponyms would be most useful. However, before we embark on that, this would be a good place to introduce a concept useful for all spinal injuries, and that is the three-column concept. First introduced 30 years ago by Denis (9), it is mainly used for lumbar spine injuries, but is equally appropriate for the cervical and the thoracic spine. Denis divided the spine into three columns: (*i*) consisting of the anterior two-thirds of the vertebral body and the attendant ligaments, etc.; (*ii*) consisting of the posterior one-third of the vertebral body, the pedicles with all the ligaments; and (*iii*) consisting of the posterior elements of the spine, the lamina, the spinous process, ligamentum flavum, and the other ligaments. If any two of these columns are violated, the injury is unstable, i.e., 1 and 2, 1 and 3, 2 and 3.

Clayshoveler's Fracture

This is usually an isolated fracture of the tip of the C7 spinous process, produced classically by an acute hyper-extension force when your shovel suddenly frees itself from the clay and you hyperextend your neck. This is a minor injury (Fig. 113A, B).

Hangman's Fracture

This fracture (more correctly, hangee's fracture) is a horizontal injury through the anterior column either through the C2-3 disc or through the base of the dens, with an oblique fracture of the lamina of C2, which may be unilateral or bilateral. This is a serious injury, which can have major side effects. It was initially inflicted by the hangman to criminals in medieval England. A large knot was placed behind the criminal's right ear, and a tight noose was placed around the neck. The trap door was opened, and the criminal would drop some 14 to 15 ft. It was actually not the fall that broke the neck, but the rotational injury received at the end of the rope that snapped the ring of C2 and usually killed the criminal (Fig. 114A, B, C, D).

Jefferson Fracture

This is a burst fracture of C1 caused by an axial loading injury, where the lateral masses are pushed outward. The

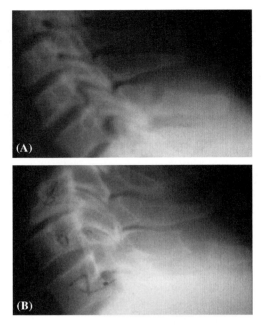

Figure 113 (**A** and **B**) Clayshovelers fractures. Note the separation of the C7 spinous process as a result of an avulsion from the nuchal ligament in two different patients.

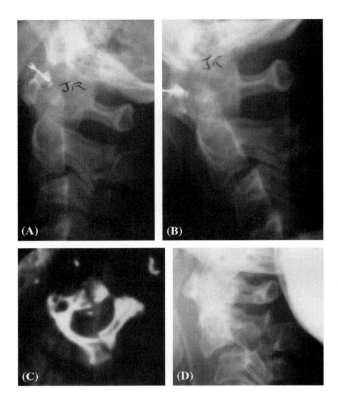

Figure 114 (**A** and **B**) Hangman's fracture. Flexion and extension views in a patient the ER didn't realize had a fracture. There is a typical hangman's fracture with a fracture through the posterior elements of C2. (**C**) This is confirmed on a CT scan showing the fractures of both the anterior process and the posterior elements. (**D**) Hangman's fracture in a different patient showing not only the fractures of the posterior element of C2 but now also with separation of the C2/C3 disc space. This patient died. *Abbreviations*: ER, emergency room; CT, computed tomography.

transverse ligament is usually also disrupted. Although potentially major, Jefferson fractures are only rarely associated with neurological sequelae (Fig. 115A, B).

Locked Facets

If bilateral, they are always associated with anterior and posterior spinal injuries, which may or may not be visible on the plain film. Look down the line of the pillars and make sure that each pillar "covers" the one below, i.e., that there are no articular surfaces that do not coincide with another articular surface. Both unilateral and bilateral locked facets are potentially very dangerous injuries (Figs. 116A, B, C and 117A, B).

Perched Facets

This is an almost complete subluxation of one or both facet joints where the anterior lip of the upper pillar is "perched" on the posterior lip of the lower pillar. More rarely, this can be reversed. In either case, this is a potentially disastrous situation if missed (Fig. 118A, B).

Rotational Injuries

These are usually unilateral and associated with a slipped or locked facet, with the contralateral facet strained, but not disrupted. These are difficult to diagnose on CT without reconstruction. They are also difficult to see on plain films, although, if you look at the space between the back of the pillars and the front of the lamina (the "lamina

space"), these should be uniform the whole way down the spine. Note that the "lamina line" is not real anatomically, since the pillars are on the lateral aspects of the spine and the lamina is situated centrally. There is also a "shark's fin" sign where one of the pillars, because it is locked, is angled. This is also a potentially dangerous situation if not diagnosed.

Teardrop Fractures—Extension

This is not a major injury; the vertical height of the fracture fragment exceeds the horizontal length, and this is often due to an avulsion fracture of the anterior longitudinal spinal ligament (Fig. 119A, B, C).

Teardrop Fractures—Flexion

This is a very major injury; the horizontal length of the fracture exceeds the vertical height and is associated with

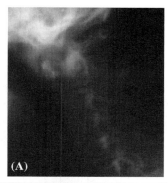

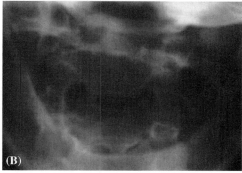

Figure 115 Jefferson fracture. (**A**) Lateral view. Note the separation of the alantoaxial joint with the dens floating freely. (**B**) AP view. This shows the marked widening of the space between the dens and the pillars of C2 bilaterally. *Abbreviation*: AP, anteroposterior.

compression of the vertebral body and retropulsion of fragments into the spinal canal. Flexion teardrop fractures are often associated with quadriplegia or, at the least, quadriparesis, and with fractures of the lamina, pedicles, and spinous process (Fig. 120A, B, C, D).

Unilateral Locked Facets

See the section "Rotational Injuries."

At least 3% of all cervical spine fractures are either combinations of the fractures described above, or none of them; i.e., isolated facet or pillar fractures are not uncommon. Isolated fractures of the uncinate process, transverse process, or of the lamina occur; lateral wedge fractures of the various vertebral bodies can be seen, as can burst fractures other than those at C1. Fortunately for us, most of these are readily visible on CT scans.

Whiplash Injuries

These were first described in the late 19th century as "Railway Spine," when it was noted that those people with their backs to the train accident had the worst neurological

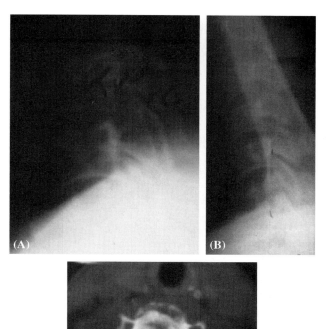

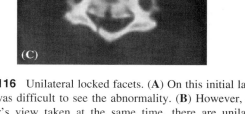

Figure 116 Unilateral locked facets. (**A**) On this initial lateral film, it was difficult to see the abnormality. (**B**) However, on a swimmer's view taken at the same time, there are unilateral locked facets at C6/C7. (**C**) CT scan confirms this finding along with the fact that there is a fracture of the C6 vertebral body with retropulsion into the spinal canal.

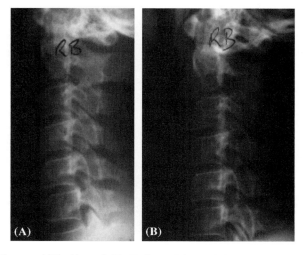

Figure 117 (**A** and **B**) Unilateral locked facets. These are quite difficult to see on the plain film, although on a subsequent film, it is relatively easy to see that the C5/C6 pillar on one side is "uncovered" and is perched on the pillar below. The other side of the cervical spine is intact.

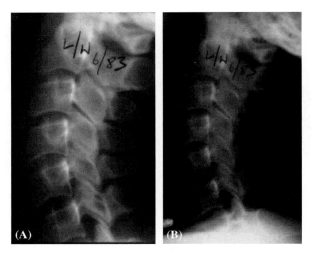

Figure 118 Perched facets. (**A**) On this initial film, the perched facets are only just seen. (**B**) However on a later lateral film the perched facets of C6/C7 can be clearly seen posteriorly.

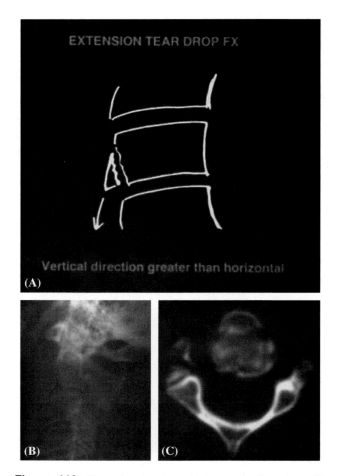

Figure 119 Extension teardrop fracture. (**A**) Drawing. (**B**) Plain film showing an anterior teardrop fracture at the body of C3. (**C**) A CT scan confirms this finding. *Abbreviation*: CT, computed tomography.

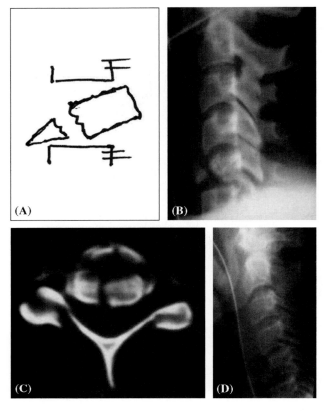

Figure 120 Flexion teardrop fracture. (**A**) Drawing of flexion teardrop fracture. (**B**) Plain film shows the typical appearance with compression and retropulsion of the C5 vertebral body with an anterior separation, which is the teardrop. (**C**) A CT scan confirms the cruciate fracture of the body of C5 with a fracture of the lamina on the right. (**D**) A later lateral film confirms these findings. *Abbreviation*: CT, computed tomography.

problems. Crowe (10), in 1928, presented eight cases of cervical spine injury to the Western Orthopedic Society in San Francisco and coined the term "whiplash injuries." Nowadays, by definition, whiplash is (*i*) a hyperextension injury to the neck, (*ii*) followed by a forward flexion injury. Thus, whiplash injuries are classically sustained when one is rear-ended in a car, often while stationary. Hence, the patterns seen on flexion films of the cervical spine are important. Recently, Bohrer (11) analyzed these patterns on flexion and extension views in 150 patients seen in the emergency room. Twenty percent were normal, i.e., there were three or more angles seen on the flexion view, usually at consecutive disc spaces. On the other hand, 25% of patients were unable to move their necks and had no angles, and this represents significant soft-tissue injury. Twenty-five percent of the patients had only one angle on flexion with the spine straight above and below the disc space, which is obviously also abnormal. Thirty percent of the patients had two angles, and

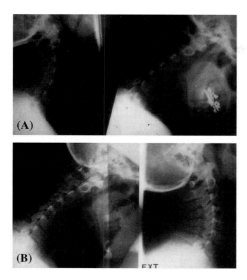

Figure 121 (A) Normal. Normal, extension, flexion, and lateral cervical spine films. (B) Whiplash. Typical whiplash with subluxation of C4 on C5 with a kink and widening of the interspinous space at C5/6 and C6/7.

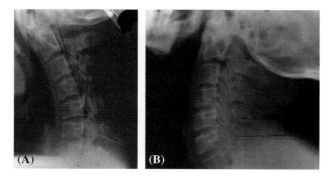

Figure 122 Whiplash. (A) Flexion. Lateral cervical spine shows how to draw the lines and take the measurements. Note the kink at C4/5 and the interspinous widening at C5/6 and C6/7. (B) Extension. Lateral cervical spine shows how to draw the lines and take the measurements. Note the kink at C4/5 and the interspinous widening at C5/6 and C6/7.

this probably represents mild soft-tissue injury and is considered within normal limits. There are various ways of ascertaining angles on spine films, but Griffiths and colleagues (12) used vertical lines drawn down the posterior end plates of each cervical vertebral body and measured the angles between them. This angulation defines the damage occurring during the hyperextension phase of whiplash and reflects damage to the anterior longitudinal ligament and, probably, the posterior longitudinal ligament (Fig. 121A, B).

To define damage done during the hyperflexion phase of whiplash, it is necessary to develop measurements for the interspinous spaces, and Griffiths and colleagues did this by measuring the separation of the spinous processes, which we termed "fanning." This is measured by drawing horizontal lines along the line of and parallel to the lower margin of each spinous process and dropping a perpendicular line down to the adjacent spinous process below.

The whole subject of whiplash injuries is extremely controversial, and many experts deny it exists! However, if you do accept it as a clinical entity, the Griffiths method of measurement has been embraced by the osteopathic and the chiropractic communities, if not by the medical ones. Thus, by definition *whiplash is (i) an isolated kinking greater than 10°, but, if a 10° angle is next to, say, an 11° angle, that is not significant. On the other hand, 12° next to 10° represents whiplash and (ii) an isolated fanning greater than 12 mm, but if 12 mm is next to 13 mm, that is not significant, although 14 mm next to 12 mm represents whiplash* (Fig. 122A, B).

THORACOLUMBAR SPINE INJURY

General Concepts

It has been estimated that there are 11,000 patients a year in the United States who have spinal cord injuries. This is approximately 53 per million population per year. Motor vehicle accidents are responsible for 50% of them, followed by falls as the next most common cause, and athletic injuries, particularly diving injuries. These mainly occur in young male adults. Looking at the statistics the other way around, 10% to 15% of spine injuries will result in spinal cord injury. Generally, the most vulnerable parts of the spine are the mid- to lower-cervical spine and the midthoracic to the upper lumbar region. The upper cervical spine is relatively spared by virtue of the anatomy of the base of the skull and the atlantoaxial joint. T2 through T11 are spared by the rib cage.

Various classifications were used, however, the classical early one is to divide injuries of the thoracolumbar spine into flexion fractures, burst fractures, fracture dislocations, shear fractures, and extension injuries. In 1982, Denis (9) introduced the three-column concept and pointed out that there is instability in the spine following trauma if two of the three columns are violated. The anterior column is approximately the anterior three-quarters of the vertebral body. The middle column is the posterior part of the vertebral body and the pedicles. The posterior column is the lamina, spinous process, transverse processes, and lateral masses (Fig. 123).

Using this classification, Gehweiler and colleagues (6) introduced a classification of thoracolumbar spine injuries, which was somewhat simpler, namely, flexion, axial compression (burst), and fracture dislocations, which may be stable or unstable. Subsequently, they modified this,

Thoracolumbar Spine Trauma:

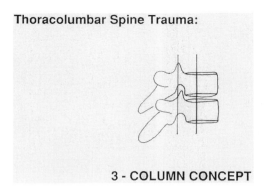

3 - COLUMN CONCEPT

Figure 123 Drawing of three-column concept.

and have more recently described six categories of injury to the thoracolumbar spine.

1. *Hyperflexion fracture dislocations.*
2. Chance and arch fractures.

    a. *Chance fractures* (seat belt injuries).
    b. *arch fractures* (Smith), posterior dislocation with avulsion

3. *Rotary fracture dislocation,* rotation around the long axis of the spine with a slice fracture of the vertebral body or a compression fracture anteriorly.
4. *Shear fracture dislocation* caused by a forward-shearing force, i.e., a blow from behind, leading to horizontal damage. There are two types of these injuries: the one in which the vertebral arch is intact and the other in which there are arch fractures ("traumatic spondylolisthesis").
5. *Hyperextension fracture dislocation.* These are rare, occurring in less than 2% of spine injuries.
6. *Isolated fractures* of the posterior elements.

In 1983, Denis (9) described the three-column spine and its significance in the classification of acute thoracolumbar spinal injuries. This paper is based on 412 thoracolumbar injuries. Denis had 132 anterior compression fractures, 59 burst fractures, 19 seat belt injuries, and 67 fracture dislocations. Denis's original paper stated that, if the middle column is involved, then the spine is unstable. However, actually, anterior compression fractures associated with posterior element fractures are also unstable.

The indications for CT scanning in suspected fractures of the thoracolumbar spine are (*i*) if there is any uncertainty about plain-film findings, (*ii*) if there is an unstable neurological picture, (*iii*) if spinal surgery is indicated, (*iv*) if the plain films are poor or inadequate, or (*v*) if the end plates are difficult to see on the plain film.

Thoracic Spine Fractures

Upper thoracic spine trauma is mainly due to flexion injuries or to axial loading without rotation. Rotational injuries in the thoracic spine are in fact rare because of the rib cage. Considerable violence is needed to produce major injuries in the thoracic region, and, should they occur, they are frequently associated with spinal cord damage.

The types of fracture seen in the thoracic spine are (*i*) compression fractures; (*ii*) burst fractures, which may be stable or unstable; (*iii*) chance or seat belt injuries, which are rare in the thoracic spine except at T12; and (*iv*) fracture dislocations.

Indirect signs of trauma to the thoracic spine include paravertebral hematomas, mediastinal widening, pleural fluid and apical capping, sternal fractures, rib fractures, and a double spinous process sign. Mediastinal widening can be caused not only by trauma to the upper thoracic spine but also following damage to the aortic arch. Thus, it is important to differentiate an aortic rupture from a thoracic spine fracture in patients with mediastinal widening. By far the quickest way to do so is to do a CT scan with contrast. This will also demonstrate any fractures that are present.

Compression Fractures in the Thoracic Spine

Denis described 132 cases of anterior compression fracture in the spine. They mainly occurred at the T6-7-8 level in the thoracic spine and at the L1-2 level in the lumbar spine.

Mild compression fractures occurring in osteopenic or osteoporotic patients are the most common type of spinal injury seen in the thoracic spine. Radiographically, these show loss of height of the anterior aspect of the vertebral body (Fig. 124A, B).

There is no involvement of the middle column, so there is no retropulsion, and the posterior elements are usually intact. A severe anterior compression injury such as

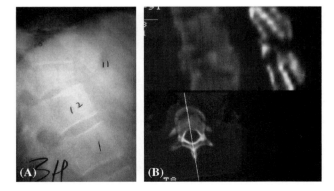

Figure 124 Compression fracture of the thoracic spine. (**A**) Plain lateral film shows a severe anterior compression fracture of T11. (**B**) CT scan in a different patient with sagittal reconstruction showing that this fracture extends through the posterior elements. *Abbreviation*: CT, computed tomography.

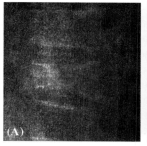
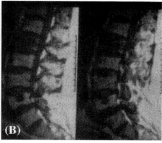

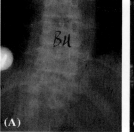
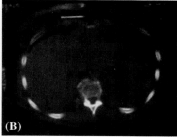

Figure 125 Osteopenia versus neoplastic collapse. (**A**) Lateral film showing a compression fracture of L2. The rest of the spine appeared normal and the patient had no evidence of cancer. (**B**) Sagittal MRI slice shows that the fracture is of low intensity on all sequences and that other end plate fractures are also present. This is all highly suggestive of a benign fracture secondary to osteoporosis. Note the huge Schmorl's node in the upper surface of L5. *Abbreviation*: MRI, magnetic resonance imaging.

Figure 126 Burst fracture of T7. (**A**) AP film showing some apparent widening of the vertebral body itself but definite widening of both paraspinal lines. (**B**) CT scan confirms that this is a "burst" fracture with anterior fragmentation. *Abbreviations*: AP, anteroposterior; CT, computed tomography.

caused by a loading injury can also distract the posterior elements. Neurological deficits are rare in simple compression fractures. Most of these fractures are due to axial loading in flexion.

Osteopenic Fractures Vs. Neoplastic Collapse

It can be difficult to differentiate metastatic collapse of a vertebral body from a fracture seen in osteopenia. Obviously, the state of the whole spinal column must be taken into account. The age of the patient is important, as well as if there is a history of a primary malignancy or multiple myeloma. If necessary, and if the plain film fails to help, then CT scanning and, more particularly, MRI scanning can be useful to exclude metastatic disease in the spine and elsewhere (Fig. 125A, B).

Burst Fractures in the Thoracic Spine

Burst fractures occur at the region of, or just below, the major curve of the thoracic kyphosis. In Denis's 59 cases, the majority in the thoracic spine were at T7 and T8. Obviously the majority of burst fractures occur in the lumbar spine, mainly from L1 through L3. Burst fractures in the thoracic spine are extremely severe injuries. They are sagittally oriented and usually are associated with a Y-shaped vertebral body fracture. They extend superiorly, often becoming comminuted, and the superior end plate can be separated and retropulsed (Fig. 126A, B).

Burst fractures are associated with posterior element fractures, and neurological damage occurs in 65% of cases. Spinal cord severance or hematoma often results in paraplegia. Burst fractures are due to axial loading. There are a number of secondary radiological signs, including paravertebral hematomas. Incidentally, in a

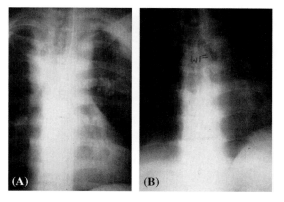

Figure 127 (**A**) Widening of the paraspinal lines in a patient involved in a severe motor vehicle accident with a steering wheel injury to his sternum. Has he an aortic rupture or not? If in doubt do an angiogram. (**B**) Widening of the paraspinal lines in a different patient with a compression fracture of T7.

normal person, the *right paravertebral line* is usually invisible, whereas the *left paravertebral line* may extend 4 or 5 mm away from the spine because of the hemizygous systems. Nowadays, most burst fractures will be further investigated using CT scanning with sagittal reconstruction. If spinal cord injury is suspected, MRI is obviously the investigation of choice (Fig. 127A, B).

Burst fractures imply that there has been an axial loading injury on the spinal column and that the spine is basically split, involving the anterior, middle, and posterior columns. If the posterior column is split, another radiological sign called the double spinous process sign can be rarely seen. This is usually more obvious on CT scanning.

Fracture Dislocations in the Thoracic Spine

Fracture dislocations in the thoracic region are rare in the upper thoracic spine. They are also regularly associated with retropulsion of the posterior part of the superior end

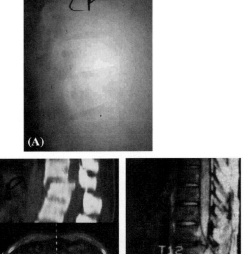

Figure 128 Fracture dislocation of T10 and T11. (**A**) Plain film, which is difficult to interpret, but discrete pencil marks have been placed on the posterior aspect of the posterior vertebral end plates. (**B**) CT scan of the same patient confirms these findings. (**C**) Sagittal MRI in a different patient showing a fracture dislocation of T12 on T11 with marked retropulsion and a severed cord. *Abbreviations*: CT, computed tomography; MRI, magnetic resonance imaging.

plate and adjacent vertebral body, resulting in spinal cord compression or severance (Fig. 128A, B, C).

Fracture dislocations in the lower thoracic/upper lumbar region are usually a result of a shear injury in which there may be superior facet fractures, posterior arch fractures, or ligamentous and disc disruption with locked facets. Finally, sternal and rib fractures, which may be seen on plain films, should lead one to investigate the thoracic spine for unexpected burst fractures or fracture dislocations.

Kümmell's Syndrome

Many people do not believe that Kümmell's syndrome exists, including this author. What the term implies is avascular necrosis of a vertebral body with collapse. I think it is much more likely that what we are actually seeing is severe osteopenia with secondary collapse.

Summary of Thoracic Spine Injuries

Compression fractures are the most common fractures in the thoracic spine and are usually stable and usually only

involve one, or rarely two, columns. Burst fractures, alone, are actually stable and only involve two columns. However, burst fracture dislocations are unstable and involve all three columns. Fracture dislocations are also unstable and involve all three columns.

The diagnostic challenges in thoracic spine trauma are (*i*) in differentiating aortic rupture from upper thoracic spine fractures, (*ii*) in differentiating osteopenic fractures from neoplastic collapse, and (*iii*) in differentiating Scheuermann's disease and physiological wedging from anterior compression fractures. This subject is dealt with later.

LUMBAR SPINE TRAUMA

Once again, basically, the types of fractures seen in the lumbar spine can be subdivided into compression fractures; burst fractures, which may be stable or unstable; Chance fractures or seat belt injuries; and fracture dislocations.

Compression Fractures in the Lumbar Spine

The same problem occurs in the lumbar spine as in the thoracic spine. Compression fractures, both at the anterior end plate and the superior end plate, are common in patients with osteoporosis. There are two intellectual difficulties with their diagnosis, however. One is to differentiate a simple compression fracture from a fracture caused by multiple myeloma or a metastasis. This is best worked out using an MRI scan (Fig. 129A, B).

A CT scan would only confirm the findings seen on plain film. A bone scan would be positive in either case, but an MRI would be able to show whether there is any actual replacement of marrow elements by metastatic disease. The second intellectual problem is to age an osteoporotic fracture. The plain film is of no use. A CT scan of the lumbar spine may be of some help if there is a localized hematoma, but this is rare in osteoporotic fractures. Nuclear medicine is no help since both old and recent fractures light up. MRI is not really of much help either. By far the best method of aging compression fractures is by having a good clinical history and previous films.

Burst Fractures

Burst fractures occur typically in the upper, rather than the lower, lumbar spine, and there are a number of classifications, including one introduced by Denis in which they were subdivided into fractures with involvement of both end plates, a fracture only of the superior

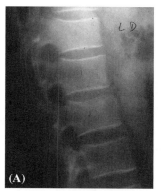

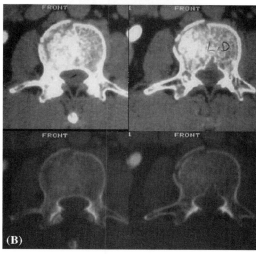

Figure 129 (A) Plain film. Discrete compression fracture of L2. (B) CT scan confirms these findings. *Abbreviation*: CT, computed tomography.

end plate, a fracture of only the inferior end plate, a burst fracture with rotation, and a burst fracture with lateral flexion (Figs. 130A, B, C and 131A, B).

In real life, these subdivisions are not particularly important. Hashimoto (13), in a very elegant paper pub-

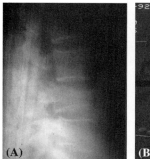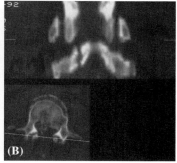

Figure 130 (A) Plain film: burst fracture of lumbar spine. (B) CT scan with coronal reconstruction confirming the burst fracture with retropulsion and a vertical fracture of the laminar. *Abbreviation*: CT, computed tomography.

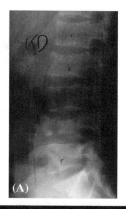

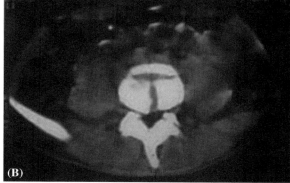

Figure 131 (A) Plain film. Burst fracture of L4. (B) CT scan confirms these findings. *Abbreviation*: CT, computed tomography.

lished in 1988, looked at no less than 112 thoracolumbar burst fractures. He and his coauthors discovered that there is a significant risk of neurological involvement if the retropulsed fragment narrowed the spinal canal to only 35% at T11-T12, to 45% at L1, and 55% at L2 and below because of the cauda equina. Of their patients, there were 17 burst fractures at T12, 48 at L1, and 25 at L2. Sixty-eight percent of their 74 patients who had three-column disruption of the vertebrae had neurological deficits.

Chance Fractures or Seat Belt Injuries

George Q. Chance (14) wrote a wonderful two-page paper in 1948 titled "*Note on a Type of Flexion Fracture of the Spine*," published in the British Journal of Radiology. He described a true flexion fracture with horizontal splitting of the vertebral body and the neural arch, and he reported on three cases with little anterior wedging and no dislocation of the facet joints. None of his three patients had cord damage. The mechanism of injury was hyperextension of the spine. Denis had 19 cases of seat belt injuries, four involving T12, four at L1, six at L2, and five at L3. By definition, a Chance fracture is a horizontal fracture

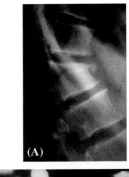

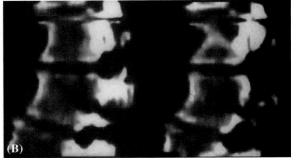

Figure 132 Chance fracture (seat belt injury). (**A**) Lateral plain film shows the horizontal disco vertebral fracture through the L1 vertebral body. (**B**) The CT scan confirms the fracture runs through all three columns of the spine. *Abbreviation*: CT, computed tomography.

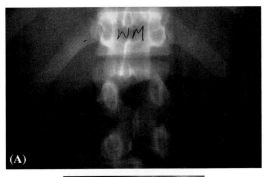

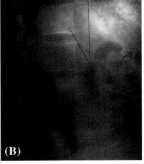

Figure 133 Chance fracture—plain film. (**A**) AP view shows the angulation of the lower part of the L1 vertebral body on the vertebra below as well as the "naked" facet sign. (**B**) The lateral view confirms these findings. *Abbreviation*: AP, anteroposterior.

through the vertebral body, usually adjacent to the upper end plate, although it may, in fact, involve the disc, or both the disc and the body (Figs. 132A, B and 133A, B).

Chance fractures also involve the pedicles, the lamina, the facet joints, and the spinous processes. Denis also looked at the distribution of two-level, seat belt–type injuries, although he only had eight cases. One involved T11 through L1 and one involved T12 through L2; however, three involved L1 through L3 and three involved L2 through L4.

There are two rarer forms of seat belt injury; namely, the Smith fracture, which is usually through the disc, with a fracture posteriorly at the junction of the lamina and the spinous process. There is also a rotational injury, which is a one-sided fracture through the posterior elements.

Fracture Dislocations

Fracture dislocations are also common in the lumbar spine. Denis had 67 cases, of which 19 occurred at the L1-2 level. Next most commonly involved were the T12 and L2 levels. Both seat belt injuries and fracture dislocations can produce another plain-film radiological sign called the naked facet sign, where there is separation of the facet. Most fracture dislocations are easy to diagnose on the plain films alone, although obviously CT scanning

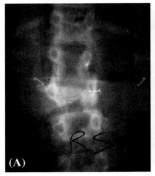

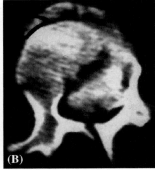

Figure 134 Fracture dislocation of L2. (**A**) AP film shows the marked widening of the L2 vertebral body with "uncovered" or "naked" facets at L1. (**B**) A CT scan confirms these findings with marked retropulsion of the posterior aspect of the vertebral body into the spinal canal. *Abbreviation*: AP, anteroposterior; CT, computed tomography.

will confirm the diagnosis nicely, particularly with sagittal reconstruction (Fig. 134A, B).

Other Fractures

Obviously, isolated fractures of the transverse processes can also be seen. These are often associated with intra-abdominal trauma such as fractures of the kidney, rupture of the spleen, large, retroperitoneal hematomas, and separation of the intestine where it dives through the peritoneum in such places as the duodenal loop and the sigmoid colon. Fractures of the spinous processes can also occur as a result of direct injuries in the lumbar region, although they are rare. Finally, fractures of the posterior margin of the lumbar vertebral bodies have been described. Most of these occur as a result of direct trauma, or even strenuous sports activity. They are obviously difficult to see since they lie within the spinal canal, although both CT and MRI can better define them.

Summary of Lumbar Spine Injuries

Denis produced his final classification of lumbar spine injuries:

1. compression fractures
2. burst fractures
3. flexion distraction fractures (seat belt injuries)
4. fracture dislocations

In the lumbar spine, compression fractures are usually stable and often only involve the proximal column. Burst fractures may be stable or unstable. The stable ones involve only the vertebral body and, at the most, two columns. Burst fracture dislocations are unstable and involve all three columns. Fracture dislocations are unstable and involve three columns, and seat belt injuries are also unstable, involving all three columns.

SACRAL FRACTURES

Sacral fractures have also been considered under the section "Pelvic Fractures," with which they are usually associated. Traumatic fractures of the sacrum are often vertical and in the sagittal plane, and may be the result of a shear injury, but one can also see compression and other types of fractures.

Insufficiency fractures of the sacrum in the elderly or in patients with severe osteopenia are vertical compression fractures, and these often have a horizontal component; thus producing the characteristic Honda sign on bone scans. Traumatic separations or diastasis of the sacroiliac joint are also commonly seen in association with major pelvic trauma; remember that separation of the symphysis pubis is usually associated with separation of one or other sacroiliac joint, and fractures of the rami are usually associated with a sacral fracture.

MYOSITIS OSSIFICANS

Although people have attempted to classify myositis ossificans, it is nearly always associated with trauma, except, perhaps, the extremely rare condition of myositis

ossificans progressiva, which is genetically predisposed. Myositis ossificans is usually seen following straightforward trauma in an athlete, but it can also be seen in patients with spinal cord injury and in patients following total joint replacement, particularly the hip.

Myositis Ossificans Following Trauma

Myositis ossificans was first described in the 17th century in the elbow of ladies, who, while riding sidesaddle, fell off their horse and landed on their elbow (a case of not knowing your posterior from one's elbow?). The elbow would be noted to stiffen up, freeze, and ossify, and, in fact, the Museum of the Royal College of Surgeons in London has such a case from 1839 in a glass pot (Fig. 135).

More recently, posttraumatic myositis ossificans has been well described in young athletes, usually aged 15 to 25 years, and usually male, and usually in the leg, more often in the buttock and upper thigh. It has two quite different appearances; in the classical type, myositis occurs as a result of the avulsion of a muscle from its insertion into the femur. The periosteum will form new bone, fanning out into the muscle, and the radiological diagnosis depends on one's ability to see a clear-cut lucent line between the myositis and the underlying bone (Fig. 136A, B).

This lucent line represents the periosteum, which is fibrous tissue and, hence, lucent. This may require oblique views to confirm the diagnosis. If no lucent line can be found on them, the differential diagnosis of a parosteal osteosarcoma also needs to be considered, and this will be dealt with elsewhere. However, usually, with a history of recent trauma, increasing pain and swelling, as well as the presence of a lucent line between the lesion and the

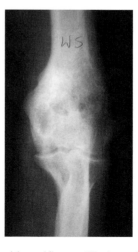

Figure 135 Myositis ossificans. AP view of the elbow. There is complete fusion of the humerus to the radius and ulna in a patient who sustained a supracondylar fracture one year earlier. *Abbreviation*: AP, anteroposterior.

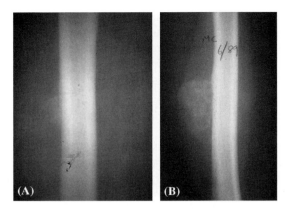

Figure 136 Myositis ossificans. (**A**) AP view of the right femur taken six weeks after a football injury, showing early soft tissue ossifcation, with a lucent line running between the ossification and the femur itself representing the periosteum. (**B**) Film taken three months later showing the classical appearance of maturing myositis ossificans. Again, note the lucent line representing the periosteum. *Abbreviation*: AP, anteroposterior.

This subsequently ossifies along its outer margins. In both of these types of myositis ossificans, plain films often show little or nothing for the first two or three weeks, but then a faint area of ossification becomes apparent, linear in the first case and circumferential in the second. On the other hand, bone scans are positive very early on (very sensitive, but nonspecific), and MRI is a good way to confirm the more circular type of myositis ossificans (Fig. 137A, B, C, D).

The pathogenesis is simple: trauma and bleeding into an area will be followed by healing with fibroblasts, which originate from the endomysium. Primitive mesenchymal cells will proliferate to promote healing and repair, and in most cases, these will turn into fibroblasts. However, in some people, they differentiate into osteoblasts, which, in turn, lay down bone rather than fibrous tissue. The reason for this is unknown. In either case, the repair process usually takes three or four months to mature, and the actual healing process to return to normal may take as long as a year.

underlying bone, the diagnosis of posttraumatic myositis ossificans can be confidently made.

The second type of posttraumatic myositis ossificans is more circumscribed and probably occurs as a result of a tear in the body of a muscle when a hematoma occurs.

Myositis Ossificans Seen in Spinal Cord Injury

This was first described in the 1920s and occurs predominantly around the hips, although in a review of over a hundred patients done when I was in Boston, we also saw

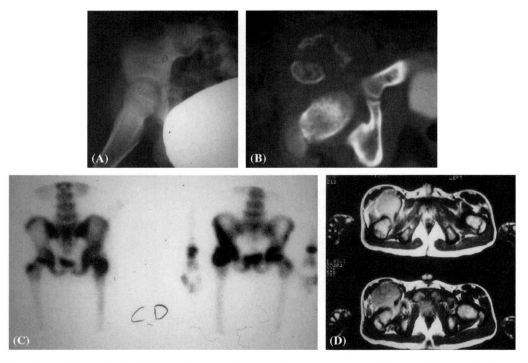

Figure 137 Myositis ossificans. (**A**) Plain film. Showing the circumferential area of ossification lying just in front of the femoral head, following a fall from a horse. (**B**) CT scan. Showing the circumferential area of ossification lying just in front of the femoral head, following a fall from a horse. (**C**) Bone scan showing increased uptake anterior to the right hip. (**D**) MRI confirms these findings. *Abbreviations*: CT, computed tomography; MRI, magnetic resonance imaging.

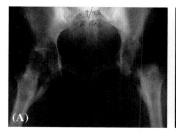
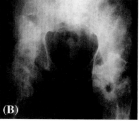

Figure 138 Myositis ossificans in two different patients with spinal cord injuries. (**A**) Around the hips in a quadriplegic 24-year-old male one year after C5 injury. (**B**) Also around the hips in a young paraplegic male with an L2 fracture/dislocation following an MVA. *Abbreviation*: MVA, motor vehicle accident.

it adjacent to the knee, elbow, and shoulder, as well as in the spine in a few patients. This form of myositis ossificans is also posttraumatic and results from too vigorous physiotherapy, causing bleeding into the muscles and, hence, myositis ossificans (Fig. 138A, B).

In these paralyzed patients, myositis ossificans takes up to 24 months to mature, and, if operated on before full maturity, it recurs. The way to follow it to maturity is by serial bone scanning, and, once mature, a transverse cut is usually made through the now-totally-ossified muscle, thus releasing the joint. However, prevention is better than cure, and today most of these patients are placed on either aspirin or low-dose ibuprofen to prevent the myositis ossificans.

Myositis Ossificans Associated with Total Joint Replacement

In the early days of joint replacement, myositis ossificans was so common that it was graded 0, I—very minimal, II—quite marked, and III—solid fusion. In these patients, it was thought also to be posttraumatic, although presence of methyl methacrylate appeared to increase the incidence of myositis ossificans in total joint replacements, markedly. It was classically seen within three months of operation and, again, took up to two years to fully mature, when it could be operated on and removed. Over the years, it was noted that it was much more common around the hip than the knee and the shoulder, and that it occurred in "bone formers," i.e., patients with a predisposition to form excess bone; young patients with ankylosing spondylitis, older patients with either hypertrophic degenerative arthritis or with diffuse idiopathic skeletal hyperostosis (DISH). Again, prevention is better than cure, and now aspirin and ibuprofen are given to this group of patients, both pre- and postoperatively. Alternatively, a course of low-dose radiation therapy can be used. As a result of these precautions, hypertrophic bone formation following total hip replacement is now uncommon.

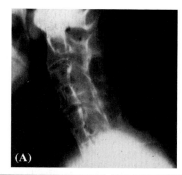
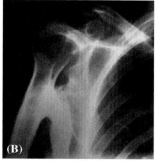
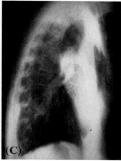

Figure 139 Myositis ossificans progressiva in a young male patient with progressive ossification of many muscle groups. (**A**) Lateral cervical spine. (**B**) Shoulder. (**C**) Lateral chest.

Myositis Ossificans Progressiva

This is a very rare hereditary condition with a pattern of autosomal dominant inheritance. The muscles slowly ossify without a history of trauma, often starting in the paraspinal and psoas muscles, and slowly progressing to involve all the muscles, including the intercostal ones, which leads inevitably to the patient's death in their late 40s or 50s. In many cases, associated congenital anomalies have been described—particularly microdactyly of the middle phalanx of the fifth toe and little finger, which can also be seen in females carrying the disorder (Fig. 139A, B, C).

REFERENCES

1. Rogers LF. Radiology of Skeletal Trauma. New York: Churchill Livingstone, 1982.
2. Young JW. Pelvic injuries. Semin Musculoskelet Radiol 1998; 2(1):83–104.
3. Weber BG. Klassifikation und Operationsindikation der Verletzungen des O.S.G. In: Verletsungen der oberen Sprunggelenkes. Bern: Hans Huber, 1965:51–65.
4. Lauge-Hansen N. Fractures of the ankle. AJR Am J Roentgenol 1954; 71:456–471.
5. Kelikian H, Kelikian AS. Disorders of the Ankle. Philadelphia: W.B. Saunders Co., 1985.

6. Gehweiler JA, Osborne RL, Becker RF. The Radiology of Vertebral Trauma. Philadelphia: W.B. Saunders, 1980.

7. Daffner RH, Brown RR, Goldberg AL. A new classification for cervical vertebral injuries: influence of CT. Skeletal Radiol 2000; 29:125–132.

8. Anderson LD, D'Alonso RT. Fractures of the odontoid process of the axis. J Bone Joint Surg 56A; 1663:1978.

9. Denis F. The three column spine and its significance in the classification of acute spinal trauma. Spine 1983; 8:817–831.

10. Crowe HE. Injuries to the cervical spine. Paper presented at the Western Orthopaedic Association Meeting, San Francisco, 1928.

11. Bohrer SP, Chen YM, Sayers DG. Cervical spine flexion patterns. Skeletal Radiol 1990; 19:521–525.

12. Griffiths HJ, Olson PN, Everson LI, et al. Hyperextension strain or "whiplash" injuries to the cervical spine. Skeletal Radiol 1995; 24:263–266.

13. Hashimoto T, Kaneda F, Abumi K. Relationship between traumatic spinal canal stenosis and neurological deficits in thoracolumbar burst fractures. Spine 1988; 13:1268–1272.

14. Chance CQ. Note on a type of flexion fracture of the spine. BJR Suppl 1948; 21:249–250.

2

Arthritis

ARTHRITIS

A traditional approach to arthritis would probably start with the most common types of disease and then go on to describe the rarer ones. However, I believe that it is more logical to subdivide arthritis into a number of different categories, of which hypertrophic and erosive are the most important. However, this does not begin to cover all the variations, and so I will subdivide the chapter into hypertrophic arthritis, erosive arthritis, the seronegative spondyloarthropathies, and the crystalline arthropathies.

HYPERTROPHIC FORMS OF ARTHRITIS

Degenerative Arthritis or Osteoarthritis

Degenerative arthritis, or osteoarthritis, is the most common form of hypertrophic arthritis seen mainly in large, weight-bearing joints in older patients. It is caused by repetitive impact on the articular cartilage and thus is more commonly seen in more active and larger patients. However, there is also a familial aspect to the condition. Obviously, any internal derangement of the joints will also lead to premature degenerative arthritis. Since we all place weight on our hips, knees, and ankles on a minute-to-minute basis, particularly while we are walking and more particularly while we are running, why do we not all get osteoarthritis in our knees by the age of 30? This is mainly because there is a continuous repair process going on, so

that any damage gets repaired quickly. The mediator for this repair is the release of cytokines, from the synovial membrane, which act on the cartilage to repair the damage by stimulating the chondrocytes to lay down new cartilage fibrils. An essential part of this repair process is an adequate blood supply to the bones through the subchondral surface of the bone and hence to the cartilage itself.

Various factors will affect the efficiency of this process, including synovial disease, poor blood supply, aging, and hereditary factors. As the process breaks down, there are attempts to repair the cartilage, which becomes thin and fragile. The chondrocytes will gather in clusters, and this will lead to loss of matrix and breakdown of the repair process and the advent of degenerative arthritis. What we see radiologically is localized loss of joint space or thinning of the cartilage, which occurs as a result of cartilaginous fibrillation. The remaining normal cartilage, which is often at the margins of the joint surface, will revascularize and enchondral ossification occurs, resulting in osteophytes. As the process continues, the loss of cartilage leads to bone articulating against bone, and new bone formation occurs on the cancellous subchondral bone, and this we see as "eburnation." This is an old pathological term implying "ivory" bone, since the eburnated bone appears very bright and shiny at autopsy or on arthroscopy. As the pressure increases in the joint, small infractions will occur in the subchondral bone, thus allowing synovial fluid to be pumped into the underlying bone (which has a lower intrinsic pressure in any case). Subchondral cysts or geodes thus occur. These are usually fibrous tissue walled mucus- or synovial fluid–containing cysts adjacent to the weight-bearing surface of the joint. They are extremely common and can be frequently seen on magnetic resonance imaging (MRI) of the knee and shoulder in older patients. Incidentally, the term "geode" is a geological term referring to a flint which, when broken open, is actually hollow and contains many quartz crystals. Finally, the osteochondral margins may fragment and fall off into the joint, where they form the basis of an interarticular loose body. Loose bodies often start from a small fragment of articular cartilage, which will metaplase into an osteochondral loose body by getting its nutrition from the synovial fluid. They were originally called joint mice in the old days because of the difficulty that surgeons had in finding them at arthrotomy.

When a joint or a disc has become markedly narrow, any stress will produce a vacuum phenomenon. This is actually release of nitrogen from the bloodstream into a potential space. Vacuum phenomena also occur in people who crack their knuckles, and, in a normal joint, if placed under enough stress. However, vacuum phenomena are routinely seen in association with degenerative arthritis in joints or disc spaces, which have lost their articular cartilage (or disc material) and are a useful pointer to help the diagnosis of degenerative arthritis. Parenthetically, a vacuum phenomenon would be extremely rare in patients with fluid or pus in the joints unless the organism is gas-forming. Thus, if a vacuum phenomenon is seen in a joint, one can effectively exclude infection.

Degenerative arthritis may be primary or secondary, although in view of the foregoing discussion, the concept of primary degenerative arthritis is difficult to understand. Rather, if degenerative arthritis is seen in a weight-bearing joint such as a hip or a knee in an elderly patient, it would usually be considered to be the primary form of osteoarthritis. If one sees degenerative arthritis in an unusual joint, such as an elbow or shoulder, then it is usually secondary. Similarly, premature degenerative arthritis in a knee or a hip is probably secondary to a mechanical derangement, old infection, old trauma, or something similar. Since this varies so much from joint to joint, I thought that I would go through the individual joints and give a brief discussion of how to image them and what to look for in patients with suspected degenerative arthritis.

The Knee

The weight-bearing surface of the knee is actually approximately 35° off the midline on the lateral view, so an anteroposterior (AP) view of the knee may be misleading. An ideal knee series is a lateral view, an AP view of both knees standing, and a 35° "notch" view, also of both knees standing. The earliest signs of degenerative arthritis in the knee are loss of cartilage posteriorly, only seen on the

notch view and primarily in the medial compartment, squaring off of the articular surfaces (in reality early osteophyte formation), and a joint effusion (Fig. 1).

As the condition progresses, narrowing of the articular surface, again, primarily medially, and increasing osteophyte formation occur.

Once the articular cartilage has been lost completely, then increasing sclerosis of the underlying subchondral bone occurs (eburnation).

Loose body formation may occur at any time, but is usually only seen in the later stages of the disease. The loose bodies usually end up in the interchondylar notch and are best seen in either the notch or the lateral view of the knee, although they may be obscured on the latter by the femoral condyles. Rarely, if the patient has a Baker's cyst, the loose bodies will end up in it (Fig. 2).

Similarly, subchondral cyst formation may occur at any time. These usually occur in the region of the ligamentous or synovial insertion into the bone. Common sites for subchondral cyst formation are at the insertion of the posterior cruciate into the posterior aspect of the tibial plateau (Fig. 3) and the insertion of the rotator cuff into the greater tuberosity of the humerus. If these appearances are seen in a patient older than 60, we might consider them to be "primary." However, if they are seen in a patient in their 30s or 40s, this will almost certainly be due to "secondary" changes, i.e., repeated bleeding (athletes, hemophiliacs), repeated trauma or internal derangement (meniscal tear, cruciate tear, postmeniscectomy, or old osteochondritis ossificans, for example), secondary to some previous insult (infection), or arthritis (juvenile chronic arthritis or rheumatoid arthritis). Classical degenerative arthritis involves the medial compartment of the knee, primarily, but will also involve both the lateral compartment and the patellofemoral joint in due course.

However, if you see a patient with primary involvement of the patellofemoral joint with loss of joint space and eburnation, but typically neither with osteophyte formation nor with involvement of the medial or lateral compartment, think of calcium pyrophosphate disease (CPPD) and look for the presence of chondrocalcinosis (Figs. 107 and 110).

The Hip

The superior aspect of the hip joint is the weight-bearing surface; hence, pure degenerative arthritis manifests itself clinically by narrowing of the superior part of the joint with sclerosis (eburnation), osteophyte formation, and lateral migration of the femoral head (Fig. 4). However, on a computed tomography (CT) scan, degenerative changes can also be seen in the medial aspect of the joint. Loose bodies are relatively uncommon in the hip, but on the other hand, subchondral cysts are very

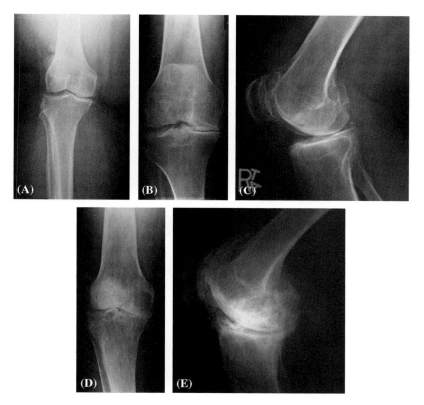

Figure 1 Different stages of degenerative arthritis in the knee. (**A**) Mild. Shows the early loss of joint cartilage with spurs on the tibial spines and squaring off of the edges of the articular surfaces. (**B**) Moderate. AP view shows more marked loss of cartilage with marginal osteophytes. (**C**) Lateral view confirms these changes. (**D**) Severe. AP view shows severe degenerative joint disease with eburnation, almost total loss of cartilage in the medial compartment and large osteophytes. (**E**) Severe. This is a lateral view of a different patient. *Abbreviation*: AP, anteroposterior.

common, particularly in the outer margin of the acetabular roof (Fig. 4).

It is also not uncommon to see "kissing" cysts, apparently opposite to each other, one in the acetabular roof and the other in the femoral head.

Interestingly, this appearance is more common in CPPD of the hip with secondary degenerative arthritis rather than in primary osteoarthritis. Premature degenerative arthritis in the hip can be seen as a result of repeated bleeding, previous infections, or arthritis, but particularly as a result of previous mechanical problems. In the hip joint these would include developmental hip dysplasia, Legg-Calvé-Perthes disease, slipped capital femoral epiphysis, old fractures, dislocations, etc. (Fig. 5).

Most of the erosive arthritides such as juvenile chronic arthritis, rheumatoid arthritis, and ankylosing spondylitis cause central destruction of the joint cartilage in the hip. Thus, when secondary degenerative arthritis occurs, the femoral head migrates medially rather than laterally, as is seen in primary osteoarthritis. In fact, if one sees medial migration of the femoral head in association with

degenerative arthritis, you need to think of an underlying secondary cause of the arthritis.

The Ankle and The Foot

Since the ankle is really only a simple hinge joint, it is unusual to see significant degenerative arthritis in the tibiotalar joint, although osteophytes from the anterior surface of the tibial plafond are not uncommon. In fact, if one sees degenerative arthritis in the tibiotalar joint, some underlying disorder should be considered, such as previous trauma or arthritis, infections, bleeding, or a neuropathic joint (Fig. 6).

Obviously, mechanical problems are also a potent cause of secondary osteoarthritis, and again, previous fractures, dislocations, and congenital anomalies should be looked for.

Degenerative arthritis in the small bones of the foot can be seen as a result of mechanical problems in the foot, such as pes planus, pes cavus, and metatarsus varus. Patients with marked disruption and severe osteoarthritis

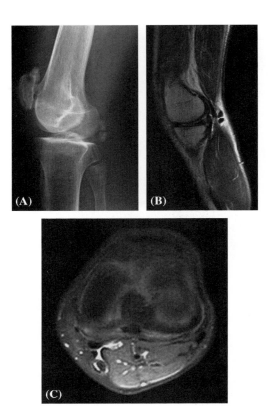

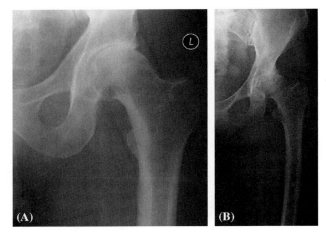

Figure 4 Degenerative arthritis. Hips. (**A**) Early changes. Note the loss of superior cartilage with sclerosis of the acetabular roof and osteophyte formation. (**B**) Subchondral cysts. There are large cysts in the acetabular roof.

Figure 2 Degenerative joint disease. (**A**) Knee with loose body formation. Note the moderate degree of joint space loss and early osteophyte formation. (**B**) Sagittal MRI to show loose bodies lying within a Baker's cyst. (**C**) Axial MRI showing loose bodies in a Baker's cyst. *Abbreviation*: MRI, magnetic resonance imaging.

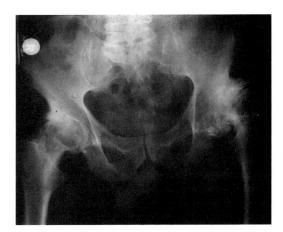

Figure 5 Degenerative arthritis. Hips in a young male patient with an old slipped capital femoral epiphysis on the left who has now developed moderate degenerative changes on the right. On the left, there is distortion of the femoral head, almost total loss of cartilage space, sclerosis, and osteophyte formation.

of some of the tarsal joints almost certainly have an underlying neuropathic disorder. Today, diabetes is by far the commonest cause of neuropathic joints in the feet. This is discussed separately.

This would also be a good place to discuss hallux valgus and hallux rigidus. Hallux valgus refers to a valgus angulation of the great toe and the first metatarsal; the mechanical disadvantage of this situation leads to secondary osteoarthritis in the first metatarsophangeal joint with loss of joint space, subchondral sclerosis, and osteophyte formation (Fig. 7).

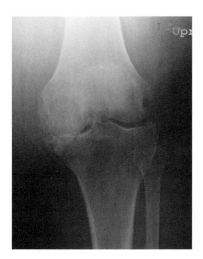

Figure 3 Degenerative arthritis. Knee with subchondral cyst formation in a 68-year-old male with moderate degenerative arthritis.

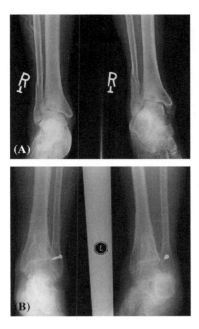

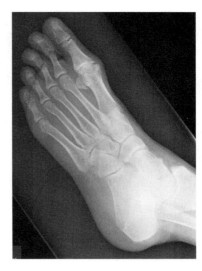

Figure 8 Hallux rigidus in a 45-year-old male patient with secondary degenerative arthritis in the first metatarsophalangeal joint.

Figure 6 Degenerative arthritis of the ankle. (**A**) AP film. There is loss of cartilage space, sclerosis, an effusion, and osteophyte formation in this patient who had a previous malleolar fracture. (**B**) Oblique films. There is loss of cartilage space, sclerosis, an effusion, and osteophyte formation in this patient who had a previous malleolar fracture.

Soft-tissue thickening also occurs on the medial aspect of the exposed metatarsal head, leading to a bunion. However, the primary cause of hallux valgus is not the metatarsophalangeal angulation, but rather the medial migration of the first metatarsal away from the second metatarsal and the rest of the foot. A normal metatarsal angle (the angle between the shafts of the first and second metatarsal) is considered to be below 10°, but hallux valgus occurs when this angle is greater than 15°, and 12° is the usually accepted cutoff for a normal angulation.

Hallux rigidus refers to a congenital anomaly of the first metatarsal, which is saddle-shaped (i.e., has shoulders), and this is a situation which renders the first metatarsophalangeal joint "rigid" and hence leads to premature degenerative arthritis (Fig. 8).

The Shoulder

Although the shoulder joint is non–weight-bearing, it is the third commonest large joint where one sees arthritis. The reason for this is that the integrity of the shoulder depends on the ligaments, tendons, and muscles that surround it—particularly the rotator cuff. Once this is compromised, so is shoulder stability, and hence the advent of degenerative change is in the glenohumeral joint (Fig. 9).

This condition is probably seen most often in older patients who have complete tears of their rotator cuff, allowing the humeral head to migrate upward and articulate with the under surface of the acromion; this is known as "impingement" (Fig. 9).

The integrity of the joint is severely damaged, and rapid degenerative arthritis ensues with narrowing, sclerosis, and

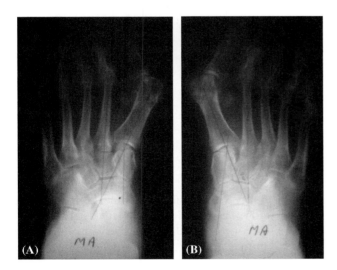

Figure 7 (**A**) Hallux valgus. Note the 45° valgus angulation of the great toe on the first metatarsal head. This should be less than 25°. Note also the increased angulation between the first and second metatarsal shafts. This should be less the 12°. (**B**) Hallux valgus. Note the 40° valgus angulation of the great toe on the first metatarsal head. This should be less than 25°. Note also the increased angulation between the first and second metatarsal shafts. This should be less the 12°.

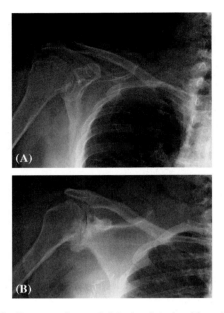

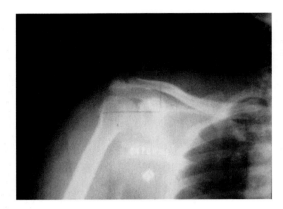

Figure 10 Degenerative arthritis of the acromioclavicular joint. Note the narrowing of the joint, sclerosis, and osteophyte formation both below where it can lead to rotator cuff damage and above where a bursa can form and present as a "mass."

Figure 9 Degenerative arthritis in the shoulder. (**A**) Early degenerative changes in the glenohumeral joint. (**B**) Marked degenerative changes in the glenohumeral joint with upward shift of the humeral head in the glenoid, leading to narrowing of the subacromial space or "impingement." The normal space should be greater than 10 mm.

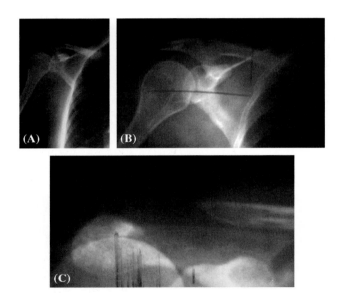

Figure 11 Posttraumatic osteolysis of the clavicle. (**A**) Initial film. (**B**) One year later. (**C**) Three years later showing progressive resorption of the distal clavicle.

osteophyte formation. On the other hand, premature secondary degenerative arthritis in the shoulder can be seen in younger patients with hemophilia and juvenile chronic arthritis, and as a neuropathic situation in young people with congenital loss of pain sensation and in older patients with syringomyelia, which may in fact go on to destroy the joint completely. Degenerative changes also occur in the acromioclavicular joint as a result of instability, and even fairly minor degrees of ligamentous laxity in the young (as can be seen in weight lifters) will lead to degenerative changes in the acromioclavicular joint, with joint space, widening, osteophyte formation, and bone irregularity (Fig. 10).

Another side effect of posttraumatic changes in the acromioclavicular joint is posttraumatic osteolysis of the clavicle. Loss of the distal clavicle can be seen in association with secondary hyperparathyroidism and renal failure, in rheumatoid arthritis and in other rheumatoid variants, as well as in posttraumatic osteolysis (Fig. 11).

Recurrent subluxation of the acromioclavicular joint leads to an inflammatory reaction in which the distal clavicle gets resorbed.

The Elbow

Degenerative changes are rare in the elbow but can be seen as an occupational disease. They can also be seen in pitchers in baseball or in fast bowlers in cricket (Fig. 12).

Otherwise, the presence of degenerative arthritis in the elbow should lead one to suspect an underlying disorder, such as hemophilia, juvenile chronic arthritis, osteochondritis ossificans (Panner's disease of the capitellum) with loose body formation.

The Wrist

Similarly, primary degenerative arthritis is rare in the wrist but often accompanies other disorders, such as chronic disability as is seen in association with dorsal intercalary segmental instability (DISI), volar intercalary segmental instability (VISI), and the scapholunate advance collapse (SLAC) wrist. It can also be seen as a secondary

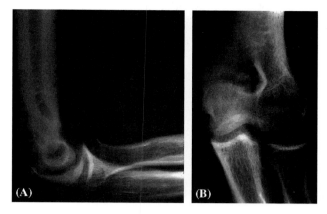

Figure 12 Degenerative arthritis in the elbow. This 28-year-old professional pitcher was complaining of pain in his elbow. There are osteophytes on many of the joint surfaces. Note also the hypertrophy of the humeral cortex secondary to his occupation. (**A**) Lateral film. (**B**) AP film. *Abbreviation*: AP, anteroposterior.

phenomenon in CPPD, rheumatoid arthritis, juvenile chronic arthritis, and in other forms of arthritis. On the other hand, degenerative arthritis of the first carpometacarpal joint is common in patients older than 50 (Fig. 13).

This disorder occurs as a result of increasing motion and instability of the joint and presents as radial subluxation, joint space narrowing, subchondral sclerosis, and osteophyte formation. This is probably the only true form of degenerative arthritis seen in the small joints of the wrist and hand. Erosive osteoarthritis of the interphalangeal joints of the fingers is discussed separately.

The Spine

Facet joint arthritis is commonly seen in both the mid-cervical region, as a secondary result of cervical spondylitis, and in the lower lumbosacral spine accompanying degenerative disc disease.

In the cervical spine, a good lateral view, with flexion and extension views as well as an oblique view, would be useful to find these changes. In the lumbosacral spine, oblique views are best to diagnose facet joint arthritis (Fig. 14).

In either site, narrowing, subchondral sclerosis, and vacuum phenomena are common, as are the presence of hypertrophic spurs, which can encroach on the nerve root, which is well seen on the oblique views and can cause a radiculopathy. In the lumbosacral spine, the hypertrophic spurs can become so large as to appear that the spine has become fused.

The Sacroiliac Joints

Obviously, the sacroiliac joints take a lot of pressure, and hence degenerative arthritis will occur in them, although not very frequently. This is no doubt because of their

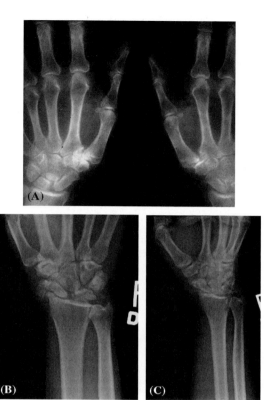

Figure 13 Degenerative arthritis in the hands and wrist. (**A**) Early. Early degenerative changes are noted in the first carpometacarpal joint with sclerosis, subluxation, and loss of cartilage space. (**B**) Moderate. Moderate changes in a different patient with narrowing of the radiocarpal joint, triscaphe joint, and the first carpometacarpal joint. (**C**) Severe degenerative changes or a scapholunate advanced collapse (SLAC) wrist.

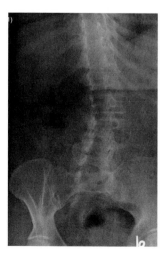

Figure 14 Facet joint arthritis in the lower lumbar spine with sclerosis, narrowing, and osteophyte formation.

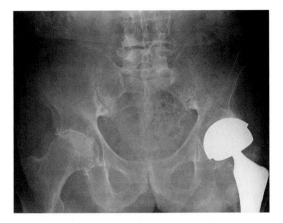

Figure 15 Degenerative arthritis in the sacroiliac joints in a 45-year-old female patient who has had several children. Note the sclerosis, narrowing, and osteophyte formation.

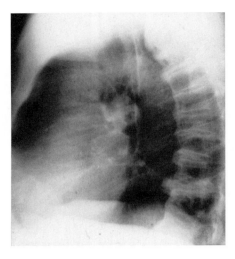

Figure 16 DISH. Spine showing the flowing syndesmophytes. Note that the disc spaces are normal. *Abbreviation*: DISH, disseminated idiopathic skeletal hyperostosis.

complex shape, which is oblique in both the coronal and axial planes, and the joint itself is a combination of both fibrous tissue and synovially lined joint space. The synovial joint is the lower two-thirds as you look at a film of the pelvis and the anterior two-thirds as you look at a CT scan. Degenerative arthritis of the sacroiliac joints manifests itself the same way as in every other joint: narrowing, subchondral sclerosis, and osteophyte formation (Fig. 15). It can be unilateral or bilateral, the former being frequently seen in association with scoliosis.

Disseminated Idiopathic Skeletal Hyperostosis or Ankylosing Hyperostosis

Although disseminated idiopathic skeletal hyperostosis (DISH) is not a true form of degenerative arthritis, I felt it should be considered in this chapter. In fact, it is difficult to classify it as a condition. If one sees a disc space with large spurs but no disc space narrowing, no sclerosis, and no vacuum phenomenon, it is almost certainly caused by DISH.

It is often helpful to remember its old name, which is: "ankylosing hyperostosis." It occurs in approximately 20% of patients older than 60 years. Remember that if there is NO loss of disc height and the patient has syndesmophytes rather than osteophytes, then DISH is probably the cause of the back pain. Osteophytes run horizontally in the spine and are associated with degenerative disc disease. Syndesmophytes run basically vertically, occur in the small intraspinal ligaments, and "flow" from one end plate to the next, but are associated with a normal disc space (Fig. 16).

DISH is a systemic condition in which new bone formation occurs at each and every enthesis i.e., at every place that a ligament or tendon originates or inserts.

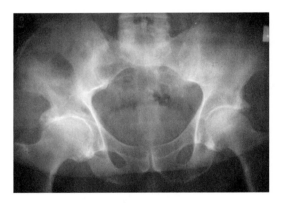

Figure 17 DISH—pelvis. There is extensive new bone formation at each ligament and tendon insertion ("whiskering") typical of this condition. Note that the joints are normal. *Abbreviation*: DISH, disseminated idiopathic skeletal hyperostosis.

This is colloquially known as "whiskering" and occurs in all of the enthesopathies (Fig. 17).

Many of the causes of exaggerated or premature degenerative arthritis have already been mentioned in the preceding paragraphs. However, I believe that they should be also considered separately.

Acromegalic Arthritis

Acromegaly is a metabolic, endocrine condition caused by excessive growth hormone either from the adrenals or the pituitary gland. It is dealt with in more detail in the chapter on metabolic disease. However, patients with

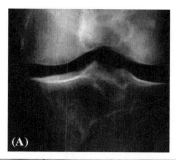

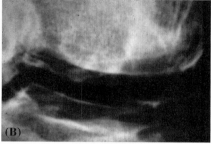

Figure 18 Acromegalic arthritis. (**A**) Standing AP knee show true widening of the joint space. (**B**) Arthrogram confirms the genuine thickening of the articular cartilage. *Abbreviation*: AP, anteroposterior.

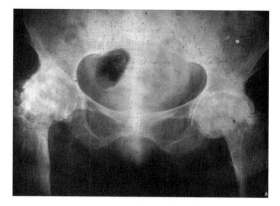

Figure 19 Acromegalic arthritis: AP view of the pelvis shows significant degenerative changes seen in both hip joints in this 38-year-old male with acromegaly. *Abbreviation*: AP, anteroposterior.

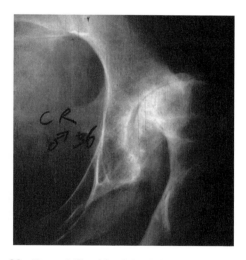

Figure 20 Hemophilia. AP of the left hip in this 36-year-old male patient with hemophilia who has had many bleeds into the left hip and has now developed severe degenerative joint disease with sclerosis, loss of joint cartilage, and osteophytes. *Abbreviation*: AP, anteroposterior.

acromegaly get premature degenerative arthritis. Once one has reached skeletal maturity, it is impossible to increase the thickness of the hyaline cartilage. But if you have acromegaly, everything that can overgrow does so, and the articular cartilage is no exception (Fig. 18).

Unfortunately, the overgrowth is due to infiltration of fibrocartilage, and this actually leads to destruction of the hyaline cartilage and hence to premature degenerative arthritis. This is typically seen in weight-bearing joints such as the hips and the knees, where there is premature and rapid loss of joint space, subchondral sclerosis, and acromegalic osteophyte formation, i.e., hugely overgrown osteophytes (Fig. 19). The other signs of acromegaly should however make the diagnosis obvious.

Hemophiliac Arthritis

Hemophilia is due to a factor VIII deficiency and occurs almost entirely in males. It is a sex-linked recessive disorder with the females carrying the genes and handing it onto their sons. Von Willebrandt's disease is due to a decrease in the factor VIII antigen level and is associated with decreased platelet aggregation, but has few musculoskeletal problems. Christmas disease (or hemophilia B) is a deficiency of clotting factor IX and is similar to hemophilia, although less severe. One of the problems with these conditions is excessive bleeding after even the most minor trauma. Although painful in the soft tissues,

recurrent bleeding into a joint will destroy the articular cartilage and lead to premature arthritis, as well to synovial hypertrophy (Fig. 20).

In most hemophiliacs, any bloody effusion is, or should be, immediately evacuated. However, if the blood is allowed to remain in the joint, the hemoglobin breaks down and releases hyaluronidase, which directly destroys the cartilage. Thus, loss of joint cartilage space without any juxta-articular osteoporosis to suggest an inflammatory arthritis is typical of early hemophilic arthritis (Fig. 21).

This will be followed by subchondral sclerosis, but usually not by osteophyte formation, since synovial overgrowth also occurs in hemophilia and thus the margins of

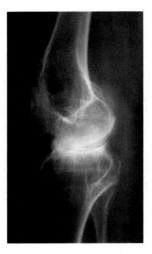

Figure 21 Hemophilia. Lateral knee. This shows the almost total loss of articular cartilage, squaring off of the epiphyses, and marked subchondral sclerosis.

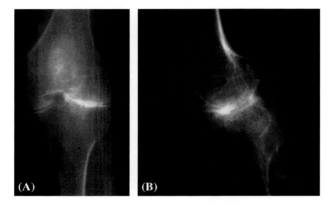

Figure 22 Hemophilia. Knee in a 53-year-old male. (**A**) AP view shows loss of cartilage space, subchondral sclerosis and widening of the intercondylar notch. (**B**) Lateral view showing squaring off of the patellar as well as the subchondral surface. *Abbreviation*: AP, anteroposterior.

the joints usually appear squared off. For instance, in the knees, there is classical widening of the intercondylar notch due to synovial overgrowth and squaring off of the femoral condyles and of the inferior pole of the patella (Fig. 22).

The recurrent bleeds into a single joint can also lead to overgrowth of the epiphyses. The differential diagnosis of widening of the intercondylar notch includes other synovial conditions such as juvenile chronic arthritis and chronic infections such as tuberculosis, and fungal infections, as well as synovial tumors such as pigmented villonodular synovitis. But if the age and sex of the patient, the lack of juxta-articular osteoporosis, and the

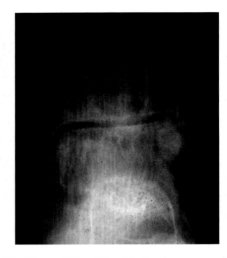

Figure 23 Hemophilia. AP ankle in the same patient as in Figure 20 showing tibiotalar slant as well as loss of joint space, subchondral sclerosis, and an abnormal trabcular pattern. *Abbreviation*: AP, anteroposterior.

frequent involvement of other joints are taken into account, this should lead to the correct diagnosis.

Many hemophilic patients have recurrent bleeds into one joint and iron (hemosiderin) may actually get deposited into the synovium, which can be clearly seen by the increased density of the joint fluid and particularly of the synovium in the suprapatellar pouch; for example, another clue to hemophilic arthritis is that it often involves an unusual joint, such as the elbow, the ankle, or the shoulder. In the ankle, one can see angulation of the tibiotalar joint (tibiotalar tilt or tibiotalar slant), and this classically occurs in hemophilia, sickle-cell anemia, juvenile chronic arthritis, and Fairbanks disease (Fig. 23).

Thus, even if one does not know that the patient is hemophilic, the diagnosis should be suspected in young male patients with premature degenerative arthritis, without significant osteophyte formation, and with involvement of unusual joints (Fig. 24).

Finally, patients with hemophilia may get massive bleeds into soft tissues, flat bones, and, occasionally, long bones, which will apparently enlarge and appear as pseudotumors (Fig. 25).

Neuropathic Arthritis

If one loses proprioception as well as local pain sensation, it is easy to place a joint or limb into an abnormal position without realizing. This places abnormal stress on the joint, but if proprioception is present, the stress is limited. On the other hand, if both proprioception and pain sensation are impaired, it is easy to place excessive stress on a joint

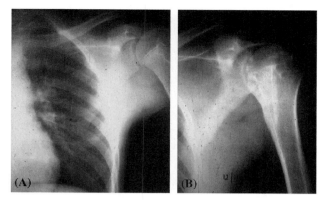

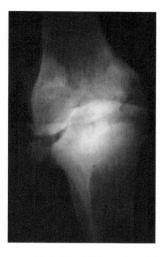

Figure 24 (**A**) Hemophilia in a 14-year-old boy. AP left shoulder shows early degenerative changes in the glenohumeral joint. (**B**) Hemophilia in the shoulder of the same patient. AP of the same shoulder taken two years later following recurrent bleeds shows more advanced degenerative joint disease. *Abbreviation*: AP, anteroposterior.

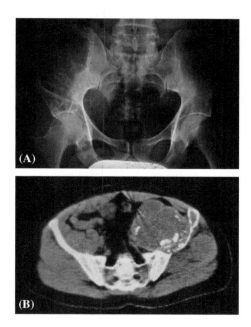

Figure 25 Hemophiliac pseudotumor. (**A**) AP of the pelvis in a 24-year-old Greek male with a large lucency in his left iliac bone. (**B**) CT scan confirms a large soft tissue mass with some bony destruction. The fact that the patient was a hemophiliac and that this occurred within the three weeks of blunt trauma makes the diagnosis relatively easy. *Abbreviation*: AP, anteroposterior.

Figure 26 Neuropathic joint. AP knee in a 58-year-old patient with tabes dorsalis showing marked disruption of the knee, sclerosis, fragmentation, and subluxation typical of a neuropathic joint. Ask yourself the question: "Would you walk on this joint?" *Abbreviation*: AP, anteroposterior.

repetitively, producing abnormal wear and tear and hence early degenerative arthritis. This situation was first described by Jean Marie Charcot, in 1859, when he found a group of patients with tertiary syphilis who had severe degenerative arthritis in their knees and ankles. This form of syphilis was called tabes dorsalis because of the damage it caused to the dorsal columns of the spine. The dorsal columns carry the nerves that control proprioception and local pain sensation. Tabes dorsalis has basically died out since the advent of penicillin. Neuropathic joints (or Charcot joints) are now mainly seen in association with two conditions that damage the dorsal columns in different ways: (1) Diabetes by small-vessel disease, primarily involves the feet and ankles. (2) Syringomyelia, usually in the cervical region, where swelling of the cord leads to damage to the dorsal columns secondarily by compressing them against the posterior elements of the spine. This type of neuropathic joint primarily involves the shoulders. However, other situations arise, and neuropathic joints can be seen in association with congenital loss of bone sensation (the elbows and the wrists, primarily), syringomyelia in the lumbar region (the hips and the knees), in such situations as the spinal cord injury and cerebral palsy, and in patients with meningomyeloceles.

The hallmark of a neuropathic joint is the almost total disruption of the joint, which can occur rapidly, but usually occurs over months, if not years (Fig. 26).

There are premature degenerative changes, as well as either subluxation or frank dislocation of the joint, often with fragmentation of some of the bone resulting in "bone dust" (Fig. 27).

Usually the patient experiences some pain, but has lost all proprioception. The characteristic radiographical appearance is of a disrupted joint with fractures, sclerosis, and fragmentation, rather than juxta-articular osteopenia. The sclerosis is a dominant part of neuropathic joints and is due to attempts at bone healing and callus formation.

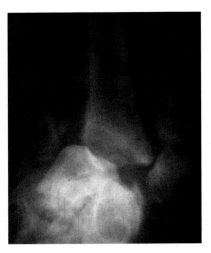

Figure 27 Neuropathic joint. AP view of the ankle in a 25-year-old male with diabetes and severe renal failure. Note the complete disruption of the normal anatomy with subluxation and "bone dust" (fragmentation).

An old, preroentgenographic description of a neuropathic joint was of a "bag of bones," and one can often literally hear the patient walking with the bones grinding against each other.

In the feet, diabetes is the most common cause of neuropathic joints and is seen primarily at the tarsometatarsal joint (Lisfranc joint) where fragmentation, increasing sclerosis, subluxation, loss of joint cartilage, and fractures can be clearly seen, but is often best appreciated on the lateral view where it appears as if the mid foot has sunk because of the subluxation (Fig. 28).

The hallmark of the diabetic foot consists of five radiographical findings:

1. Neuropathic joints
2. Vascular calcification
3. Periosteal reaction along the shafts of the third and fourth metatarsals
4. Patchy lucencies in the metatarsal heads
5. Osteomyelitis

In the shoulders of patients with syringomyelia, there is total disruption of the glenohumeral joint with loss of joint cartilage, fragmentation, sclerosis, and subluxation or actual dislocation; similar changes occur in the hip (Fig. 29).

However, diabetic Charcot joints also occur in the calcaneocuboid, talarnavicular (Chopart joint), tibiotalar, and subtalar joints, and more peripherally (Fig. 28).

The humeral head will often apparently dissolve. Some years ago, an attempt was made to subdivide neuropathic joints into those where all the bone fragments dissolved (atrophic) and those where the bone fragments appear to actually increase in density, size, and number (hypertrophic).

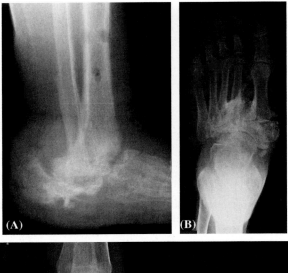

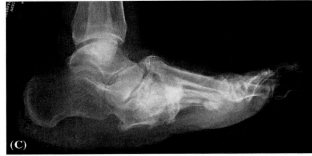

Figure 28 Neuropathic foot—two different patients. (**A**) Neuropathic hindfoot of the first patient showing complete disruption of the talocalcaneal joint with collapse and fragmentation as well as rotation of the talus into a near vertical position. Subluxation of the talonavicular and calcaneal-cuboid joint has also occurred. (**B**) AP view. (**C**) Lateral view in the second patient showing collapse and fragmentation of many of the intertarsal and tarsometatarsal joints.

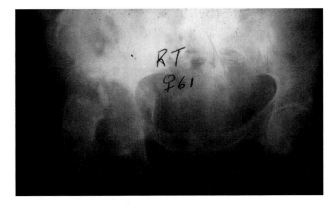

Figure 29 Neuropathic joint. AP pelvis in a 61-year-old female with tertiary syphilis, showing disintegration of the right hip joint with destruction of the acetabulum, protrusio acetabuli, and loss of much of the femoral head and neck as well as "bone dust" and fragmentation.

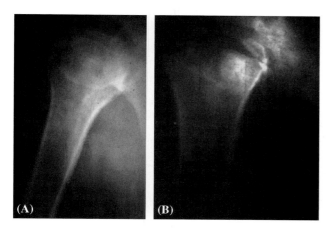

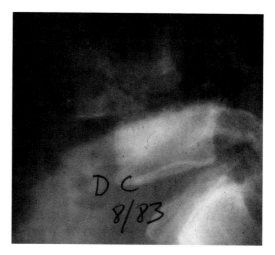

Figure 30 Neuropathic joint. Rapid onset of a Charcot joint in a 58-year-old male patient with syringomyelia. (**A**) On May 3rd, an AP view of his left upper humerus suggested avascular necrosis with a crescent sign. (**B**) On May 30th, the destruction and fragmentation of the humeral head becomes typical of a neuropathic joint. *Abbreviation*: AP, anteroposterior.

Figure 32 Neuropathic joint in a young female diabetic with painless fragmentation, loss of disc height, and subluxation of the L4-5 disc space.

This was supposedly related to the adequacy of the blood supply, but I find this classification spurious. Another way to look at these joints would be to subdivide them into those with a good or a poor blood supply, and, again, I believe this is unnecessary. Occasionally, one can see a very rapid onset of a neuropathic joint. There are several cases quoted in the literature of a joint that went from normal to complete disintegration in 5 to 10 days (Fig. 30).

In the spine, because of the marked disruption of the normal anatomy, the old description was of "tumbling bricks" and was classically seen in tabes dorsalis (Fig. 31).

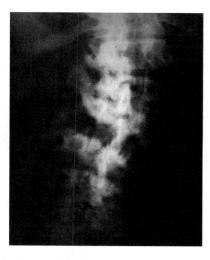

Figure 31 Neuropathic joint in a young male patient with tabes dorsalis showing typical "tumbled bricks" appearance of the lumbar spine.

However, today, diabetic neuropathy can produce similar changes, with loss of disc height, increasing sclerosis, fragmentation, and disruption of the normal alignment of the spine in both the AP and lateral views (Fig. 32).

This process never seems to be as severe as was seen in tabes dorsalis, where the spine basically collapsed and fragmented, looking like a brick wall that had fallen down.

Hemochromatosis

The last of what I call the "hypertrophic arthritides" is hemochromatosis. This is a metabolic disorder, which may be primary or secondary. In children, it is thought that hemochromatosis is due to an enzymic deficiency. In adults, hemochromatosis is caused by biliary cirrhosis. In either case, the patient develops liver failure and iron gets deposited in various tissues: in the liver, where it leads to further damage and cirrhosis; in the skin, where the patient develops an interesting orange color; and in the articular cartilage, where the deposition of iron basically leads to cartilage breakdown, chondrocalcinosis, and premature degenerative arthritis (Fig. 33).

In the soft tissues and fibrocartilage, the iron deposition leads to obvious chondrocalcinosis. In time, the liver disease becomes profound and the liver's ability to synthesize vitamin D is impaired, leading to rickets in children and osteomalacia in adults. Thus, a patient with severe osteoporosis, chondrocalcinosis, and a curious form of hypertrophic arthritis should suggest hemochromatosis.

In the hands, apart from chondrocalcinosis (seen in the triangular fibrocartilage, as well as in the articular cartilage of many of the metacarpal heads) hypertrophic changes are seen in the metacarpophalangeal joints, with

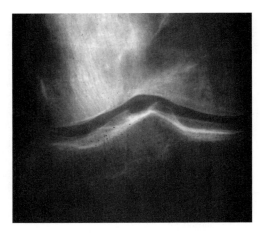

Figure 33 Hemochromatosis. AP knee in a 45-year-old male with early degenerative change and chondrocalcinosis. *Abbreviation*: AP, anteroposterior.

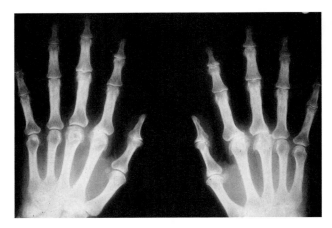

Figure 35 Hemochromatosis. AP hands in a different patient shows similar changes although without the osteopenia. *Abbreviation*: AP, anteroposterior.

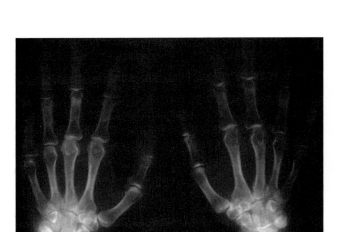

Figure 34 Hemochromatosis. AP hands show subchondral sclerosis in many of the joints but particularly in the second through fifth metacarpophalangeal joints and the interphalangeal joints. Chondrocalcinosis is present in the triangular fibrocartilage and the patient is noted to be osteopenic. *Abbreviation*: AP, anteroposterior.

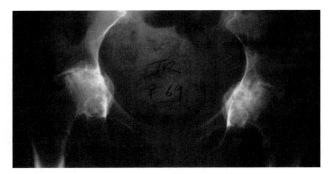

Figure 36 Hemochromatosis. AP pelvis shows bilateral protusio acetabuli, degenerative arthritis in both hips, chondrocalcinosis in the symphysis pubis, as well as profound osteopenia in a patient with hemochromatosis and osteomalacia secondary to biliary cirrhosis. *Abbreviation*: AP, anteroposterior.

squaring off of the metacarpal heads, loss of joint space, and hypertrophic spur formation (Fig. 34).

Attempts to separate the appearance of hemochromatosis from that of CPPD, depending on the distribution of the arthritis, largely fail, although, on the whole, CPPD predominantly involves the second and third metacarpophalangeal joints, whereas hemochromatosis involves all of them as well as many of the interphalangeal joints (Fig. 35).

However, osteoporosis does not occur in CPPD, and hypertrophic spur formation is much more common in hemochromatosis than in CPPD. In the spine, patients with hemochromatosis develop disc calcification as well as marginal spur formation. In the knee, although chondrocalcinosis is widespread in both conditions, specific narrowing of the patellofemoral joint only occurs in CPPD and osteoporosis only occurs in hemochromatosis. The appearance of hemochromatosis in the pelvis is quite characteristic, with chondrocalcinosis in the symphysis, bilateral protrusio acetabula, profound osteopenia, loss of joint cartilage space, and central hypertrophic arthritis with marked subchondral sclerosis in both the hips (Fig. 36).

However, it is the hand X-ray that has the most characteristic appearance in hemochromatosis, so remember, squaring off of the metacarpal heads, chondrocalcinosis, hypertrophic changes in the metacarpophalangeal and interphalangeal joints, as well as joint space narrowing and subchondral sclerosis should lead you to the correct diagnosis.

Occupational Arthritis

This subject is not dealt with at all in most textbooks on musculoskeletal disease; however, increasing interest with problems associated with repetitive motion, such as seen in factory workers, people who spend their time on computers, and professional musicians has at last caught the interest of the politicians. However, occupational arthritis was first described in Finnish lumberjacks using chain saws continually in their work of felling trees. It manifests itself primarily with large subchondral cysts and early degenerative change. This no doubt occurs because of the constant vibration of the chainsaw, leading to small infractions through both the cartilage and the subchondral bone, allowing synovial fluid to be pumped from the joint through the crack and into the bone. Occupational arthritis was also seen, in this country, in jackhammer workers, but is now rare, no doubt due to new safety regulations (Fig. 37).

It can still be seen in the hands and wrists of people during repetitive manual labor such as in tire shops and in people who work on a line in a factory doing such menial tasks as tightening lids on jars (Fig. 38).

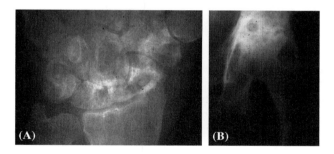

Figure 37 Occupational arthritis in a jackhammer worker. (**A**) Wrist: Note the many subchondral cysts in the carpal bones with loss of much of the joint cartilage space. (**B**) Left hip: There is severe degenerative joint disease with loss of cartilage but the main findings are the large subchondral cysts.

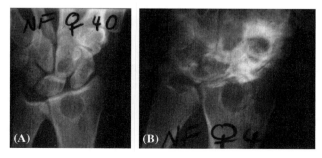

Figure 38 Occupational arthritis in the hand of a line worker at a ketchup factory where her job was to tighten lids on ketchup bottles. (**A**) Plain film shows a large subchondral cyst in the distal radius. (**B**) A wrist arthrogram showing the contrast entering the cyst from the joint.

EROSIVE ARTHRITIS

This disorder was called "erosive osteoarthritis," which is really a misnomer, although it is an arthritis and it is erosive, but there is no relationship to osteoarthritis elsewhere in the skeleton. It was initially described by Heberden in 1820 when he noted small nodes adjacent to the distal interphalangeal (DIP) joints in middle-aged ladies. He dissected several of these nodes and found a cyst with an osteophyte protruding into it. Later in the 18th century, Bouchard described similar changes at the proximal interphalangeal joint (PIP). It is also known as Kellgrens arthritis.

Erosive arthritis is bilateral and symmetrical, often familial, and involves the PIP and DIP joints sparing the metacarpophalangeal joints and carpus. It has an equal sex incidence and occurs over the age of 50, although many patients are in the 60s and 70s. It starts with loss of joint space and central erosions (which appear like a child's drawing of seagulls), classically involving the DIP (Fig. 39).

There is no juxta-articular osteoporosis, and so with these findings, erosive arthritis can be differentiated from rheumatoid arthritis. If also seen in younger female patients (mainly younger than 30), then systemic lupus erythematosus needs to be considered. If it is seen in a patchy form with some carpal involvement and new bone formation, then psoriatic arthritis is in the differential diagnosis. There is another formal of erosive arthritis occurring in middle-aged ladies of Anglo-Saxon origin where the arthritis almost uniquely involves only the DIP joints (Fig. 40).

Thus, if you see an older patient with a symmetrical erosive arthritis involving the DIP and PIP joints, sparing the carpus and MCP joints, think of erosive arthritis.

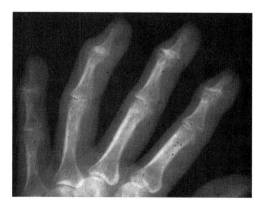

Figure 39 Classical erosive arthritis with bilateral symmetrical arthritis involving the DIP and PIP joints in this 73-year-old female patient with no evidence of arthritis elsewhere. *Abbreviations*: DIP, distal interphalangeal; PIP, proximal interphalangeal.

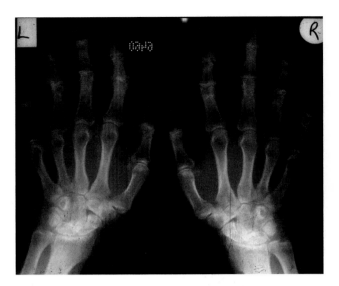

Figure 40 Erosive arthritis. "Heberden's" arthritis, involving predominantly the DIP joints in a 53-year-old female. *Abbreviation*: DIP, distal interphalangeal.

RHEUMATOID ARTHRITIS

Rheumatoid arthritis is a common form of arthritis, often closely related to a systemic disease. It is basically an autoimmune disease, and the patients are rheumatoid factor–positive, antinuclear antibodies (ANA)-negative, and have elevated α-2 and γ-globulins. Classically, rheumatoid arthritis affects young females, but it may occur in either sex and at any age. The female-to-male ratio is 3:1. Although the median age of presentation is 33, a juvenile form of rheumatoid arthritis occurs in children as young as five years and is discussed later in this chapter. In male patients, rheumatoid arthritis can appear as almost a different disease, and in black male patients, it may present like gout.

Typically, rheumatoid arthritis has an insidious onset and starts with fatigue and malaise, and the patient will complain of diffuse musculoskeletal pain. Over the course of time, this goes on to morning stiffness, with symmetrical involvement of the hands and wrists, spreading to the feet, elbows, shoulders, and other joints in time. There will be soft-tissue swelling and muscle atrophy around the affected joints, and the patient will experience decreasing strength and low-grade fever, and chills can also occur. At this stage, the diagnosis is often difficult to confirm. The American Rheumatism Association has developed criteria for the diagnosis of rheumatoid arthritis, but these are usually considered too cumbersome for everyday use; a simpler set of criteria was developed in New York City.

From here the disease may become progressive, may cease, may become intermittent, or may have long

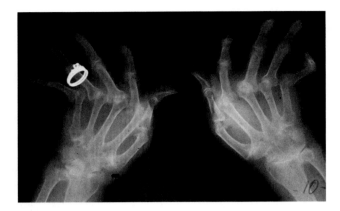

Figure 41 Severe rheumatoid arthritis: both hands showing the typical and serious late changes of the disease with ulnar deviation, subluxation of many of the metacarpophalangeal joints, fusion of some of the carpal bones, and widespread osteoporosis.

remissions. Rheumatoid arthritis can exhibit a number of unusual patterns, such as adult Still's disease, palindromic rheumatism (which resembles gout), and various curious manifestations in older patients, particularly men. Pathologically, rheumatoid arthritis is an inflammatory polyarthritis, which produces a "pannus" which starts in the bare area of the bone between the hyaline cartilage and the synovium. This pannus usually grows into and destroys the synovium in rheumatoid arthritis, and hence marginal erosions are the hallmark of early rheumatoid arthritis. When the pannus grows into the articular cartilage, thereby destroying it, it causes loss of joint cartilage, narrowing of the joint, and, ultimately, central erosions.

To get back to the radiology of rheumatoid arthritis, the classical presentation is in the hands and wrists, although many authorities claim that the feet are involved earlier and in a more severe manner than the hands. The classical presentation in the hands is with symmetrical erosions of the carpal bones and the metacarpophalangeal and, possibly, the interphalangeal joints of the fingers. This is usually associated with severe juxta-articular osteoporosis and ulnar deviation of the fingers at the metacarpophalangeal joints in the later stages of the disease (Fig. 41).

However, in the earliest cases, the erosions may be very difficult to see and the diagnosis may be very difficult to make, radiologically. For some reason, rheumatoid arthritis appears to affect the ulnar aspect of the wrist and fingers; so look at the ulnar aspect of the base of the fifth metacarpal where the ulnar collateral ligament inserts, or at the adjacent ulnar surface of the hamate, or either at the very tip of the ulnar styloid or at its base where the synovium of the distal radioulnar joint is inserted (Fig. 42).

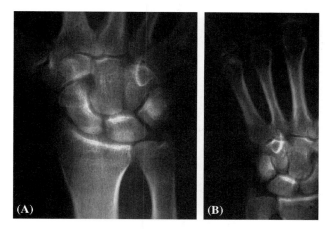

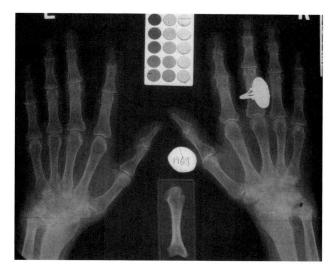

Figure 42 (**A, B**) Early rheumatoid arthritis in two different patients. There is discrete juxta-articular osteoporosis, particularly at the bases of the metacarpals. Note the very early erosions of the ulnar aspect of the base of the fifth metacarpal where the ulnar collateral ligament inserts. Figure 42A is somewhat less advanced than Figure 42B.

Figure 44 More advanced rheumatoid arthritis with quite severe bilateral and symmetrical disease in the carpus with loss of joint cartilage space and erosions.

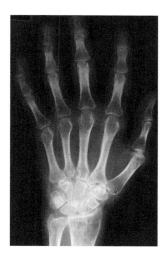

Figure 43 Early rheumatoid arthritis with juxta-articular osteoporosis, erosions of many of the carpal bones and distal radius as well as the ulnar aspects of the fourth and fifth metacarpophalangeal joints.

Look at the ulnar aspect of the bases of the proximal phalanges, particularly the fourth and third fingers (in that order of frequency). Do not glance from a long distance, but look carefully and close-up (if you are shortsighted, take off your spectacles), and follow the bone around the corner. The bone should be a continuous cortical line from the subchondral bone of the joint, around the corner (the bare area of the bone), and into the metaphyseal, and, ultimately, the diaphyseal cortex (Fig. 43). This should be a continuous white line, although quite narrow in normal

bones, but it gets eroded and destroyed in early rheumatoid arthritis. These are the so-called "marginal erosions."

As the disease progresses, erosions may be seen in any part of the hand and wrist, and they are usually remarkably symmetrical (Fig. 44). Apart from erosions on the ulnar aspects of the proximal phalanges, early erosions can also be seen under the necks of the metacarpals, and an oblique or "ball-catcher" view may be useful to emphasize these erosions, which are seen end-on on a true AP film and hence appear as circular "cysts," whereas they are in fact also marginal erosions.

There is obvious and increasing juxta-articular osteoporosis. Erosions will start appearing in the interphalangeal joints, in the other carpal joints, in the distal radioulnar joints, and basically anywhere else in the hands. At this stage, with the lack of motion, the patient also develops generalized, disuse osteoporosis on top of the juxta-articular changes.

The metacarpophalangeal joints will sublux, usually anteriorly and radially, as a result of increasing ligamentous laxity, but they can sublux in any direction and get boutonniére (see Chapter 1, Fig. 45) and swan-neck deformities. Since rheumatoid arthritis is a systemic disease and the soft tissues get involved as well as the joints at this stage, the pull of the ulnar-sided ligaments overcomes the normal balance of the joints, so ulnar deviation occurs and the patient becomes severely handicapped (Fig. 45).

Thus, this could be considered to be the endpoint of severe rheumatoid involvement of the hands, severe osteoporosis, ulnar deviation of the metacarpophalangeal joints, many of which are subluxed, severe erosive involvement of

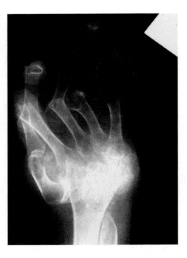

Figure 45 Severe rheumatoid arthritis with bilateral and symmetrical involvement, marked osteoporosis, subluxation, and a boutonniere deformity of the fifth finger.

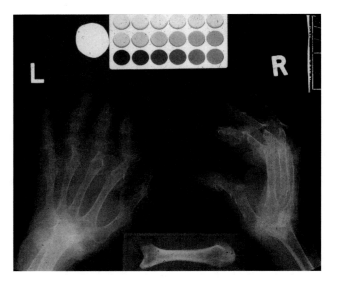

Figure 46 Severe rheumatoid arthritis with both carpal fusion and destruction, marked ulnar deviation, and widespread osteoporosis as well as destruction of many of the metacarpal joints. There are also cup and pencil deformities more reminiscent of psoriatic arthritis, although this young patient had aggressive rheumatoid arthritis.

the wrists and interphalangeal joints, as well as actual fusion of some, if not all, of the carpals (Fig. 46).

The fusion occurs because the pannus removes the hyaline cartilage and, thus, bone is exposed to bone, and with the profound hyperemia, immobilization occurs and then one bone can fuse to another. End-stage rheumatoid arthritis has been described in the old literature as arthritis mutilans.

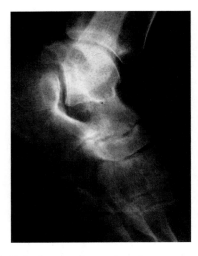

Figure 47 Palindromic rheumatism in a young black male with erosive arthritis involving the mid tarsal joints of one foot only. The differential diagnosis would include any form of inflammatory arthritis, including gout.

In men, the involvement of the hands is similar, although osteopenia is less obvious; in fact, it is frequently absent, which can make the diagnosis of rheumatoid arthritis in men quite difficult. Also, men will often have degenerative changes in some of the joints, which can precede the onset of rheumatoid arthritis. Thus, men may present with a combination of what looks like erosive disease and hypertrophic changes, and this can resemble erosive osteoarthritis, which was discussed earlier.

However, erosive osteoarthritis spares the metacarpophalangeal joints and wrists, whereas, obviously, rheumatoid arthritis involves these areas primarily (Fig. 58). In black patients, rheumatoid arthritis may present as very localized erosive changes, resembling an acute inflammatory arthritis, such as infection or even gout. This form of rheumatoid arthritis has a very old name—palindromic rheumatism (Fig. 47).

The feet have similar changes to the hands, with erosions of the metatarsophalangeal joints, particularly involving the metatarsal heads, where marginal erosions undermine the neck of the bone. Erosions are seen in both the medial and lateral corners of the proximal phalanges, and, unlike in the hands, there appears to be no predilection for either side of the interphalangeal joints of the feet. Although the tarsal joints become as severely involved as the carpal joints, we do not often see this aspect of rheumatoid arthritis, mainly because rheumatologists choose to x-ray the hands rather than the feet. However, erosions, loss of joint cartilage space, and fusion will occur, particularly in the subtalar joints, the calcaneocuboid joint, and the talornavicular joint. In the periphery, hammertoes and valgus deformities of the metatarsophalangeal joints can also occur.

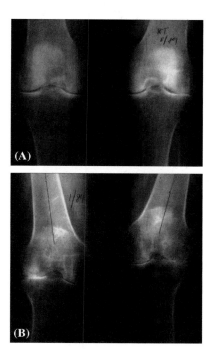

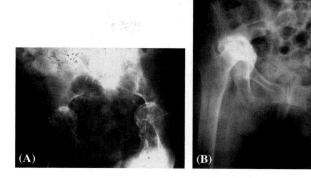

Figure 48 Rheumatoid arthritis of the knee. Two standing views in the same patient with severe rheumatoid arthritis. (**A**) AP view. These films show the bilateral symmetrical loss of joint cartilage as well as the erosions in the intercondylar notch. (**B**) Thiry-five-degree flexed view. These films show the bilateral symmetrical loss of joint cartilage as well as the erosions in the intercondylar notch. *Abbreviation*: AP, anteroposterior.

Figure 49 Rheumatoid arthritis of the hips in two different patients showing the marked bilateral and symmetrical protrusio acetabulae that can occur. (**A**) Both hips in a 52-year-old female who had rheumatoid arthritis for 20 years with medial and upward subluxation of both femoral heads. Note that there appears to be an articular space and this is caused by the formation of fibrocartilage acting as a buffer between the femoral head and the destroyed acetabulum. (**B**) A more advanced case where there is now added secondary degenerative arthritis with subchondral sclerosis, osteophyte formation, and loss of this space.

In the ankle, early erosions can be seen at the synovial insertion into the distal tibia on the lateral view, often in association with a joint effusion. Erosions can also be seen on the lateral and medial sides of the talus on the AP view. Loss of joint cartilage space, with erosions in the distal tibiofibular syndesmosis also occurs, although the ankle rarely fuses. Because it is a weight-bearing joint, secondary degenerative arthritis of the ankle is common, with subchondral sclerosis and eburnation.

The characteristic appearance of rheumatoid arthritis in the knees is bilateral, symmetrical loss of joint cartilage space, unlike in primary degenerative arthritis, where the medial compartment is involved first (Fig. 48).

On the lateral view, an effusion and early erosions are apparent at the synovial insertions in the intercondylar notch and at the margins of the tibia (often best appreciated on oblique views). As the disease progresses, osteoporosis will occur, but not to the extent seen in the hands. Similar to the ankle, secondary degenerative arthritis occurs early because the knees are weight bearing, so that subchondral sclerosis and osteophyte formation can be seen in the earlier stages.

The hallmark of rheumatoid arthritis in the knees is bilateral, symmetrical loss of joint cartilage space, without squaring off of the articular surface or of osteophyte formation.

In the hips, rheumatoid arthritis also has a characteristic appearance with medial loss of joint space, compared with the superior joint space narrowing seen in primary degenerative arthritis.

Erosions can be difficult to see in the hips, although synovial pits (erosions seen on end) may be apparent in the femoral neck. However, as the disease progresses, erosions of the medial wall of the acetabulum lead to increasing protrusion of the femoral head centrally into the acetabulum. This is known as protrusio acetabula, with the femoral heads migrating medially into the pelvis (Fig. 49).

This is normally associated with profound osteopenia, as well as erosions of the sacroiliac joint and symphysis pubis. There are many causes of unilateral protrusio acetabula, including trauma, infection, Paget's disease, metastases, and rheumatoid variants (particularly ankylosing spondylitis). There are only two causes of bilateral protrusio acetabula: rheumatoid arthritis and the constellation of conditions associated with osteomalacia, such as renal bone disease, rickets, and hemochromatosis. In severe cases of Paget's disease with bilateral involvement of the pelvis, bilateral protusio acetabula can also be seen. The endpoint of severe rheumatoid arthritis in the hips is never seen today because of the use of total joint replacements at a much earlier stage than was done in previous years.

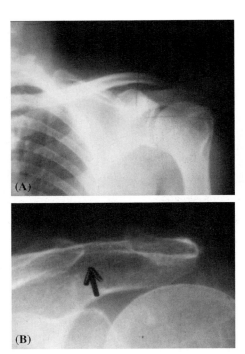

Figure 50 (**A**) and (**B**) Rheumatoid arthritis of the shoulder showing the typical erosions involving both sides of the acromioclavicular joint with "pointing" of the distal clavicle.

In the shoulder, rheumatoid arthritis also has a fairly characteristic appearance, even in its early stages, with erosions of the acromioclavicular joint as well as in the line of the insertion of the synovium in the humeral head, best seen on the external oblique AP view of the shoulder.

In the acromioclavicular joint, rheumatoid arthritis involves both the distal clavicle and proximal acromion, unlike hyperparathyroidism (both primary and secondary), which only involves the distal clavicle, and unlike recurrent trauma or posttraumatic osteolytis of the clavicle, in which the patient has a history of weight lifting and is associated with acromioclavicular joint separation. This process also involves only the distal clavicle. In rheumatoid arthritis of the glenohumeral joint, there is progressive loss of joint cartilage space, increasing osteoporosis, increasing erosive changes, until secondary degenerative arthritis also occurs, leading to secondary sclerosis, osteophyte formation, and marked distortion of the joint itself (Fig. 50).

In the elbow, rheumatoid arthritis can be very destructive, although initially the erosions are subtle and best seen on the lateral view where an associated joint effusion is common. As the disease progresses, the erosions destroy the intercondylar notch from both sides and undermine the capitellum and trochlear in the distal humerus, as well as eroding the olecranon notch, the coronoid process, and the radial neck (Fig. 51).

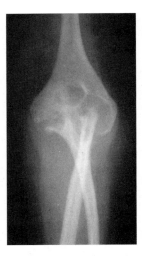

Figure 51 Rheumatoid arthritis of the elbow with severe destruction of all three subchondral surfaces and "pointing" of the proximal radius.

This eventually leads to loss of the radial head, with pointing of the proximal radius, and a cup-shaped appearance to the intercondylar region of the distal humerus. With the advent of more aggressive forms of therapy, this appearance is rare in primary rheumatoid arthritis today, although it can still be seen as the end result of both juvenile chronic arthritis and hemophilia.

In the spine, one of the best-known complications of rheumatoid arthritis is atlanto-axial separation. The odontoid or dens, which is embryologically the body of C1, is held in place by a transverse ligament which has a synovially lined bursa between it and the underlying dens itself. As the rheumatoid arthritis progresses, synovial overgrowth and hypertrophy of this bursa causes the ligament to weaken and eventually rupture. This allows the dens (the axis) to separate from the atlas (Fig. 52).

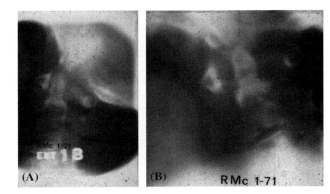

Figure 52 Rheumatoid arthritis atlantoaxial joint. (**A**) Neutral. (**B**) Flexion. These two old-fashioned tomograms show a somewhat eroded odontoid in the neutral view with alantoaxial separation in the flexion view. The normal subdental space should never measure more than 2 mm.

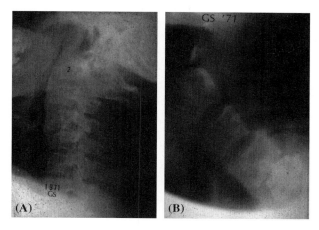

(A)   (B)

Figure 53 Cervical spine in severe rheumatoid arthritis. (A) Lateral view. In the lateral view, the dens appears to be missing. Note the subluxation at C4/5 and the facet joint arthritis throughout the spine. (B) Tomogram confirming these findings.

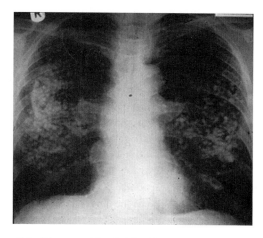

Figure 54 Rheumatoid arthritis. Chest X-ray in a patient with long-standing disease. This film shows multiple pulmonary nodules and interstitial pulmonary fibrosis related to the disease.

Similarly, there are synovial bursa on top of and in front of the dens, and synovial overgrowth in these bursae will also cause erosions and loss of bone, so that the odontoid may become pointed or even disappear altogether, which leads to severe atlanto-axial separation or rocking (Fig. 53).

This is very important to all patients with advanced rheumatoid arthritis, but, in those patients who are about to undergo anesthesia, it is life-threatening, since the anesthesiologist will have to extend the neck to intubate the patient, thus pithing the patient if this diagnosis has been missed. So flexion and extension views of the cervical spine should be mandatory in patients with severe rheumatoid arthritis who are about to undergo surgery.

Rheumatoid arthritis involves mainly synovially lined joints, so it involves the facet joints in the spine rather than the disc spaces. Narrowing of the facet joints in the cervical spine is a fairly common consequence of early rheumatoid arthritis (Fig. 53).

Although similar changes occur in the thoracic spine, what is usually seen is a generalized osteoporosis, which underlies the whole disease. However, facet-joint arthritis can be seen in the lumbar region, where it is usually accompanied by secondary degenerative changes, particularly in the lowermost facet joints.

Once again, rheumatoid arthritis does not really involve the disc spaces in the lumbar region. Finally, bilateral symmetrical involvement of the sacroiliac joints in rheumatoid arthritis has been described, but appears to be quite rare. More often, one will see asymmetrical erosions associated with generalized osteopenia, as well as protrusio acetabula and erosions of the symphysis pubis.

Soft-tissue involvement in rheumatoid arthritis is also common, but usually presents clinically rather than

radiographically. Apart from the ulnar deviation seen at the metacarpophalangeal joints, tendonitis may occur anywhere in the body. Bursitis can also be seen, particularly in areas of maximum use, such as the wrists and elbows. Rheumatoid nodules, which are inflammatory granulomatous nodules, can be seen subcutaneously in the arms and legs. Involvement of the chest in rheumatoid arthritis is not uncommon, with rheumatoid nodules as well as interstitial pulmonary fibrosis occurring (Fig. 54).

The most common manifestation of rheumatoid disease in the chest is interstitial pneumonitis with fibrosis. In its initial stages, this may be very subtle, but, as the fibrosis progresses, a reticular, nodular pattern may be seen throughout the lung fields. Rheumatoid nodules can be seen in the chests of 1% to 2% of patients with rheumatoid arthritis and are usually multiple, occurring classically in the periphery of the lung field. They frequently cavitate. Caplan's syndrome was first described in coal miners, in Wales in 1953, who had both pneumoconiosis and rheumatoid arthritis. Radiologically, Caplan's syndrome resembles the presence of multiple rheumatoid nodules. Various other pulmonary disorders have been described in association with rheumatoid arthritis including pleuritis, pleural effusions, pneumothorax, obliterative bronchiolitis, and bronchiectasis.

Thus, to summarize, rheumatoid arthritis is a generalized disorder with both local and systemic manifestations. The findings in the hand and wrists have been well documented. Involvement of the hips with protrusio acetabula and involvement of the upper cervical spine with atlanto-axial separation is well known. However, rheumatoid arthritis can involve any synovially lined space, bursa, or joint in the body.

JUVENILE CHRONIC ARTHRITIS

This is a complex subject, since the term "juvenile chronic arthritis" actually covers several different entities. Incidentally, the old term "juvenile rheumatoid arthritis" is still preferred in some countries, but, in fact, less than 5% of patients with juvenile chronic arthritis are actually rheumatoid factor–positive, and since the remaining 95% are rheumatoid factor–negative, I will use the term "juvenile chronic arthritis" for this book. Depending on how one subdivides the condition, there are four or five major types of arthritis under this heading: juvenile rheumatoid arthritis (a polyarthritis in which the patients are rheumatoid factor–positive), Still's disease (patients present with a systemic illness, but a delayed onset of arthritis), oligo-arthritis, or pauci-arthritis (in which not more than four joints are involved), poly-arthritis (in which there is involvement of five or more joints), and an enthesitis type of arthritis (i.e., juvenile onset, ankylosing spondylitis, or psoriatic arthritis). The age of onset of juvenile chronic arthritis is variable, but over 80% of children become symptomatic by the age of seven years.

The incidence of juvenile chronic arthritis varies from the United States, where it is 5 of 100,000, to Britain (10 of 100,000), to developing countries where it can be as high as 65 of 100,000 children. Thus, criteria have been developed for the diagnosis of juvenile chronic arthritis and these include a minimum of three months disease duration and onset before 16 years of age.

Juvenile Rheumatoid Arthritis

By definition, this is juvenile polyarthritis in patients younger than 15 years who are rheumatoid factor–positive. This presents as early-onset rheumatoid arthritis in somewhat older children and adolescents. It is usually symmetrical and involves both small and large joints, particularly the wrists, hands, ankles, feet, hips, and knees. One relatively characteristic appearance is of interphalangeal joint involvement with marked juxta-articular osteoporosis and hyperemia, leading to "dumbbell"-shaped phalanges (Fig. 55).

Juvenile rheumatoid arthritis is highly destructive and often goes on to joint fusion by the late teenage and early twenties, and this is particularly seen in the large joints such as the hips, knees, ankles, and wrists (Fig. 56).

The disease will often become quiescent for a time before reemerging 10 to 20 years later as adult-type rheumatoid arthritis. Juvenile rheumatoid arthritis is the most destructive form of juvenile chronic arthritis and has the second highest morbidity and mortality rate associated with it.

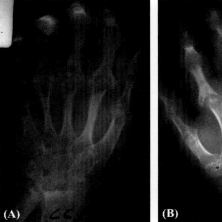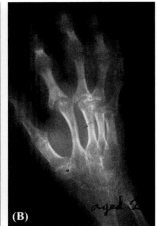

Figure 55 Juvenile chronic arthritis in two young patients. These figures show the typical "dumbbell"-shaped phalanges as well as the widespread destructive erosive changes and the carpal fusion. (**A**) AP hand. (**B**) Oblique. *Abbreviation*: AP, anteroposterior.

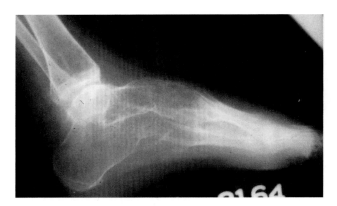

Figure 56 Juvenile chronic arthritis lateral foot showing the fusion of much of the mid and hindfoot (this is the same patient as Fig. 55A).

Still's Disease or Systemic Arthritis

This condition usually presents with a systemic illness before the onset of arthritis in very young children (often younger than five years), making the diagnosis somewhat difficult to substantiate. The children present with generalized malaise, hepatosplenomegaly, and other constitutional symptoms, which grumble on for months, if not years. Then, a polyarthritis sets in, with a clinical presentation ranging from minor arthralgias to joint swelling to major destructive arthritic changes. As the arthritis becomes increasingly prominent, the systemic features will gradually regress, usually within three to four years of onset. Children with Still's disease may also have cervical spine involvement, which is rare in other forms of juvenile chronic arthritis. Initially, neck pain and stiffness will occur, going on to fusion of the posterior elements and facet joints. In about 1% of patients with Still's disease, atlanto-axial instability will occur. The prognosis for this group of patients is generally poorer than in those patients with rheumatoid-negative polyarthritis without systemic symptoms. In Still's disease, 25% of patients will only have a mild form of arthritis, systemic manifestations will not recur, and the disease will die out. Twenty-five percent will manifest a more active form of arthritis with more destructive changes, but will also remit and not recur. However, 50% will develop a progressive, unremitting, destructive arthritis, and the systemic illness will recur, leading to high morbidity and mortality.

Felty's syndrome refers to a rare form of juvenile chronic arthritis (usually rheumatoid factor–positive), which is associated with splenomegaly and neutropenia. The systemic manifestations of the disease are serious, including recurrent infections, as well as a severe, destructive arthritis.

Pauci-Articular Arthritis or Oligoarthritis

This condition also has other names, such as monarthritis in which only one joint is involved, which is not uncommon, and oligoarthritis in Britain. By definition, these patients are rheumatoid factor–negative and have not more than four joints involved over the course of the disease. This disease does not have systemic manifestations. If the disease extends to involve more than four joints, it automatically falls into the category of polyarticular disease. Classically, the knee is the first joint involved, although the wrist or ankle may be the first joint involved. Pauci-articular arthritis is more common in girls and frequently seen before the age of five years and often as young as three years. Characteristically, it is associated with chronic anterior uveitis, and the antinuclear antibody is positive, leading some authorities to speculate that it is indeed an autoimmune disease or, possibly, a collagen vascular disease. The classical presentation is of a swollen, painful knee in a young child, and the differential diagnosis must include infection, so aspiration is essential to exclude this (Fig. 57).

If more than one joint is involved, they are very rarely involved synchronously, and so the patient will have one knee involved at age three years, the hip at age five years, and the wrist at age nine years, until the condition dies out.

Although uveitis is commonly seen in association with pauci-articular arthritis, it is rare to have any other generalized systemic manifestation. Finally, a few cases of pauciarthritis grumble on, and the disease can become the polyarticular type of juvenile chronic arthritis. Also, a

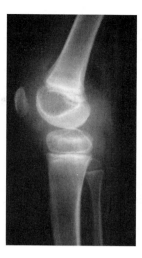

Figure 57 Juvenile chronic arthritis. Monarticular or pauciarticular involvement of the knee. Note the soft-tissue swelling and the effusion, although the bones are normal at this stage.

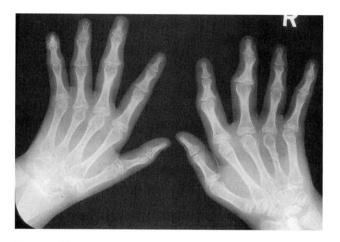

Figure 58 Juvenile chronic arthritis. Still's disease in a 45-year-old female patient with a long history of juvenile chronic arthritis but who now has systemic disease. The hands resemble rheumatoid arthritis.

few cases will go on to develop an arthritis that resembles adult rheumatoid arthritis, but the patients remain rheumatoid factor–negative. This is what the clinicians refer to as seronegative rheumatoid arthritis (Fig. 58).

Polyarticular Arthritis

This type of juvenile chronic arthritis also presents early (usually by age five years) but with five or more joints involved at the time of presentation. However, it is often a less destructive form of the condition, and the joint changes are clinical rather than radiological; joint stiffness, pain, arthralgias, and contractures. This, again,

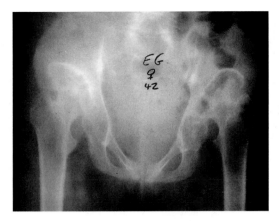

Figure 59 Juvenile chronic arthritis. Long-standing polyarticular arthritis has led to this unusual appearance in this 42-year-old female with the femoral heads apparently migrating upward.

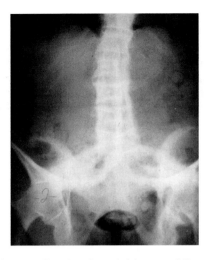

Figure 61 Juvenile chronic arthritis resembling ankylosing spondylithisis in the spine. Which came first?

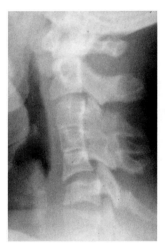

Figure 60 Juvenile chronic arthritis. Long-standing polyarticular arthritis in a different patient leading to spinal fusion and deformity of C3, C4, and C5.

would suggest some form of collagen vascular disease or, at the least, some degree of overlap between juvenile chronic arthritis and collagen vascular disease. The joints involved may be large or small; it is somewhat more common in boys than girls and uveitis and other systemic manifestations are rare. Unlike the pauciarticular type of juvenile chronic arthritis, polyarticular disease has a poor outcome, with marked destructive changes involving many of the joints (Figs. 59 and 60).

ENTHESOPATHIC ARTHRITIS

The juvenile onset of ankylosing spondylitis, Reiter's syndrome, and psoriatic arthritis is uncommon, particularly the latter. Each of these diseases will be considered

more fully later in this chapter. Most of the patients with juvenile-onset ankylosing spondylitis are human leukocyte antigen (HLA)-B27-positive, male (over 80%), and aged 12 to 15 years, and have acute anterior uveitis. They will often present with a pauciarticular peripheral arthritis before the onset of sacroiliitis and spinal changes, which are equivalent to adult-onset ankylosing spondylitis. However, occasionally, juvenile ankylosing spondylitis (as I prefer to call it) will start in the mid- to lower-thoracic spine, rather than the sacroiliac region, and I believe that this accounts for those rare patients with ankylosing spondylitis who have fusion of their thoracic spine but sparing of their lumbar region (Fig. 61).

Juvenile-onset Reiter's syndrome is not uncommon and is seen almost entirely in boys older than 12 years, who also present with anterior uveitis but who, in addition, have some form of nonspecific urethritis. It has the same clinical presentation, radiological appearance, and course as adult Reiter's syndrome (see later) (Fig. 62).

Finally, juvenile-onset psoriatic arthritis may in fact be a separate entity than adult psoriatic arthritis. The HLA subtyping is different, and the disease is rapidly progressive, starting with an inflammatory arthritis involving the fingers and toes, going on to a severe destructive polyarthritis involving large and small joints. There is usually either some psoriasis in the child or a very strong family history of the condition.

Overlap Syndromes

In real life there is often some overlap among these various, carefully defined subgroups, although usually patients with Still's disease are easily separated out. The commonest form of juvenile chronic arthritis is still

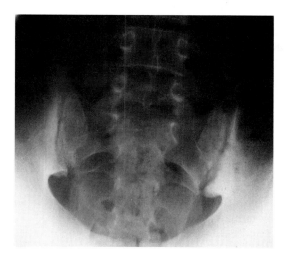

Figure 62 Juvenile chronic arthritis or Reiter's syndrome. There is bilateral, symmetrical sacroilitis in this young male patient with typical polyarticular juvenile chronic arthritis.

monarticular or pauciarticular arthritis, and this can also be separated from the rest. The overlap syndromes largely involve the patients with polyarticular disease who may or may not have spinal involvement or various clinical problems, particularly acute anterior uveitis.

Radiological Features

Obviously, most patients with juvenile chronic arthritis present with arthralgias and soft-tissue swellings. The first radiological manifestation is juxta-articular osteoporosis. Unlike in adult rheumatoid arthritis, the next finding is loss of joint space, which occurs within the first two years, particularly in those patients with Still's disease (Fig. 55). Growth and modeling deformities occur frequently in the younger patients (younger than five) and largely consist of overgrowth of the affected epiphyses due to the marked hyperemia. If the process continues, premature fusion of the epiphyses will result in shortening of the bone or limb, often accompanied by valgus or varus deformities, particularly in weight-bearing joints such as the knee and ankle. In contrast, the diaphyses of the bones are frequently gracile or narrowed (Fig. 63).

Erosive changes are a late finding in juvenile chronic arthritis and occur mainly after significant cartilage loss has occurred. This is because, in juvenile chronic arthritis rather than adult rheumatoid arthritis, the synovium becomes invaded by T lymphocytes and macrophages, which produce cytokines, which, in turn, lead to pannus formation. The pannus formation releases proteolytic enzymes, which initially destroy the articular cartilage before eroding the underlying bone.

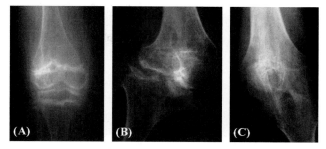

Figure 63 Juvenile chronic arthritis showing the progression of the disease in the knee in a young male patient. (**A**) Fairly early with overgrowth of the epiphyses and early erosive changes. Note the severe osteopenia. (**B**) Note the marked destructive changes in the joint in this film taken some years later. (**C**) Finally, fusion occurs approximately 10 years after the initial film.

On the whole, erosions are seen earlier in rheumatoid factor–positive juvenile chronic arthritis (juvenile rheumatoid arthritis) than in the other forms of juvenile chronic arthritis, usually in the first two years of onset. In the other types of polyarticular disease where 55% of patients get erosions and the systemic-onset disease where 45% get erosions, erosions usually occur between ages two and five years. In the pauciarticular disease, erosions are uncommon (30%), and, if they do occur, are seen five years or later after onset.

Two final radiological features are relatively unique to this group of arthritides: bony fusion and periostitis. Bony fusion has now become fairly rare because of the advent of more advanced therapy, including the use of large doses of anti-inflammatory drugs, chemotherapy (usually methotrexate), and the use of active physiotherapy. In the old days, the joints were often immobilized for long periods of time, allowing fusion to occur (Fig. 64). This is not done today. Periostitis is unusual in any other form of

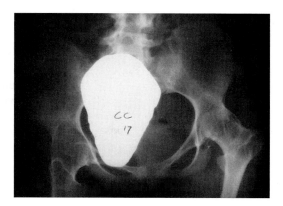

Figure 64 Juvenile chronic arthritis. Bony fusion in both hips in a 17-year-old female patient. This is the same patient as shown in Figure 55A and Figure 56.

arthritis, even in severe, adult rheumatoid arthritis, presumably because these forms of arthritis are predominantly destructive and not bone forming. However, periostitis along the metaphyses and diaphyses of the short, tubular bones of the hands and feet can be seen in polyarticular juvenile chronic arthritis. Presumably, it is some form of reaction to the synovitis in the adjacent joint, or possibly occurs as a result of synovitis in the tendon sheath in the adjacent fingers and toes.

Lupus Erythematosus

There are a number of different forms of arthritis associated with systemic lupus erythematosus as well as some musculoskeletal sequelae of the disease. Many of the appearances overlap with those seen in pure arthritis, although there are some variants, and there appear to be two or three types of arthritis associated with lupus that are relatively pathognomonic.

Of the specific types of arthritis, "mouse-ear" erosions are relatively pathognomonic of all the collagen vascular diseases, but particularly lupus. They occur usually in the DIP joints, but occasionally in the PIP joint, with discrete erosions occurring in the base of the distal phalanx of the joint. These are more central than the peripheral marginal synovial erosions that are typically seen in pure rheumatoid arthritis (Fig. 65).

Mouse-ear erosions occur because the pannus grows in so rapidly that it destroys the subchondral bone on both the radial and ulnar aspect of the phalanx, producing an

effect like a child's drawing of Mickey Mouse—hence the name. They can be also seen in rapid-onset rheumatoid arthritis but are rare. As the destruction continues, marginal erosions and complete loss of joint cartilage as well as subluxation will occur.

Jaccoud's arthritis was first described in inpatients following rheumatic fever many years ago, but is seen more frequently nowadays in patients with systemic lupus erythematosus. It starts as periarticular swelling involving the small joints of the hands and feet, but, specifically, seems to involve the metacarpophalangeal joints. As the condition progresses, there is progressive ulnar deviation, probably as a result of fascial and peritendinous fibrosis, leading to marked ulnar deviation.

Erosions are rare, although flexion deformities can occur, and "hook-like" erosions have been described on the radial aspect of the metacarpal neck. However, the hallmark of Jaccoud's arthritis is a marked ulnar deviation of the metacarpophalangeal joints, without obvious erosive disease (Fig. 66).

Loss of the soft tissues in the extremities also occurs in systemic lupus erythematosus, with loss of the thenar and hypothenar eminence, as well as the tufts of the fingers. This loss of soft tissues will be accompanied ultimately by acro-osteolysis, with loss and pointing of the tufts of the distal phalanges. This can be also seen in Raynaud's disease and phenomenon (Fig. 67).

Arthritis in systemic lupus erythematosus may rapidly progress into a form indistinguishable from pure rheumatoid arthritis, although the patients are usually rheumatoid factor–negative and ANA-positive. At this stage, the patient will get erosions, subluxations, boutonniere, and swan-neck deformities.

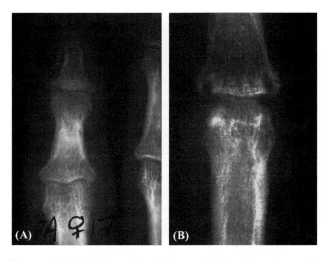

Figure 65 (**A**) Finger in a 17-year-old female patient with lupus who has typical "mouse-ear" erosions of the proximal aspect of the distal phalanx of the index finger. Note the juxtarticular osteopenia. (**B**) Finger in a more advanced and older case in a patient with lupus with typical erosions—more central than those seen in rheumatoid arthritis.

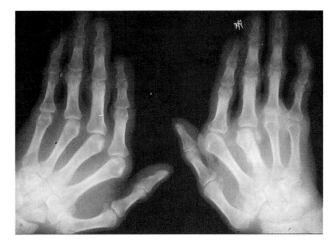

Figure 66 Jaccoud's arthritis. This 53-year-old man had rheumatic fever at age 9 and has now developed the classical ulnar deviation seen in Jaccoud's arthritis. Apart from an old fracture of the right second metacarpal, there are no obvious erosions.

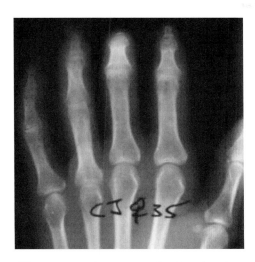

Figure 67 Lupus erythematosus showing the characteristic loss of both the tuft and soft tissues over the terminal phalanx, typically seen with Raynaud's disease.

Both atlantoaxial subluxation and sacroiliitis have been described in association with lupus: the former occurring quite early in the disease, and the latter, although usually bilateral and erosive, occasionally presenting unilaterally.

Finally, systemic lupus erythematosus is a small-vessel disease and is associated with an increased incidence of avascular necrosis, particularly in the femoral and humeral heads. However, many patients with lupus are treated with high doses of steroids, which markedly increase the risk of avascular necrosis.

This is discussed more fully under the section on avascular necrosis in the chapter on trauma. Similarly, the high doses of steroids required to control lupus lead to steroid-induced osteoporosis, which may be severe and associated with fractures of the femoral neck and wrist, as well as compression fractures of the vertebral bodies. This is also discussed more fully in the chapter on metabolic bone disease.

Septic Arthritis

Although not usually included in a chapter on arthritis, septic arthritis is indeed a form of inflammatory arthritis. Obviously, it is dealt with in much greater detail in chapter 3 on infectious diseases. However, a brief description of septic arthritis seems appropriate in this context. The characteristic radiological findings in acute septic arthritis are of juxta-articular osteopenia, synovial erosions, and a blurring of many of the subchondral bony margins. In this respect, it is indistinguishable from other forms of inflammatory arthritis, such as juvenile chronic arthritis, rheumatoid arthritis, psoriatic arthritis, and gout, depending on the age of the patient.

In younger children, the only manifestation of septic arthritis may be a joint effusion, in which case it is difficult to distinguish from juvenile chronic arthritis. In older patients and in a small joint, it is difficult to separate septic arthritis from gout. In any case, by putting a needle directly into the joint, the diagnosis of septic arthritis can be easily substantiated. In patients with a chronic septic arthritis, the diagnosis can be much more difficult to make without a careful history and a joint aspiration. Both tuberculous and fungal infections of joints produce little in the way of juxta-articular osteoporosis but are associated with large synovial erosions and ultimately with destruction of the joint cartilage.

My final comment is, "Always remember septic arthritis if there is involvement of only one joint in a patient who does not appear to have any other manifestations of an inflammatory arthritis."

SERONEGATIVE SPONDYLOARTHROPATHIES

This is a group of four conditions, which have a number of biochemical, clinical, and radiological features in common. All the patients are rheumatoid factor–negative, HLA-B27-positive, and usually have, as a major manifestation, sacroiliitis with or without spinal involvement. The conditions, in approximately chronological order of presentation, are

- Ankylosing spondylitis
- Reiter's syndrome
- Enteropathic arthritis
- Psoriatic arthritis

If one excludes psoriatic arthritis for the moment, sacroiliitis is the most significant feature of the other three seronegative spondyloarthropathies. Remember that the synovial part of the sacroiliac joint is the inferior two-thirds on radiographs and the anterior two-thirds on CT scans. Sacroiliitis may be bilateral, unilateral, symmetrical, or asymmetrical, and remember that there are other causes of sacroiliitis than the seronegative spondyloarthropathies (Table 1).

The diagnosis of very early sacroiliitis is controversial, with some people arguing that CT is more sensitive than MRI and that both are more sensitive than plain film. Personally, I believe that in many patients a CT scan is just as sensitive as MRI, and a lot cheaper.

In the spine in patients with seronegative spondyloarthropathies, a number of different findings may be seen, although syndesmophytes are the most commonly seen change in Reiter's syndrome, enteropathic arthritis, and psoriatic arthritis. Syndesmophytes are large, curving spurs, which originate either 2 mm above the lower end plate of a vertebral body or 2 mm below the upper end plate (Figs. 68 and 69).

Table 1 Sacroiliitis

1. Bilateral, symmetrical
   a. Ankylosing spondylitis
   b. Enteropathic arthritis
   c. Reiter's syndrome
   d. Hyperparathyroidism
2. Bilateral, asymmetrical
   a. Reiter's syndrome
   b. Psoriatic arthritis
   c. Rheumatoid arthritis
3. Unilateral
   a. Infection (particularly tuberculosis)
   b. Psoriatic arthritis
   c. Gout
   d. Degenerative arthritis

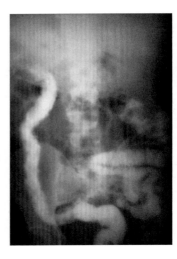

Figure 69 Syndesmophytes in enteropathic arthritis, similar findings are seen in this young female patient with ulcerative colitis.

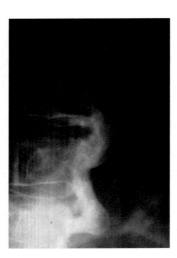

Figure 68 Syndesmophytes: this male patient with severe psoratic arthritis has large "flowing" syndesmophytes going in a vertical direction from one vertebral body to the next.

Figure 70 Ossification of Sharpey's fibers seen in a 34-year-old male with ankylosing spondylitis. Note that the ossification is in the line of the spine and lies under the anterior longitudinal ligament.

They follow the course of a small, intraspinous ligament and occur not only in the seronegative spondyloarthropathies but also in disseminated idiopathic skeletal hyperostosis (DISH or ankylosing hyperostosis), which affects 20% of men and 15% of women older than 60. Thus, syndesmophytes are most commonly seen in patients with DISH, rather than in those with seronegative spondyloarthropathy (Fig. 16).

Patients with ankylosing spondylitis do not, on the whole, develop syndesmophytes, although there is a possibility. Usually these patients ossify the outer fibers of the annulus fibrosis of their discs (known as Sharpey's fibers), and this finding is pathognomonic of ankylosing spondylitis (Fig. 70).

There are several other causes of spinal ligament calcification and ossification (Table 2). It can be seen in association with degenerative disc disease with osteophyte formation and loss of disc height. Osteophytes originate at the outer margins of the end plate and usually run horizontally away from the disc space, similar to osteophytes, say, in the knee joint. Syndesmophytes originate 2 mm above or below the end plate and run in a curved but vertical fashion toward the next vertebral body and without loss of disc height. Spinal ligament calcification can also be seen in hypervitaminosis A, which occurs nowadays when patients overdose with Retin A, which is used in the treatment of acne (Fig. 71).

Table 2 Spinal Ligament Ossification and Calcification

- Ankylosing spondylitis
- Reiter's syndrome
- Enteropathic arthritis
- Psoriatic arthritis
- DISH
- Degenerative arthritis
- Retin A
- Ossification posterior longitudinal ligament
- Ochronosis
- Fluorosis
- Diabetes

Abbreviation: DISH, disseminated idiopathic skeletal hyperostosis.

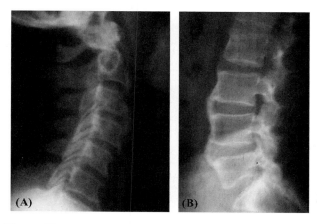

Figure 71 Syndesmophytes seen in a young male patient with acne who has been treated with Retin A. (**A**) Cervical spine. (**B**) Lumbar spine.

These patients develop early syndesmophytes throughout their spine, although the cervical region is often the most involved. Calcification can also be seen in a number of dystrophic disorders, such as ochronosis, fluorosis, and diabetes, all of which are described elsewhere (Table 2).

Ossification of the posterior longitudinal ligament (OPLL) appears mainly to involve the cervical spine in patients of Japanese origin (Fig. 72). Its etiology is unknown, but it can cause quite severe symptoms with cord compression. It is, however, seen occasionally in the caucasian population, possibly as a result of trauma.

Ankylosing Spondylitis

Classically, ankylosing spondylitis starts in the late teenage with low back pain and is mainly in males who initially have no radiographic findings, although their sacroiliac joints are tender and their backs are stiff on clinical examination. There is a large spectrum of age, sex, and clinical presentation. For instance, ankylosing spondylitis can start as late as the thirties and the forties, and in some series, approximately 30% of the patients are females. However, in nearly every patient, ankylosing spondylitis starts with erosions in the sacroiliac joints, ultimately leading to fusion, and then inexorably climbs the spine from the lumbosacral junction up the atlanto-axial joint (Figs. 73–75). Frequently, this will take between 10 and 20 years before the whole spine becomes solidly fused.

In ankylosing spondylitis, the sacroiliac joints show early erosions involving both sides of the joint and are not particularly associated with the dense iliac sclerosis that can be seen in both Reiter's syndrome and in enteropathic arthritis (Fig. 108). In ankylosing spondylitis, the synovial part of the sacroiliac joint will then fuse solidly, often followed by fusion of the fibrous tissue of the upper part of the joints. Since ankylosing spondylitis is an inflammatory form of arthritis, the acute inflammation surrounding each disc space will lead to localized bone resorption and to osteoporosis of the vertebral bodies, as well as to marginal erosions of the vertebral bodies. In fact, many people think that the first radiological sign of early ankylosing spondylitis is the presence of osteoporosis in the lower lumbar

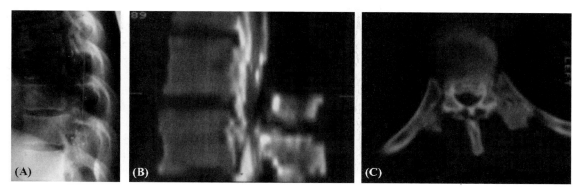

Figure 72 (**A, B, C**) Ossification of the posterior longitudinal ligament. This occurred in a young Abyssinian princess who developed stiffness of her neck.

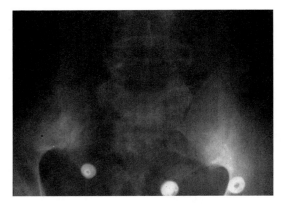

Figure 73 Sacroiliitis in ankylosing spondylitis. This young male patient shows bilateral symmetrical sacroilitis with erosions on both sides of both sacroiliac joints. Note the relative lack of osteosclerosis.

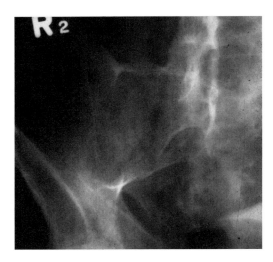

Figure 75 Sacroiliitis in ankylosing spondylitis. There is total fusion of the sacroiliac joint in the same patient five years later.

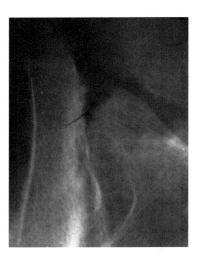

Figure 74 Sacroiliitis in ankylosing spondylitis. This close-up view of the left sacroiliac joint in another patient with ankylosing spondylitis shows the erosions as well as the early new bone formation, which will ultimately lead to fusion.

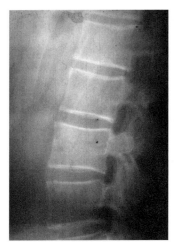

Figure 76 Spine changes in ankylosing spondylitis. Note the early squaring off of many of the lower lumbar vertebral bodies with a suggestion of early osteopenia.

vertebral bodies, with characteristic squaring off of the anterior end plates (Fig. 76).

The normal anterior end plate is somewhat curved, but, in ankylosing spondylitis, it becomes vertical by virtue of discrete marginal erosions occurring in the same region as the insertion of the small interspinous ligament. These erosions have been termed Romanus lesions or the "shiny corner" sign because, in some patients, they are associated with an underlying bony sclerosis, no doubt representing healing (Figs. 77 and 78).

Classical ankylosing spondylitis only involves the spine and sacroiliac joints, although some 25% of patients will get peripheral joint involvement. This is most often seen in large joints rather than small and in proximal joints

rather than distal joints. The hip is most often involved, and, strangely, this is usually unilateral in a disease that is otherwise symmetrical and bilateral (Fig. 79).

The joint will show central joint space narrowing, central and marginal erosions, which involve both the superior and medial joint spaces, often with surrounding osteopenia, all suggesting an infectious or inflammatory etiology. This will often go onto fusion of the hip and the necessity for a total hip replacement. However, any other peripheral joints may be involved, usually unilaterally, and often with the appearance of an inflammatory arthritis reminiscent of that seen in either Reiter's syndrome or enteropathic arthritis, for instance, in the hands or feet,

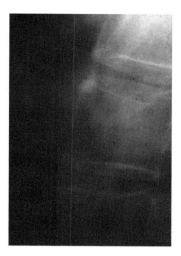

Figure 77 Romanus lesion in early ankylosing spondylitis. There is rounding off of the edge of the vertebral bodies with some sclerosis anteriorly on the upper surface of L3 (*shiny corner sign*).

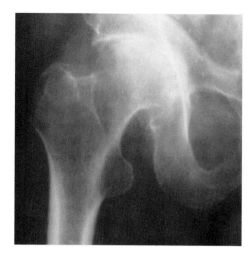

Figure 79 Hip involvement in ankylosing spondylitis. There is narrowing and loss of cartilage in the right hip joint in this 46-year-old male patient with long standing ankylosing spondylitis.

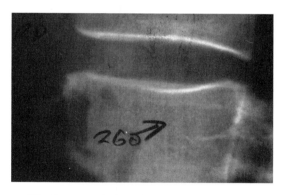

Figure 78 Romanus lesions in early ankylosing spondylitis. A discrete erosion can be seen at the corner of the upper end plate of L5 in a 26-year-old male with early ankylosing spondylitis.

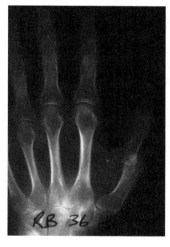

Figure 80 Peripheral joint involvement in ankylosing spondylitis. There is subluxation and erosive change in the left first metacarpophalangeal joint in this patient with ankylosing spondylitis (same patient as shown in Fig. 79). This is the typical appearance of an inflammatory arthritis but is seen more commonly in Reiter's syndrome.

with erosions, joint destruction, subluxation, as well as new bone formation (Fig. 80).

As the spinal fusion progresses upward, the whole spine becomes osteoporotic, as well as fused. This fusion involves not only the longitudinal spinal ligaments but also the facet joints posteriorly (Fig. 81).

Usually the disease stops at the atlanto-axial joint, although this too can be involved, which is probably better for the patient. Otherwise atlanto-axial instability can obviously lead to quadriplegia or death. Patients with ankylosing spondylitis may also get a number of specific complications, including upper-zone pulmonary fibrosis, aortic regurgitation, and conjunctivitis, uveitis, or iritis in the eye. Upper-zone pulmonary fibrosis is presumably

caused by the involvement of the costovertebral joints in the thoracic spine.

Aortic regurgitation is of unknown etiology but is possibly due to a rheumatoid nodule occurring in the aortic valve ring and suddenly rupturing, causing severe aortic insufficiency and pushing the patient into catastrophic congestive cardiac failure and death. Fortunately, this complication is rare. Conjunctivitis, uveitis, or iritis in the eye is very similar to that seen in Reiter's syndrome.

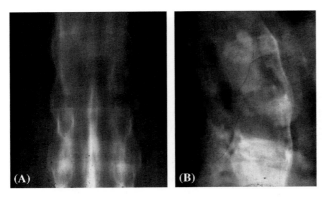

Figure 81 Classical ankylosing spondylitis in the spine. Note the ossification of Sharpey's fibers, the complete fusion of the vertebral bodies, as well as the porterior elements and facet joints. (**A**) AP view. (**B**) Lateral view. *Abbreviation*: AP, antero-posterior.

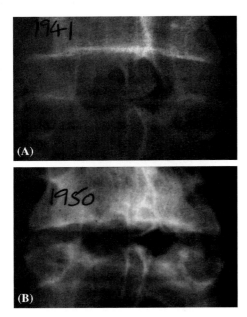

Figure 82 Anderson lesion with nine year follow up. (**A**) Normal disc space in 1941. (**B**) Sclerosis, narrowing of the disc space and fragmentation seen in 1950, typical of a disco-vertebral lesion.

Anderson lesions are unique to ankylosing spondylitis and occur as a result of trauma to a spine that is already weakened with severe osteoporosis, usually due both to the severity of the disease and to disuse. An Anderson lesion is a disco-vertebral fracture, and these lesions occur characteristically in the mid-thoracic spine at the apex of the kyphosis (T6). They were first described in 1937 and occur in 3% to 5% of all patients with severe ankylosing spondylitis (Fig. 82). However, Anderson lesions can be seen at multiple levels in a single patient as well as at any

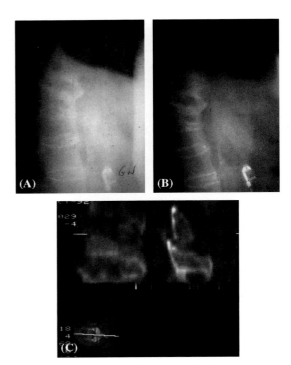

Figure 83 Anderson lesion. Ten-year follow-up. (**A**) Initial lateral view of the thoracolumbar spine, which shows typical findings of ankylosing spondylitis. (**B**) Follow-up film 10 years later shows typical discovertebral fracture (Anderson lesion) between T10/T11/T12. (**C**) A CT scan confirms these findings with destruction and fragmentation of the disc spaces between T10/T11 and T11/T12. Note the fracture line (and fragmentation) posteriorly. Hence the name disco-vertebral lesion.

level in the spine from the mid-cervical region to the lower lumbar spine (Fig. 83).

Unfortunately, the patient will often relish the additional motion they appear to have been granted and often a simple Anderson lesion becomes a disco-vertebral pseudarthrosis with repeated motion. Obviously, there is a major risk of severe spinal cord injury and paralysis, and it is necessary to refuse the spine at the earliest opportunity.

The differential diagnosis between ankylosing spondylitis and the other spondyloarthropathies is often not as easy as it sounds; however, patients with Reiter's syndrome usually have urethritis, whereas those with ankylosing spondylitis do not. Patients with enteropathic arthritis have bowel problems and patients with psoriatic arthritis are older and usually have visible psoriasis. Even so, in some patients, one is left with the diagnosis of an "overlap" syndrome.

In summary, ankylosing spondylitis is a progressive disease characterized by fusion of the spine, starting with bilateral, symmetrical sacroiliitis. In its early stages, it is also characterized by localized osteoporosis of the lower lumbar vertebral bodies, with squaring off of the anterior vertebral end plates, particularly at L4 and L5. As it progresses inexorably up the spine, the spine fuses, with ossification of the outer part of the annulus fibrosis (Sharpey's fibers) as well as the facet joints. Ossification occurs in all of the paraspinal ligaments. The complications of late-stage ankylosing spondylitis include peripheral arthritis (classically, the hip), which occurs in 25% of patients; disco-vertebral fractures (Anderson lesions), which occur in 3% to 5%; atlanto-axial instability (5%); pulmonary fibrosis; and acute onset aortic regurgitation, which is a surgical emergency since many of these patients die undiagnosed.

Reiter's Syndrome

Although this condition was actually first described in a young male patient with knee swelling and gonorrhea, in the 16th century, it was not until 1917 that Reiter described a case and the eponym, Reiter's syndrome, was first used. This syndrome consists of a triad of conditions—sacroiliitis, urethritis, and uveitis. However, not all patients have all three, and, in fact, many only have two of them and rarely at the same time. For instance, it is common for a patient to develop nonspecific urethritis, be treated and cured, and six months later develop sacroiliitis, and then six months later, eye problems.

However, before we start the discussion on Reiter's syndrome, this is a good place to bring in the whole concept of reactive arthritis. By definition, "reactive arthritis" is an aseptic arthritis that follows an episode of infection elsewhere in the body, often preceding it by months, if not years (take Lyme disease as an example). In the case of Reiter's syndrome, the nonspecific urethritis will often precede the sacroiliitis and other joint changes by three to six months. Other examples of reactive arthritis include enteropathic arthritis and psoriatic arthritis, which will be discussed next. Then, there is a whole group of arthralgias and frank arthritides that follow specific infections, finally ending up with a group of rare conditions that are being called "alphabet soup"! These conditions include PPLO, CRMO, and SAPHO—can you guess what these acronyms stand for? If not, I will discuss these later in this subsection.

To return to Reiter's syndrome, usually following an episode of nonspecific urethritis, which is seen in approximately 80% of patients, or uveitis (seen in over 60% of patients), the patient who is almost invariably young (younger than 25) and male (98%) will develop low back pain centered over the sacroiliac joint. Thus, the first radiological finding is of sacroiliitis, which is invariably bilateral but may be either relatively symmetrical or somewhat asymmetrical, and occurs in about 100% of patients with Reiter's syndrome. In this case, there are erosions on both sides of the joint, but there is more sclerosis on the iliac side than is seen in ankylosing spondylitis (Fig. 84).

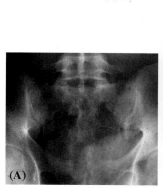
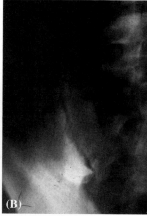

Figure 84 (A) Reiter's syndrome. Sacroiliitis. Twenty-six-year-old male patient with back pain and urethritis. The sacroiliitis is bilateral, symmetrical, and shows erosive change but also some sclerosis. (B) Reiter's syndrome. Close-up of the right sacroiliac joint in a different patient showing erosions and sclerosis mainly on the iliac side of the joint.

This rarely goes onto fusion, and, in fact, unlike ankylosing spondylitis, most patients with Reiter's syndrome undergo remission with complete disappearance of both their clinical symptoms and their radiological appearance of sacroiliitis. However, a small number, probably as low as 5% to 10%, go onto other musculoskeletal manifestations, including sacroiliac joint fusion, syndesmophyte formation in the spine, and a peripheral, erosive, inflammatory arthritis that is characterized by longitudinal periosteal reaction, particularly seen in the periphery (Fig. 85).

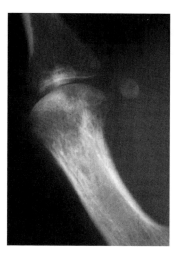

Figure 85 Reiter's syndrome. Perisosteal reaction and erosive changes in the left first metacarpophalangeal joint in a 34-year-old male patient with Reiter's syndrome.

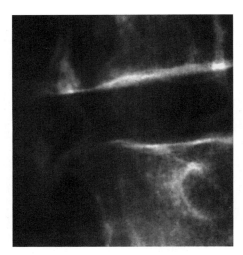

Figure 86 Reiter's syndrome. Spine in a young male patient showing a vertical syndesmophyte between L2 and L3.

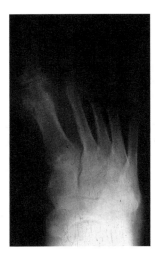

Figure 87 Reiter's syndrome. Foot with an erosive arthritis in the first metatarsalphangeal joint with sclerosis and periosteal reaction, typical of one of the seronegative spondyloarthropathies.

In the spine (which is involved in 25% of patients with Reiter's syndrome), the characteristic finding is of syndesmophytes, but these are rarely symmetrically placed, rarely progressive, and are most often in the mid- to lower-lumbar region, rarely involving L5-S1 and virtually never involving the facet joints (Fig. 86).

The ossification of Sharpey's fibers and vertebral osteoporosis that is seen in ankylosing spondylitis does not occur in Reiter's syndrome. In the more peripheral joints, it the feet and hands that appear to be involved the most frequently, and, although the books state that over 50% of patients with Reiter's syndrome develop a peripheral arthritis, I believe that it is, in fact, quite rare. Feet are more frequently involved than hands, large joints rarely, although the ankles and heel pads are quite frequently involved, at least clinically (Fig. 87).

The characteristic peripheral arthropathy seen in 5% of patients with Reiter's syndrome consists of marginal erosions with subluxation of a metatarsophalangeal joint (or a metacarpophalangeal joint), often with a discrete parallel, linear, periosteal reaction or periostitis (Fig. 85). The juxta-articular osteoporosis is a major constituent of this condition. Another relatively characteristic finding in all of the seronegative spondyloarthropathies is of an enthesopathy involving the calcaneus, both where the Achilles tendon inserts on its upper surface and where the plantar fascia originates on its lower surface. A mixture of erosions and sclerosis can be seen at both these sites, though particularly on the under surface (Fig. 88).

Both ankylosing spondylitis and rheumatoid arthritis are associated with a predominantly erosive picture, whereas Reiter's syndrome, enteropathic arthritis, and psoriatic arthritis are all associated with erosions and underlying sclerosis (representing bony healing), where

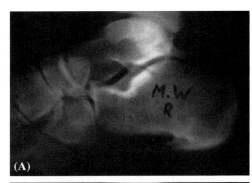

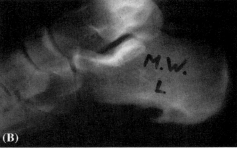

Figure 88 Reiter's syndrome. Enthesopathy involving the calcaneus bilaterally and symmetrically with erosions and new bone formation at the insertion of the plantar fascia. (**A**) Right foot. (**B**) Left foot.

the sclerosis and new bone formation is often the predominant finding.

The differential diagnosis between Reiter's syndrome and the other seronegative spondyloarthropathies is mainly based on the associated clinical findings, for they are rare in the other conditions. Reiter's syndrome has patchy involvement of the spine, similar to that seen in psoriatic arthritis, but does not have the associated skin condition. Reiter's syndrome is almost always seen in young male patients, similar to ankylosing spondylitis, whereas psoriatic arthritis is of equal sex incidence in patients predominantly older than 40. If one takes the sacroiliac joint appearance alone, the differential diagnosis is between Reiter's syndrome and either ankylosing spondylitis or enteropathic arthritis. Once again, with a characteristic clinical history, this is usually easy, but without one, enteropathic arthritis and ankylosing spondylitis are predominantly bilateral and symmetrical; ankylosing spondylitis is not associated with sclerosis, and enteropathic arthritis has marked iliac sclerosis, whereas Reiter's syndrome is classically bilateral and asymmetrical with iliac sclerosis.

In summary, Reiter's syndrome is the first of the group of reactive arthritides that we have discussed. The classical triad is of urethritis, uveitis, and sacroiliitis, and, although they do not all occur at the same time, the patient, who will be young and male, will develop at least two of them in sequence. He will be HLA-B27-positive, ANA-negative, rheumatoid factor–negative, and have bilateral, asymmetrical sacroiliitis with sclerosis on the iliac side of the joint. This is usually associated with nonspecific urethritis and uveitis and occasionally with patchy syndesmophytes in the spine and a sporadic patchy inflammatory arthropathy. Reiter's syndrome is by and large a transient condition, and once the inflammation has settled down, often taking months or years, all the symptoms and radiological features will disappear, leaving the majority of patients in complete remission.

Enteropathic Arthritis

Although the term "enteropathic arthritis" is predominantly used for the arthritis seen in association with both regional enteritis (Crohn's Disease) and ulcerative colitis, occasionally arthralgias, if not frank arthritis, can be seen in nearly any inflammatory condition of the abdomen such as cholecystitis, hepatitis, pancreatitis, nephritis, and so on (in fact anything ending in "itis"). It has also been described in association with biliary cirrhosis, Whipple's disease, and Yersinia, but, in the majority of these patients, there are few if any radiological findings. Incidentally, once again, the majority of these patients are HLA-B27-positive, rheumatoid factor–negative, and ANA-negative. However, in approximately 10% of patients with both regional enteritis and ulcerative colitis, sacroiliitis will occur, occasionally associated with spinal changes and rarely with a peripheral arthritis. This group of conditions is also another example of reactive arthritis.

Classically, the patient is young and either male or female with established regional enteritis or ulcerative

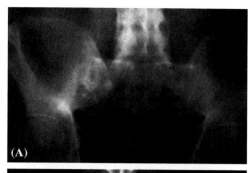
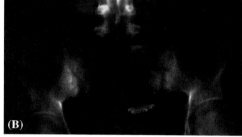

Figure 89 Enteropathic arthritis. Two examples of sacroiliitis. (**A**) Young male patient with regional enteritis. (**B**) Young female patient with ulcerative colitis. Note the bilateral symmetrical erosions with varying degrees of sclerosis and fusion.

colitis and will present with low back pain. Sacroiliitis is found radiographically. This is characteristically bilateral and symmetrical and has intense sclerosis on the iliac side of the joints (Fig. 89).

It rarely goes onto fusion, but has been seen to do so on very rare occasions; in which case, many rheumatologists would consider this a case of ankylosing spondylitis in association with regional enteritis or ulcerative colitis. Spinal involvement occurs rarely and is patchy, similar to that seen in Reiter's syndrome, often only presenting with one or two syndesmophytes (Fig. 90).

Rarely, this will go onto total spinal fusion, but, once again, this probably represents a case of ankylosing spondylitis associated with inflammatory bowel disease. Peripheral joint involvement is rare in enteropathic arthritis, but, when it does occur, resembles that seen primarily in Reiter's syndrome. The enthesopathy seen at the insertion of the Achilles tendon and origin of the plantar fascia can also be seen in enteropathic arthritis (Fig. 91).

Erosions as well as new bone formation occur similar to that in Reiter's syndrome. It is said that as the patients experience remissions and exacerbations of their bowel disease, they get remissions and exacerbations of their arthritis.

In a group of 22 patients with colitic arthritis, 18 had radiographical changes. Eighty-three percent had sacroiliitis, 11% spinal changes, and 28% peripheral changes,

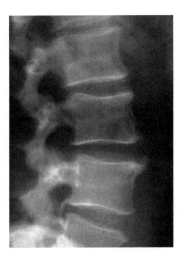

Figure 90 Enteropathic arthritis. Spine in a young male patient with regional enteritis. Note anterior syndesmophytes on the upper surface of L4.

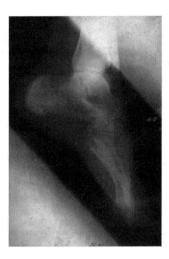

Figure 91 Enteropathic arthritis. Heel showing erosions and new bone formation in a young female patient with ulcerative colitis.

mainly migratory and involving the knees and ankles predominantly.

Once again, the differential diagnosis between enteropathic arthritis and the other seronegative spondyloarthropathies is usually easy and based on the clinical presentation rather than the radiological features. Thus, in summary, enteropathic arthritis is a form of reactive arthritis occurring in approximately 10% of patients with inflammatory bowel disease (either regional enteritis or ulcerative colitis, classically) in whom a form of bilateral symmetrical sacroiliitis is seen, complete with erosions and often with marked sclerosis on the iliac side of the joints. Syndesmophytes may

occur in the spine, and a peripheral arthritis similar to that experienced in Reiter's syndrome may also occur. The arthritis has remissions and exacerbations in conjunction with the activity of the disease, and, once the inflammatory bowel disease has been treated (by either drugs or surgical removal), the arthritis will subside, rarely leaving any permanent sequelae.

Overlap Syndromes

It is already obvious that these three conditions appear to overlap in many ways, although it is usually possible to separate out ankylosing spondylitis because of its progressive, relentless course and because of its fairly characteristic radiographical appearance. If one accepts the concept of reactive arthritis, which almost totally excludes ankylosing spondylitis from the picture, then, obviously, both Reiter's syndrome (with its 90% association with nonspecific urethritis) and enteropathic arthritis (with its exclusive association between arthritis and inflammatory bowel disease) are examples of reactive arthritis. It is of interest that some of the older textbooks referred to primary and secondary ankylosing spondylitis, the primary form being what we now know as ankylosing spondylitis and the secondary form being what we now know as Reiter's syndrome with urinary tract inflammation or enteropathic arthritis with bowel inflammation. I have separated psoriatic arthritis out of this a little, not only by this paragraph but also because peripheral arthritis is the predominant feature of psoriatic arthritis and the spinal and sacroiliac joint involvement is much less common. However, psoriatic arthritis is yet another form of reactive arthritis and will be discussed next. One final comment: to some extent all of these conditions are enthesopathies, which are conditions which have both erosions and new bone formation.

Although this is less true of ankylosing spondylitis, psoriatic arthritis is a classical example of an enthesopathy, followed by both Reiter's syndrome and enteropathic arthritis. The calcaneal changes of erosions associated with underlying bony sclerosis and new bone formation typify these three conditions. It also typifies DISH, which is yet another example of an enthesopathy.

Psoriatic Arthritis

Although generally considered as one of the seronegative spondyloarthropathies, psoriatic arthritis is probably more correctly considered under the term of reactive arthritis. It is a much more separate entity than the three previous forms of arthritis, although it does overlap with them in some ways. Apparently 2% of the population have some form of psoriasis, and approximately 1% to 2% of these develop a peripheral arthropathy, which may take a number of forms. Psoriatic arthritis occurs in older patients than the other types of seronegative spondyloarthropathies, usually in patients older than 40, although it can be seen in patients in their 20s and 30s. A juvenile type of psoriatic arthritis has been described, although this appears to be very uncommon. The sex incidence is approximately equal and the patients are largely HLA-B27-positive, rheumatoid factor–negative, and ANA-negative. Psoriatic arthritis predominantly involves the peripheral skeleton, particularly the hands (Figs. 92 and 93), but can involve large joints such as the

knee, ankle, and shoulder. It will occasionally involve the sacroiliac joints, where it is unilateral or bilateral but very asymmetrical (Fig. 94).

It will rarely involve the spine, where patchy syndesmophytes form characteristically in the upper lumbar region without any paraspinal ossification or involvement of the facet joints (Fig. 95). However, it is as a predominantly peripheral form of arthritis that psoriatic arthritis should be considered.

The hallmark of psoriatic arthritis is new bone formation and this may take a number of forms. However, the classical type is the formation of "bosses," or lumps on adjacent bones, just where the synovium inserts into the bone (Fig. 93). These are characteristically seen on the radial aspect of the metacarpal heads or in a juxta-articular

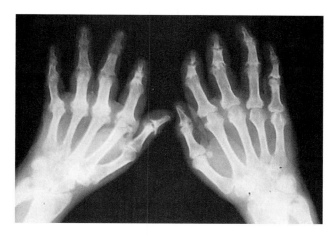

Figure 92 Classical psoriatic arthritis in a 63–year-old female with long-standing psoriasis. Note the erosions, cup-and-pencil deformities and lack of juxta-articular osteopenia.

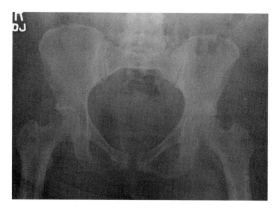

Figure 94 Psoriatic arthritis. Sacroiliitis. Note that the sacroiliitis is asymmetric although bilateral and that there are both erosions and sclerosis.

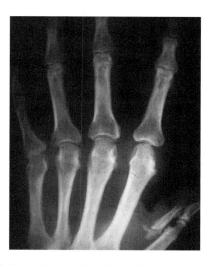

Figure 93 Psoriatic arthritis. Hands. This older lady presented with psoriasis and a remarkable total dislocation of the proximal phalanx of the left thumb with a pseudoarthrosis between the first metacarpal head and the base of the distal phalanx. Note the periosteal reaction and erosive changes as well as the typical "bossing" of many of the other metacarpal heads.

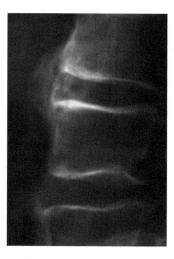

Figure 95 Psoriatic arthritis. Spine with large syndesmophytes in an older man with psoriasis.

position on the phalanges of the hand. However, fluffy perpendicular new bone formation can also occur adjacent to an involved joint, and, more rarely, a peripheral linear periosteal reaction reminiscent of Reiter's syndrome can be seen in the long bones of the hands and feet.

The other hallmarks of psoriatic arthritis are a lack of juxta-articular osteoporosis (although there is one form of the disease where this is not true) and a destructive form of arthritis with more central erosions, similar to those seen in rheumatoid arthritis, for example.

However, all is not this simple: it is widely taught that there are at least five characteristic presentations of psoriatic arthritis.

1. The classical form, with a patchy, asymmetrical, centrally destructive arthritis without juxta-articular osteoporosis, but with new bone formation involving predominantly the interphalangeal joints of the fingers. This is by far the commonest form of psoriatic arthritis (Figs. 94 and 95).
2. The solitary involvement of a large joint, with peripheral and central erosions, but without juxta-articular osteoporosis and with significant new bone formation in a patient with psoriasis. The new bone formation is often the predominant feature of this form of psoriatic arthritis. This can be seen in virtually any joint in the body, but is apparently most often seen in the knee, elbow, wrist, and ankle, and this type of psoriatic arthritis is not uncommon (Fig. 96).
3. Involvement of the whole ray in the hand in what clinically has become known as sausage fingers, with involvement of the metacarpophalangeal and both interphalangeal joints of one finger, with marked soft-tissue swelling, central and marginal erosions, and with marked juxta-articular osteoporosis as a

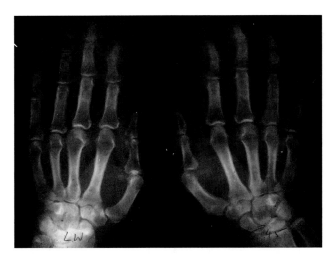

Figure 97 Psoriatic arthritis. Classical appearance in a 45-year-old male patient with bad psoriasis. Note that there is extensive involvement and soft-tissue swelling of the third and fourth rays on the right, typical of sausage fingers. There is discrete periosteal reaction as well as soft tissue swelling. Note the abnormal nail on the right thumb, typical of psoriasis.

result of the profound inflammatory nature of this type of arthritis (Fig. 97). This form of psoriatic arthritis is relatively rare and needs to be distinguished from an acute infection, which it closely resembles.

4. A form of arthritis that resembles rheumatoid arthritis with bilateral, symmetrically destructive changes and juxta-articular osteoporosis, but the patient has psoriasis and is HLA-B27-positive and rheumatoid factor–negative.

    In many rheumatologists' minds, this is what accounts for the so-called seronegative type of rheumatoid arthritis, and this type of psoriatic arthritis is relatively rare.

5. Spinal involvement in patients with psoriatic arthritis is rare, and although both sacroiliitis and syndesmophyte formation have been described, they are also not common. The sacroiliitis is usually predominantly erosive, either bilateral but very asymmetric or unilateral (Fig. 95).

    The syndesmophyte formation is variable and resembles that seen in enteropathic arthritis. Spinal involvement in psoriatic arthritis has been described as occurring, either alone or in association with any of the other forms of arthritis.

    However with advances in modern medicine, we can add two more:

6. There is also a form of psoriatic arthritis in which the characteristic joint changes are seen, particularly with the new bone formation, but in which the patient does

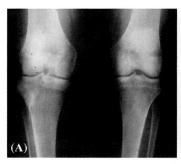 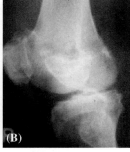

Figure 96 Psoriatic arthritis. This 45-year-old man presented with swelling and decreased range of motion in his right knee. No other joints were involved. (**A**) Standing AP view showing a normal left knee but a right knee with new bone formation and discrete erosions. (**B**) An oblique view confirms the new bone formation and erosions as well as loss of joint cartilage space. This is the typical finding of psoriatic arthritis in a large joint. *Abbreviation*: AP, anteroposterior.

not appear to actually have psoriasis. This is known as apsoriatic psoriatic arthritis, but, if one looks very carefully behind the elbows or ears, for example, discrete flecks of psoriasis can usually be found. In any case, these patients invariably go on to develop psoriasis within the next 10 years or so.

7. Arthritis mutilans is an old self-explanatory term for a very destructive form of peripheral arthritis, which can be either applied to late-stage rheumatoid arthritis or to a peculiarly aggressive form of psoriatic arthritis.

In the former, juxta-articular osteoporosis is characteristic of rheumatoid arthritis, and, in the latter, the lack of juxta-articular osteoporosis is characteristic of psoriatic arthritis. In either case, the use of high-dose steroids and/or chemotherapy will often slow the progression of the disease.

To return to the conventional form of psoriatic arthritis, the erosions are often central and very destructive, leading to a sea gull or gull's-wing appearance in the first place similar to that seen with either erosive osteoarthritis or in association with lupus erythematosus (Fig. 98).

As I said when we discussed erosive osteoarthritis, its etiology is unknown, and so one could perhaps put erosive arthritis into the category of psoriatic arthritis, yet the patients are older, the disease is symmetrical and appears familial, and the patients do not have psoriasis and are HLA-B27-negative. The central erosions in psoriatic arthritis continue to enlarge on one side of the joint with increasing marginal erosions on the other, producing what is known as a cup and pencil deformity. This is not associated with juxta-articular osteoporosis and is very characteristic, if not pathognomonic, of psoriatic arthritis. These deformities occur mainly in the DIP and PIP joints of one finger or another; they are not symmetrical or even

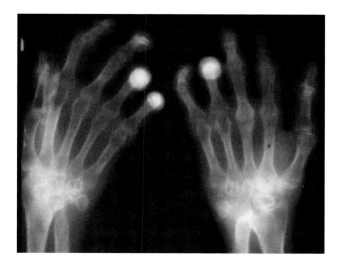

Figure 98 Seagulls.

bilateral, and, once again, the two hallmarks of psoriatic arthritis are the lack of juxta-articular osteoporosis and the presence of new bone formation. Ultimately, this peripheral arthritis will slowly extend to involve the metacarpophalangeal joints and the carpus, again usually unilaterally or bilaterally and asymmetrically. Other joints can also become involved, and, once again, involvement with psoriatic arthritis has been described in virtually every joint in the body, including the temporomandibular joint, atlanto-axial joint, and the facet joints of the spine. In the heel, erosions with new bone formation adjacent to the insertion of the Achilles tendon and the origin of the plantar fascia are quite common and resemble those seen in both Reiter's syndrome and enteropathic arthritis. Psoriatic arthritis is probably the most destructive arthritis that we see today after rheumatoid arthritis, but, again, the hallmark of psoriatic arthritis is the concomitant new bone formation. One final clue to the presence of psoriatic arthritis can be occasionally found on a hand X-ray of a patient with psoriasis. Patients with severe psoriasis also have nail involvement and the nail bed becomes lifted and eroded, and these changes can be seen on the radiograph overlying the tufts of the fingers, particularly the thumbs where this intense inflammatory reaction may actually produce fluffy new bone formation in the underlying phalanx.

Reactive Arthritis

Reactive arthritis is defined as an acute, subacute, or chronic arthritis following an infection elsewhere in the body. Although the term "reactive arthritis" is relatively new, the concept is not.

The pathophysiology is based on infection-producing antibodies, which enter the joint and affect the cartilage either by DNA-specific immune complexes (for example, seen in Yersinia) or actual particles (for example, seen in chlamydia). These complexes or particles release macromolecules which act as antigens in the synovial fluid. In turn, these affect type II collagen fibers, proteoglycans, and cartilage oligomeric matrix proteins (COMP). In most people, the antigens neutralize the antibodies and the process reverses itself with complete recovery. But, in some conditions such as rheumatoid arthritis, for example, the system breaks down, producing severe cartilage damage.

Of the types of reactive arthritis, psoriatic arthritis, Reiter's syndrome, and enteropathic arthritis have already been discussed, and these are obviously the best-known examples of reactive arthritis. These three types of arthritis all have something else in common: about 80% of the patients are HLA B27-positive. The incidence of HLA B27-positive within the normal population is only about 6%. There is a group of rare conditions that are associated with reactive arthritis and these include other interspinal infections, such as Yersinia, campylobacter, and salmonella. Whipple's disease, which is now known to be cased by an organism, Tropheryma whippelii, is also associated with reactive arthritis. There are also a number of unusual conditions, such as pyoderma gangrenosa and multicentric reticular histiocytosis in which both arthritis and skin lesions exist. Another unusual condition that may be related to reactive arthritis is known as chronic recurrent multifocal osteomyelitis (CRMO), which occurs mainly in children and adolescents, often involves the shafts of long bones, and can be associated with palmar/plantar pustulosis. Some of these patients also develop pyoderma gangrenosa, and this condition will be further discussed in the chapter on infection.

The most unusual of the syndromes associated with reactive arthritis is now known by the acronym SAPHO, which stands for synovitis, acne, pustulosis, hyperostosis, and osteitis. This primarily involves the sternoclavicular joint but may involve any of the upper ribs, clavicle, and proximal sternum. There are varieties of this condition, including PAO (which stands for pustulotic arthro-osteitis and is similar but related directly to psoriasis). PPP stands for palmar/plantar pustulosis and is probably the same disease as PAO and involves the same bones. It is considered to be a subtype of psoriatic psoriasis vulgaris. Finally, a similar condition involves the mandible, rather than the sternoclavicular joint, and is known as DSOM, which stands for diffuse sclerosing osteomyelitis of the mandible.

Thus, reactive arthritis is an interesting and complex subject of which the common conditions include psoriatic arthritis, Reiter's syndrome, and enteropathic arthritis. However, there is a large group of conditions in which reactive arthritis can follow an intestinal or generalized infection elsewhere in the body.

THE CRYSTALLINE ARTHROPATHIES

This is a group of three major conditions, with a couple of minor ones, which have little in common, although they are all caused by the abnormal deposition of crystals in or around a joint. They all occur in older patients and are all associated with either chondrocalcinosis or soft-tissue calcification. Before we begin, we should be reminded of the causes of chondrocalcinosis (Table 3).

Gout

Everyone is aware of the picture of Henry VIII with his leg up in the air and his foot heavily bandaged with clean, white bandages; at least it was in Charles Laughton's portrayal of the wily monarch. Gout occurs as a primary

Table 3 Causes of Chondrocalcinosis

1. Common causes
• CPPD
• Renal failure (secondary hyperparathyroidism)
2. Uncommon causes
• Gout
• Primary hyperparathyroidism
• Hemochromatosis
• Acromegaly
3. Extremely rare causes
• Wilson's disease
• Ochronosis

Abbreviation: CPPD, calcium pyrophosphate disease.

condition, which is familial and caused by an inherited enzyme defect. This is mainly seen in male patients older than 40. However, there are actually a number of enzymic defects, which can lead to primary gout, so that it is really not one condition. Absence or defects in glucose 6 phosphatase, glutathione reductase, and glutamine ribose amido transferase, for example, all can lead to gout. Perhaps secondary gout is nearly as common today as the primary condition, and this is seen in patients with either rapid breakdown of tissue such as aggressive cancer, lymphoma or leukemia, or in patients with various renal problems such as renal tubular acidosis and renal failure. Secondary gout has also been described in polycythemia, myelofibrosis, glycogen storage disease, for example. Uric acid is a byproduct of the oxidation of xanthine, which eventually breaks down to form allantoin, which is secreted by the kidneys. If too much uric acid is produced, the kidneys are unable to handle the extra uric acid, and it gets deposited in the tissues as sodium monohydrate monourate. The tissues usually involved are of the joints, the kidneys, and the heart. In the joints, crystals are deposited in the synovium, where they enter the synovial fluid, producing an acute inflammatory reaction with marginal erosions in the first instance. Incidentally, the crystals of urate are birefringent, which makes them unique among the crystals that cause arthritis. Outside the joints, urate deposits produce tophi, which are localized collections of crystals that occur in soft tissues, muscles, cartilage, bursae, synovium, ligaments, and tendons. Gout usually affects males older than 40, although 10% of the cases are female, and it has been rarely described also in children, almost always as a result of a major enzymic abnormality. Primary and secondary gout are indistinguishable on radiographical features alone.

Clinically, gout produces a red-hot, exquisitely tender, swollen joint. Although the first metatarsophalangeal joint is classically the first joint involved, gout may involve virtually any joint in the body, including those of the

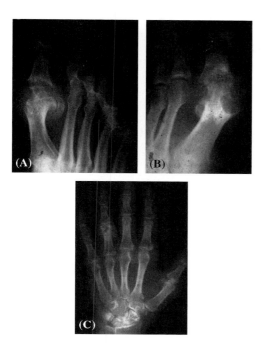

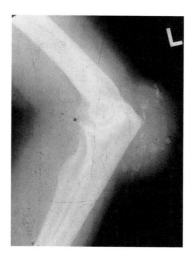

Figure 100 Gout. A large soft-tissue tophus in the olecranon bursa with internal calcifications. The bones appear intact.

Figure 99 Gout. (**A**) The foot in a 50-year-old male patient with familial gout shows typical destructive changes in the first metatarsophalangeal joint with erosions, overhanging edges, and a soft-tissue typhus. Note the similar changes in the fifth metatarsophalangeal joint. (**B**) The first metatarsophalangeal joint in another patient with typical changes of severe gout, overhanging edges, erosions, and loss of articular cartilage. (**C**) The hand in the same patient showing punched out erosions in the carpal bones and typical gouty changes in the fourth proximal phalangeal joint.

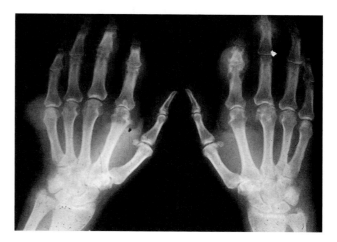

Figure 101 Gout. Soft tissue and bony erosive disease. Note the many soft-tissue tophi, which are somewhat denser than normal soft tissue. There are also typical gouty changes in many of the interphalangeal joints.

hands, wrists, knees, and elbows, as well as such unusual joints as the sacroiliac joints, atlantoaxial joints, and facet joints in the spine. Radiographically, the hallmark of gout is marginal erosions with overhanging edges and new bone formation with buttressing, but without juxta-articular osteoporosis (Fig. 99).

Initially the erosions are at the synovial insertions into the margins of the bone, but eventually the destruction will spread into the hyaline cartilage itself, and cause narrowing of the joint space. The synovial erosions can also undermine the subchondral bone, which will also cause bone destruction, but, once again, this is a relatively late finding. Overhanging edges are said to be pathognomonic of gout and occur because of the acute inflammatory nature of the condition—with bone destruction occurring centrally and new bone formation occurring peripherally, giving rise to these spurs, hooks, or curved points of bones, which are known as "overhanging edges."

Soft-tissue tophi can occur anywhere, but are commonest in the soft tissues of the hands and in the olecranal bursa of the elbow, for example (Fig. 100).

Tophi represent localized deposition of urate crystals, and they are usually very tender and inflamed. Radiographically, they appear denser than the surrounding soft tissues and are often fairly sharply demarcated from them. However, many tophi elicit a response in the underlying bone, producing spurs or even periosteal new bone formation (Fig. 101).

Interosseous tophi also occur, and these represent either gouty ganglion cysts or may be an extension of the inflammatory reaction from the synovial insertion into the bone (Fig. 102).

Osseous tophi may also be seen almost anywhere, but one of the most common sites is in the carpal bones and in

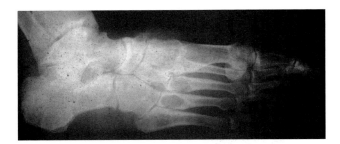

Figure 102 Gout. Punched out intraosseous gouty tophi away from the joint at the base of the third, fourth, and fifth metatarsals.

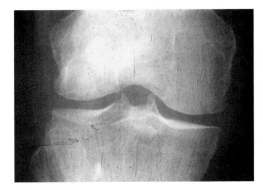

Figure 104 Gout. Chondrocalcinosis in the knee. This is the same patient as shown in Figure 100.

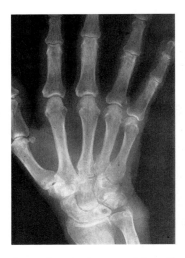

Figure 103 Gout. Carpal changes with well circumscribed lucent areas in many of the carpal bones, a soft-tissue tophus over the ulnar styloid and chondrocalcinosis.

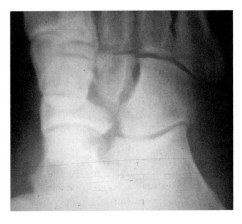

Figure 105 Gout in the foot of a young black male. The diagnosis was made by aspiration. The differential diagnosis would include any of the inflammatory arthritides including infections.

the metatarsals. They appear as central, rounded, "punched-out" lucent lesions, usually with well-defined sclerotic margins, and are indistinguishable from ganglion cysts seen in other conditions (Fig. 103).

However, the differential diagnosis of gout from other forms of arthritis is usually straightforward, with the presence of overhanging edges and soft-tissue tophi and the lack of juxta-articular osteoporosis. However, the presence of intraosseous cysts or tophi away from the joint is a useful radiographical sign to differentiate gout from other conditions. Chondrocalcinosis is commonly seen in association with secondary gout but only rarely in occurs primary gout (Fig. 104).

Clinically, the patient will characteristically have repeated attacks of acute arthritis involving the first metatarsophalangeal joint and other small peripheral joints. The affected joint is exquisitely painful, swollen, and red, and without treatment, the condition subsides

within six to eight weeks, only to recur again and again, leading to a progressive destruction of the affected joint. If not treated, the patient will form uric acid stones and eventually go into renal failure. Cardiac involvement also occurs, and the patient will often go into congestive cardiac failure. However, nowadays, preventive treatment is widely available and the acute attacks can be managed by large doses of specific anti-inflammatory drugs.

Finally, a rarely seen form of gout may occasionally occur in the black population in whom primary gout is rare. It presents as an acute inflammatory arthritis, with both the clinical and radiological picture resembling an acute septic arthritis. Often a joint aspiration or an actual synovial biopsy is the only way to differentiate between these two conditions. The finding of uric acid crystals in such a joint makes the diagnosis of gout easy (Fig. 105).

Calcium Pyrophosphate Deposition Disease (CPPD)

This is the commonest of the crystalline arthropathies and, in its asymptomatic form, involves perhaps 5% of the population older than 50. However, it is a relatively new diagnosis, and if you try to look it up in books over 20-years old, you will not find it under this heading. It was originally known as "pseudogout," and this presentation describes the nature of the condition: it presented like gout, although it primarily involved large joints, was bilateral and symmetrical, and the crystals were weakly birefringent. CPPD is caused by the deposition of calcium pyrophosphate crystals into joints, where they can remain quiescent for years or produce an acute synovitis. There is also a more chronic recurrent form of the condition. Calcium pyrophosphate is a normal constituent of the plasma and soft tissues and, in most people, gets broken down to orthophosphate and excreted. However, it appears that in some older patients this does not occur and hence an excess of calcium pyrophosphate gets laid down, particularly in the cartilage, where it causes chondrocalcinosis (Fig. 106).

As an aside, in virtually every disease or condition where chondrocalcinosis occurs, calcium pyrophosphate crystals are found, so some authors considered that there are two forms of CPPD; the primary form, which is of unknown etiology, and the secondary form, which can be associated with such conditions as renal failure, diabetes, osteoarthritis, and even gout.

The hallmark of CPPD is chondrocalcinosis, and this can be seen in both fibrocartilage (triangular fibrocartilage in the wrist, in the symphysis pubis, and in the menisci of

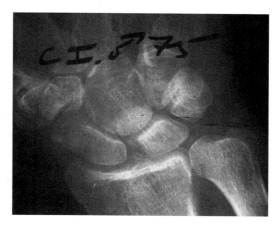

Figure 107 CPPD. Chondrocalcinosis in both the triangular fibrocartilage and the scapholunate joint in this 75-year-old male. *Abbreviation*: CPPD, calcium pyrophosphate disease.

the knee, for example) and in hyaline cartilage (in the knee, shoulder, and hips, for example) (Fig. 107).

However, once the chondrocalcinosis becomes widespread, it can be seen in every joint and has even been described in the temporomandibular joints. The condition is classically asymptomatic, but, when it presents clinically, it is usually bilateral, fairly symmetrical, and in patients older than 60 (with an approximate equal sex incidence), and classically involves the knee and the wrist (Fig. 108).

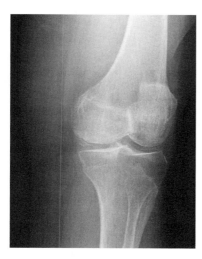

Figure 106 CPPD. Chondrocalcinosis seen in the knee: Note that it involves both the hyaline cartilage and the fibrocartilage (menisci). *Abbreviation*: CPPD, calcium pyrophosphate disease.

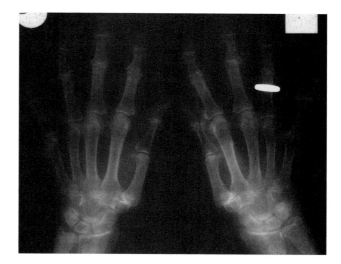

Figure 108 CPPD. Classical findings in both hands and wrists, including chondrocalcinosis in the triangular fibrocartilage and secondary degenerative changes in the radial aspect of both wrists. Note that the patient also has erosive arthritis in the proximal interphalangeal and distal interphalangeal joints. The two conditions are not related. *Abbreviation*: CPPD, calcium pyrophosphate disease.

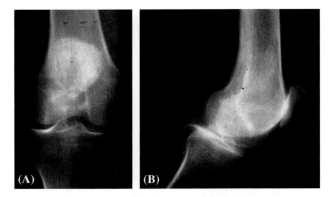

Figure 109 (**A, B**) CPPD. Knee: Note the chondrocalcinosis and the marked narrowing of the patellofemoral joint, which has lost all its articular cartilage. This is pathognomic of CPPD.

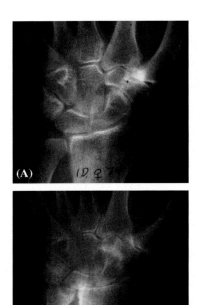

Figure 110 (**A, B**) CPPD. Both hands in a 74-year-old female patient with typical bilateral changes in the wrists including chondrocalcinosis and degenerative changes involving the radio-carpal joint, triscaphe joint, and first carpometacarpal joint. Note that the right hand is more advanced with subluxation of the lunate and worse degenerative changes. *Abbreviation*: CPPD, calcium pyrophosphate disease.

The diagnosis of CPPD depends on its involving unusual joints such as the patellofemoral joint in the knee and the radiocarpal joint in the wrist; there is also an absence of hypertrophic spur formation and an absence of juxta-articular osteoporosis. In the initial phases of the disease, there is also no joint-space narrowing. In the knee, chondrocalcinosis is obvious in the medial and lateral compartments, but the patellofemoral joint becomes markedly narrowed and painful (Fig. 109) in the wrist. Chondrocalcinosis can be seen in the triangular fibrocartilage, and there is narrowing of the radioscaphoid joint, which progresses to involve other carpal joints. Brower has pointed out that CPPD in the wrist progresses in a "stepladder"-type way involving first, the radiosca-phoid joint, next the lunatecapite joint, next the triscaphe joint, and finally the first carpometacarpal joint. With the joint space narrowing occurring, the lunate slides in an ulnar direction off its radial fossa, producing a radio-graphical subluxation (Fig. 110).

In the acute phase, this can be associated with erosions because CPPD can also produce an inflammatory type of arthritis. The differential diagnosis between CPPD and gout in the hands depends on the finding of chondrocalcinosis in the former and overhanging edges and intraosseous cysts in the latter. The differential diagnosis between CPPD and a chronic infection is the presence of calcification in the triangular fibrocartilage in the former and juxta-articular osteopenia and erosions in the latter. CPPD can involve other joints, although it is not usually as destructive as it is in the wrist and knee. Often, chondrocalcinosis is the only radiological sign, although the patient may have presented clinically with pseudogout (Fig. 111).

In the old days, people blamed CPPD as the cause of calcific bursitis and calcific tendinitis. However, it has been shown recently that, although the calcium pyrophos-phate crystal is present in these conditions, the underlying crystal responsible is the hydroxyapatite crystal.

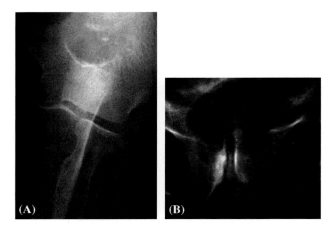

Figure 111 CPPD chondrocalcinosis elsewhere. (**A**) Elbow. This is the same patient as shown in Figure 107. (**B**) Symphysis pubis. This is the same patient as shown in Figure 107.

Hydroxyapatite Disease (HADD)

Here is yet another newly described condition; yet it really is not. Everyone has heard of calcific bursitis and calcific tendinitis, and for a long time the underlying cause of

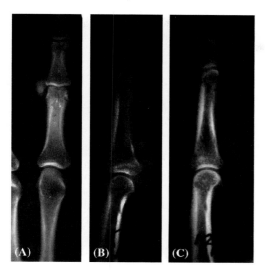

Figure 112 Calcific tendonitis adjacent to a PIP joint in a young 37-year-old anesthesiologist. (**A**) The initial film was taken in January 1993. (**B**) Film taken in May 1993. (**C**) Film taken in December of the same year, showing the slow progression from dense calcifications to a more indistinct appearance to a "toothpaste" appearance. *Abbreviation*: PIP, proximal interphalangeal.

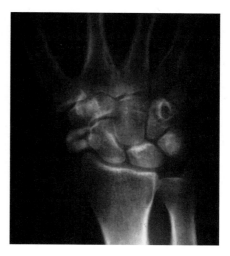

Figure 113 Calcific tendonitis in the wrist of another patient. The dense calcifications adjacent to the scaphoid styloid suggests that this is chronic.

these two conditions was thought to be the calcium pyrophosphate crystals. However, that is not so. Hydroxyapatite is an essential component of bone, ligaments, synovium, and tendons. If a tendon becomes torn, hydroxyapatite crystals get released and, in normal people, actually help with the healing process. In fact, hydroxyapatite is used as a "glue" for porous coated joint prostheses, where it is actually sprayed onto the outside of the prosthesis to aid in fusion between it and the underlying bone. And yet, no one fully understands what goes wrong in some people; when the tendon tears, blood and hydroxyapatite get deposited into the joint space and, in some people, apparently an inflammatory response ensues, which leads to calcification (and the presence of calcium pyrophosphate crystals, incidentally). This process is usually painful and is clinically known as calcific tendonitis (Fig. 112).

Classically, this condition is seen in the shoulder (rotator cuff tendon), elbow (biceps, brachio-radialis, or triceps tendon), heel (Achilles tendon), and wrist (various tendons), although it may occur anywhere in the body. Similarly, calcific bursitis probably also recurs as a result of trauma or minor inflammation. In most of us, this settles down with anti-inflammatory drug therapy. However, in some patients, the process becomes chronic, with the presence of hydroxyapatite crystals leading to further inflammation and ultimately calcification (Fig. 113). (Once again, calcium pyrophosphate crystals will also be found in the bursa.). The commonest site for calcific bursitis is the shoulder (subdeltoid bursa), but this has also

been seen virtually everywhere in the body. In a unique but similar situation, posttraumatic changes in a joint capsule can cause calcification in the lining of the joint, and this is best seen in the interphalangeal joints of the fingers (or toes) where it rejoices in the old name of "peritendonitis calcarea." Resnick has alerted us to the situation of chronic tendonitis or, more properly, tendonosis, in which the laying down of calcification is more likely to occur than an acute tendonitis. In some experimental studies, it has been shown that there are a number of stages of hydroxyapatite deposition: (1) the acute tear of a ligament, (2) an inflammatory response, (3) laying down of dense calcification, (4) dilution of the calcification with serous fluid producing an appearance like toothpaste, (5) resorption of the calcification, (6) and healing. In experimental animals, this process takes four to eight weeks; in man, a similar process appears to take four to eight months (Fig. 113).

Four elderly women in Milwaukee developed an acute destructive arthropathy in their shoulders in which the causative crystal was found to be hydroxyapatite. All the patients had severe rotator cuff tears, which were probably acute and resulted in the release of hydroxyapatite crystals directly into the joints. This disease became known as "Milwaukee shoulder" (Fig. 114).

Presumably, the immune system in these patients was unable to cope with the added insult of hydroxyapatite crystals and, hence, the destructive nature of the arthritis. In the vast majority of patients with torn rotator cuffs, no such arthritis occurred, even in elderly patients with severe, acute tears. A further 11 patients with the same condition, which was found to be often bilateral, were later described. Although occurring mainly in elderly women, it does occur in elderly men. Since that description, we have all seen the

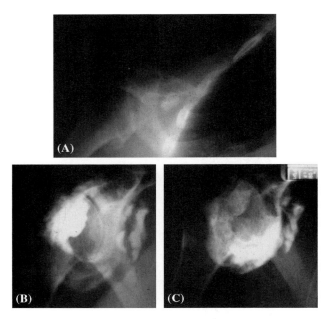

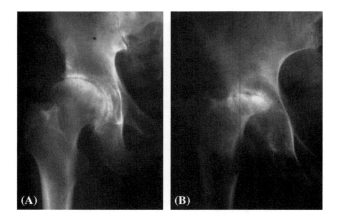

Figure 114 Hydroxyapatite disease. (**A**) The initial plain film shows widespread destruction of the glenohumeral joint as well as the acromioclavicular joint. (**B, C**) Two films taken from an arthrogram showing multiple loose bodies, capacious joint capsule, and destruction of much of the anatomy typical of a "Milwaukee Shoulder."

Figure 115 HADD in an elderly patient complaining of hip discomfort. (**A**) The initial film shows early degenerative changes in a patient with coxa magna, possibly secondary to previous slipped capital femoral epiphysis. (**B**) Three months later there has been extensive destruction of the femoral head and neck. This has the appearance of a Charcot joint except that it was extremely painful. *Abbreviation*: HADD, hydroxyapatite disease.

disease, and, although it primarily involves the shoulder, it can also occur in the hip, knee, and elbow, where a rapidly destructive arthritis occurs following trauma in elderly patients (Figs. 115 and 116).

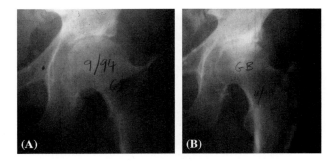

Figure 116 HADD. Similar changes in another elderly male patient. (**A**) September of 1994. (**B**) November of 1994, showing the rapid destruction of the femoral head secondary to HADD crystals. *Abbreviation*: HADD, hydroxyapatite disease.

On aspiration in these patients, both hydroxyapatite and calcium pyrophosphate crystals can be found, although there was no evidence of either infection or of urate crystals. Thus, we believe that an acute and rapidly destructive arthritis caused by hydroxyapatite crystals genuinely exists.

Ochronosis

Unfortunately, every medical student learns about this extremely rare, familial condition, which occurs as a result of a defect in the enzyme homogentisic acid oxidase, which is important in the metabolic oxidation of phenylalanine. Patients without this enzyme develop pigmentation of their skin, chondrocalcinosis, and the characteristic finding of urine, which blackens on exposure to air. The urine takes eight hours to oxidize and turn black; this finding was described in Victorian England, where people who had to urinate at night did so in a chamber pot, which was placed under the bed. The next morning the urine had turned black.

Radiographically, the vertebral discs start calcifying, usually in the 20s, starting in the thoracolumbar region but eventually spreading throughout the spine. Ultimately, this leads to disc degeneration, narrowing, and collapse, and to severe spondylosis (Fig. 117).

In the peripheral joints, although the damage is less severe, chondrocalcinosis and premature degenerative arthritis will occur. The most commonly involved peripheral joints are the larger ones, such as the shoulders, hips, and knees. However, the vertebral disc calcification is the most characteristic finding in ochronosis.

Wilson's Disease

This is the other rarely seen crystalline arthropathy, and is due to an enzyme defect which produces a build-up of copper in the patient with a characteristically green

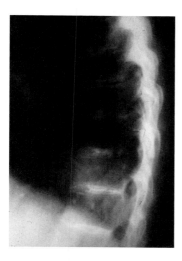

Figure 117 Ochronosis showing the dense white calcifications in all the discs in this 24-year-old man. *Abbreviation*: HADD, hydroxyapatite disease.

Kaiser-Fleischer ring, which is seen in the eye. Copper also gets deposited in the articular cartilage of the joints and tends to present as chondrocalcinosis, although, more commonly, Wilson's disease will present as premature degenerative arthritis in the hips and knees. The disease is progressive, and the patients often go into intractable renal failure and die.

SUMMARY

Gout is the best-described condition of the crystalline arthropathies, and has a typical clinical course with characteristic radiographical changes. CPPD is also fairly well understood, and calcium pyrophosphate arthritis is now better defined, although why some patients with chondrocalcinosis never go onto develop the clinical picture of pseudogout is not understood. Similarly, hydroxyapatite disease is a rare form of crystalline arthropathy, yet calcific tendinitis and bursitis are common and rarely lead to any form of arthritis in the majority of patients. Again, this is not fully understood. But, as you can see, taken together as a group of conditions and with different presentations, the crystalline arthropathies are not uncommon.

3

Musculoskeletal Infection

MUSCULOSKELETAL INFECTIONS

Virtually any part of the musculoskeletal system can get an infection, from the soft tissues to the bone (where it is known as osteomyelitis) to the joints (septic arthritis) to the spine (disc infection). Although the pathophysiology and, to some extent, the radiographic appearances are similar, the effect of an infection is different in each of these places. Initially an inflammation will occur, which will either be taken care of by the body's defense system or will worsen, often leading to a more chronic phase with abscess formation. Clinically, the patient will have pain, swelling, and fatigue, as well as redness if the infection is superficial. The old Latin terms were "color," "rubor," "tumor," and "dolor," and these refer to the clinical findings. Unfortunately, much of the musculoskeletal system is deep to the subcutaneous tissues, and hence, the pain may often be of a dull, gnawing variety, the swelling and redness do not occur, and, apart from a somewhat elevated white blood count and sedimentation rate, there are few clinical findings with infected disc spaces or the larger joints, such as the hip and sacroiliac joints, for example, which makes the diagnosis difficult. Plain films are often not useful in the initial stages of infection; nuclear scanning techniques, particularly those using indium-111-labeled white cell counts, are useful but expensive. CT scanning is not very useful. On the other hand, magnetic resonance imaging (MRI) is both sensitive and specific, so it can be extremely useful in both the diagnosis of early and the confirmation of late infection. Finally, ultrasound is also useful in the diagnosis of early

superficial infection, often outlining the pus or the abscess clearly.

Soft-Tissue Infections

With the exception of the findings in diabetic foot infections, which are discussed separately at the end of the chapter, there is little written about the radiological features of soft-tissue infections. As mentioned above, ultrasound is useful in determining if an actual abscess is present in superficial infections (Fig. 1A, B).

Nuclear medicine studies can be useful, although occasionally an abscess may appear "cold" rather than "hot," and, in any case, radionuclide studies, although sensitive, are not very specific (Fig. 2A, B).

Both CT scans and MRI will be able to show soft-tissue abscesses, particularly in the deep soft tissues such as the psoas muscle or the glutei. The magnetic resonance (MR) appearances are of a "target" lesion seen on both T1-weighted and fat saturation T1-weighted images. On the T1 image, the pus is dark, and this is surrounded by a ring of granulation tissue, which is slightly higher in intensity and has recently been described as a "penumbra" sign (Fig. 3A, B).

This is, in turn, surrounded by an area of generalized inflammation, which is also of low signal on the T1. On the fat-saturated T1 images, this is reversed, producing a "target" appearance, with the high-intensity pus surrounded by a ring of lower-intensity granulation tissue, surrounded, in turn, by an area of inflammation, which is also of high signal (Fig. 3C, D).

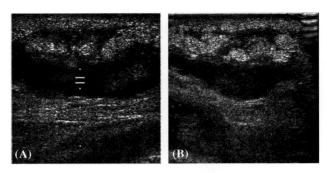

Figure 1 (**A, B**) Two ultrasound images that show the extent of a subcutaneous abscess in the upper arm.

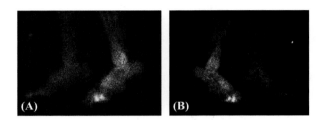

Figure 2 (**A, B**) Two delayed bone scans taken of the feet to show increased uptake involving the fourth metatarsophalangeal joint. This is typical of infection.

CT scanning is not as sensitive or as specific as MRI, but once the area of inflammation and the abscess has been identified, a CT-guided needle biopsy will confirm the diagnosis and allow the antibiotic sensitivity of the organism to be determined.

Osteomyelitis

Classically, osteomyelitis is subdivided into acute, subacute, and chronic, although it is often difficult to make this distinction in an individual patient. For instance, are Brodie's abscesses examples of subacute or chronic osteomyelitis? Once we have diagnosed septic arthritis, which is usually later rather than early, is this acute or subacute? On the other hand, the diagnosis of acute osteomyelitis can usually be substantiated following a blow or an open injury to a body part, with osteomyelitis occurring within 10 to 14 days.

Acute osteomyelitis

In the old days, acute osteomyelitis classically occurred 10 to 14 days after open or closed trauma to the metaphyseal region of a long bone. Classically, the radiographic appearances are of soft-tissue swelling at 5 days, loss of the fat planes at 10 days, and early periosteal reaction at 10 to 14 days, with patchy destruction of cancellous bone occurring shortly after (Fig. 4A, B).

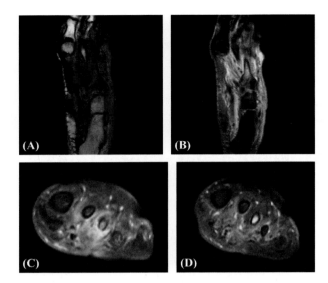

Figure 3 (**A**) MRI of a foot infection. Four slices taken from different sequences. Note the bone marrow signal of the base of the third metatarsal is abnormally dark on this coronal proton density sequence. (**B**) Note that the signal is now higher than the surrounding bone marrow signal on this fat-saturated T1 sequence typical of active osteomyelitis. (**C**) The axial slice shows the typical "penumbra" or target sign surrounding the shaft of the third metatarsal in this T1 fat-saturated sequence. (**D**) Following use of contrast, the bone marrow signal in the third metatarsal lights up considerably, which is typical of active osteomyelitis.

In fact, this is probably true today, although many cases of acute osteomyelitis are diagnosed by Technetium-99m (Tc99m) bone scans at about seven days before any radiological signs become apparent.

About 95% of all cases of acute osteomyelitis are caused by *Staphylococcus aureus,* although this percentage drops to about 70% to 75% in drug addicts or in people who are severely immunologically compromised. About 95% of all cases of acute osteomyelitis occur in the metaphysis and are more commonly seen in the distal femur and distal tibia and fibula in patients with hematogenous spread, but are quite common in the small bones of the hand and feet in patients who have direct spread from an open injury. The reason why many cases of primary hematogenous osteomyelitis are metaphyseal is said to be that there is an end capillary network that occurs in the metaphysis, with loops between the arterioles and venules that do not penetrate the growth plate, which has its own blood supply, but rather turn back on themselves. This produces sluggish flow, and if a patient sustains minor trauma to this region while having a bacteremia, the blood may sludge and pus will accumulate in this rich capillary bed (Fig. 5).

The bacteremia may be due to a minor chest or skin infection or a recent visit to the dentist. Hence, it is the metaphyseal site for many cases of acute osteomyelitis.

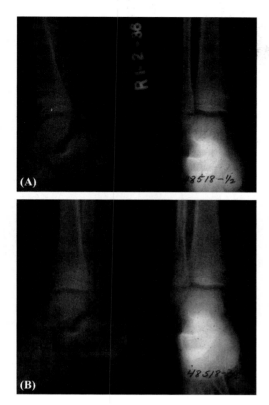

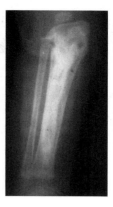

Figure 6 Typical chronic osteomyelitis with sequestrum as well as an involucrum.

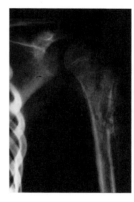

Figure 7 Subacute osteomyelitis showing patchy destruction of the proximal humeral metaphysis, a sequestrum and a lucuna.

Figure 4 (**A**) Classical early osteomyelitis seen in the year that sulphonamides were introduced. Initial film shows soft tissue swelling over the distal fibula without bony involvement. (**B**) Two weeks later there is patchy destruction of both cortical and trabecular bone in the distal fibular metaphysis.

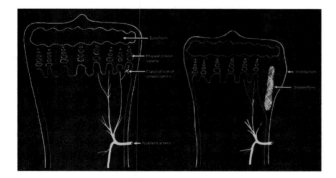

Figure 5 Drawing to explain the pathogenesis of early osteomyelitis.

Plain films should be taken in all cases of suspected acute osteomyelitis, but a Tc99m bone scan needs to be performed regardless of plain film findings. CT and MRI are of no use in this situation, and ultrasound will only be of limited use, possibly picking up periosteal elevation before it is visible radiologically. Once the diagnosis has been made, the patient is put on the appropriate antibiotic, usually parenterally at first, and the infection will heal. However, for a number of reasons, this may fail, leading to a situation known as chronic osteomyelitis.

Chronic osteomyelitis

Chronic osteomyelitis occurs because either treatment of an acute osteomyelitis failed or the infection was missed in the first place. Radiographically, the periosteal reaction becomes larger and more intense, and wraps around the area that is infected. This has an old Latin term "involucrum." The underlying bone becomes increasingly destroyed by the infection, and an abscess forms, often surrounding dead trabeculae and bone spicules. The dead bone floating in this abscess is known as a "sequestrum," which is from an old English term "to be secluded." Both the involucrum and sequestrum are obvious on plain films (Figs. 6 and 7).

Ultrasound and Tc99m scans are of no use now; however, CT does have a limited use in looking for sequestra (Fig. 8A, B).

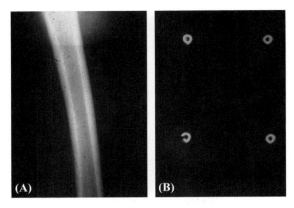

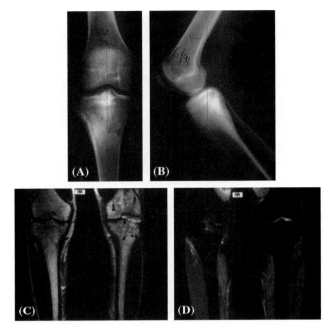

Figure 8 (**A**) Osteomyelitis of the midshaft of the femur following a fall out of the stirrups during childbirth. Plain film shows a discrete periosteal reaction running laterally in the midshaft of the right femur. (**B**) Four consecutive CT slices show the presence of a sequestrum in the intramedullary canal and a lucuna laterally in the right femur.

Figure 10 (**A, B**) Chronic osteomyelitis: Plain film showing increase sclerosis in the proximal tibia with some discrete lucency. (**C**) Coronal PD sequences showing the abnormal marrow signal in the proximal tibia. (**D**) Coronal fat saturation sequences showing the abnormal high signal in the soft tissues in the fat suppressed images.

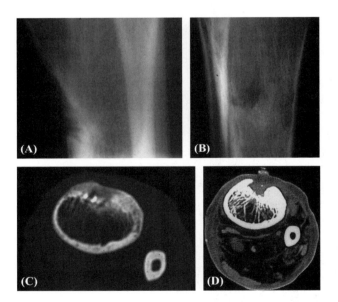

Figure 9 (**A**) Lateral film (**B**) AP film of a proximal tibia in a young patient three weeks after a puncture wound in the same area. (**C, D**) CT slices showing the chronic appearance of the defect in the proximal tibia with soft tissue swelling, discrete calcifications, and the "proud flesh" typical of an acute on chronic osteomyelitis.

It is conventional wisdom, borne out by clinical experience, that it is necessary to remove any sequestra before you can eradicate the infection, and CT is very useful in this search (Fig. 9A–D).

MRI is of little use in this situation, apart from identifying the site and the size of the abscess (Fig. 10A–D).

As the chronic osteomyelitis goes untreated or unmanaged, the pus that is walled off by the involucrum will need to escape, and a hole (or lacuna) will be eroded through the cortex, often below the area of obvious infection, and a chronic sinus tract to the outside world will be produced (Fig. 11).

At this stage, we have an imaging dilemma: how can we diagnose an acute flare-up of osteomyelitis on the background of chronic disease. Ultrasound, CT, and Tc99m scans are useless, and MRI has only limited use. However, the advent of both gallium scanning and, more particularly today, of indium-111-labeled white cell scanning is very useful in identifying an acute osteomyelitis on a background of chronic osteomyelitis.

Complications of chronic osteomyelitis. There are three complications of chronic osteomyelitis, and one, that is, the occurrence of acute osteomyelitis within the area of chronic disease, has been discussed above and is undoubtedly most common. The second complication is the appearance of amyloidosis as the result of chronic inflammation. Remember that amyloidosis also occurs in patients with long-standing rheumatoid arthritis and in patients who have been on renal dialysis for over 10 years. Amyloidosis in patients with chronic osteomyelitis is usually visceral, involving the kidneys, heart, and liver rather than the musculoskeletal system. The third

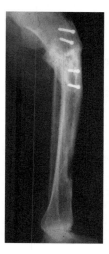

Figure 11 Chronic osteomyelitis in the proximal tibia in a patient following a wound sustained in the Korean War. Note the lacuna in the anterior/distal tibia and the chronic osteomyelitis in the proximal tibia.

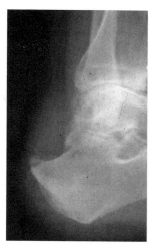

Figure 12 Squamous cell carcinoma in the same patient as Figure 13. The radiograph was taken approximately 14 years later and shows a soft tissue mass behind the ankle joint, which proved to be a squamous cell carcinoma.

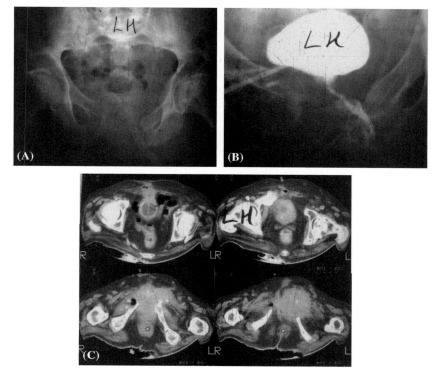

Figure 13 (**A**) Plain film, cystogram, and CT scan in a patient who is paralyzed and has bedsores with chronic osteomyelitis in the left ischium. Eight years after the original injury, a mass was discovered and the patient developed a fistula from the bladder to the skin. (**B**) A cystogram showing a fistula from the bladder to the skin. (**C**) A CT scan shows a large mass destroying the anterior part of the left ischium. This also proved to be a squamous cell carcinoma.

complication is the formation of squamous cell carcinomas in or close to the sinus tract as a result of the chronic inflammation (Fig. 12).

These are often clearly seen by the clinician and appear as a superficial mass of increasing redness and swelling adjacent to the drainage of the chronic infection (Fig. 13A–C).

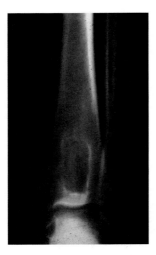

Figure 14 Typical Brodie's abscess with a well-marginated lucency lying on the growth plate of the distal tibia. This is an example of a more chronic abscess.

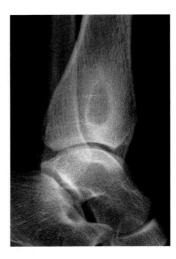

Figure 15 Typical Brodie's abscess in its more acute form with poorly defined margins and sclerosis but also lying on the growth plate of the distal tibia.

They usually occur 15 to 20 years after the chronic osteomyelitis was first diagnosed, and necessitate amputation. Many of these patients have passed away already since this situation was often seen as a result of war injuries suffered in France, Germany, and Korea, for example.

Brodie's Abscess

In 1832, Sir Benjamin Brodie described a case of primary subacute pyogenic osteomyelitis in a 24-year-old man who was treated by amputation since Brodie, who was a surgeon at St. George's Hospital in London, thought that the patient had a tumor. His original description still stands today, although he did not have the benefit of X rays. The patients with Brodie's abscesses are usually adolescent, invariably healthy, and the organism is a non-virulent *Staphylococcus* in over 99% of patients. Brodie's abscesses also occur often as a result of a mild bacteremia caused, for example, by a recent visit to a dentist and possibly following minor trauma. The patient will present with a mild, aching pain, but rarely with the signs and symptoms of an abscess. Radiologically, Brodie's abscesses are fairly characteristic: a centrally placed lucency lying adjacent to the growth plate, with well-defined, sclerotic margins, usually in the distal tibia (in approximately 90% of cases) (Figs. 14, 15, and 16A–F).

The differential diagnosis of a Brodie's abscess would include aneurysmal bone cyst, which lies away from the growth plate and is eccentric not central; giant-cell tumor, which would either grow through the growth plate or lie adjacent to it, but again be eccentric and not central; and a nonossifying fibroma, which could be more central but

would migrate away from the growth plate as the bone grows.

In younger children, the abscess may occur away from the growth plate, in which case a serpiginous tract can be seen going down to the growth plate from the abscess. Sometimes the margins are more irregular and poorly defined, and the Brodie's abscess does indeed look more like a chronic abscess (Fig. 17).

Occasionally, a Brodie's abscess can be seen as a sequel in a patient with chronic osteomyelitis in the diaphysis of the long bone, and then the Brodie's abscess will occur in the distal metaphysis, particularly if this occurs in the tibia (Fig. 18).

The plain film findings are characteristic; however, MRI is able to demonstrate the abscess clearly and will also show the serpiginous tract, if present (Fig. 16A).

Two MRI signs have already been described in association with bone abscesses: the "double ring," the "target," or the "bull's-eye" sign, which occurs on fat-saturated T1 images, with the central pus being of high signal, an outer layer of granulation tissue being darker, and the outermost bone reaction being of high signal once again (Fig. 16F).

A recent article has now described the appearance seen on a T1 image as the "penumbra" sign, where the pus is dark, the granulation tissue has a high signal, and the circumferential outer bony reaction is also of low signal (Fig. 19A, B).

Incidentally, both of these appearances can be seen in association with abscesses elsewhere in the body. The treatment of Brodie's abscess is antibiotics, usually intravenous at first and then oral, as well as curettage of the actual abscess.

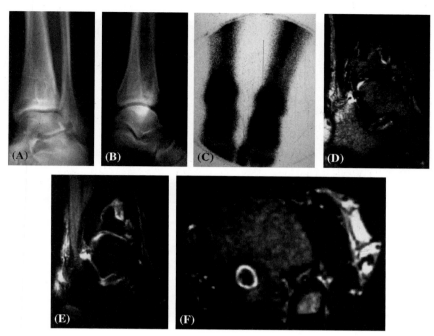

Figure 16 (**A, B**) Plain films. Brodie's abscess in the distal tibia showing the typical appearance. (**C**) Bone scan showing nonspecific increase uptake in the left distal tibia. (**D, E**) Sagittal image MRI showing the characteristic "bull's-eye" lesion with a sinus tract running down into the ankle joint as well as a joint effusion. (**F**) Axial image MRI showing the characteristic "bull's-eye" lesion in the distal tibia.

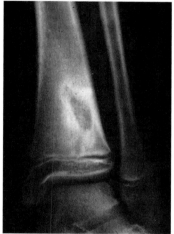

Figure 17 Brodie's abscess. This younger patient shows the characteristic sinus tract apparently running between the abscess in the metaphysis and the growth plate.

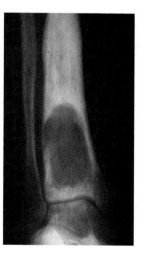

Figure 18 Chronic Brodie's abscess occurring in a distal tibia probably as a result of chronic osteomyelitis in the distal metaphysis.

Primary Epiphyseal Abscess

Although much rarer than a metaphyseal lesion, a Brodie's abscess can occur within the epiphysis. It has an appearance similar to a Brodie's abscess in its more usual location. In the original article on the subject, Green et al. (1) described eight children aged two to four who presented with pain and limp and who had well-defined lytic area in the epiphysis. The radiographic appearances are usually characteristic with a well-defined lucency within the epiphysis (Fig. 20). A bone scan often confirms the diagnosis of infection (Fig. 21); an MRI can also be useful (Fig. 22A, B).

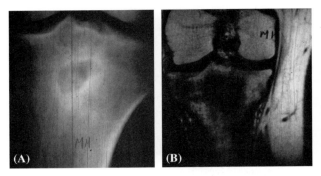

Figure 19 (**A**) A chronic abscess crossing the growth plate in a 21-year-old woman. The plain film shows a relatively well-defined lucency with some surrounding reaction. (**B**) A coronal MRI showing a typical "bull's-eye" or target appearance.

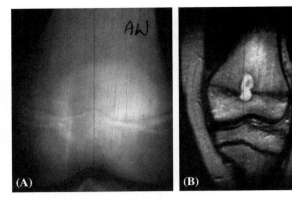

Figure 22 (**A**) Plain film of a transphyseal abscess extending from the metaphysis into the epiphysis. Plain film shows a discrete central lucency. (**B**) Coronal T2-weighted MRI shows a bilobed abscess.

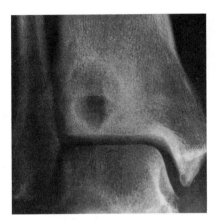

Figure 20 An epiphyseal abscess in the distal tibia probably having extended from a more typical Brodie's abscess higher up.

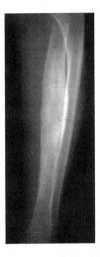

Figure 23 Sclerosing osteomyelitis of Garre. Note the thickening and increased density of the midshaft of the radius in this young child.

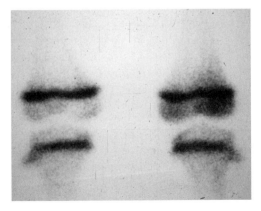

Figure 21 A bone scan in a different patient with an epiphyseal abscess of the lateral condyle of the left femur.

The bacterium found is usually a nonpurulent *S. aureus* or *Streptococcus,* although in approximately half of the cases, the pus is found to be sterile. The classical differential diagnosis of an epiphyseal lesion in a child is

infection, eosinophilic granuloma, and chondroblastoma. Azouz et al. (2) described eight children with epiphyseal abscesses, of whom five had abscesses in the distal femoral condyle and three had abscesses in the greater trochanter. Six of these had abscesses which were associated with septic arthritis. These authors also found that CT was useful to show the sequestrum.

Sclerosing Osteomyelitis of Garre

Some young children will present with a painful, swollen limb and have fusiform swelling of one bone, often a radius or ulna. The bone is widened and sclerotic, but usually has well-defined borders without evidence of an acute periostitis (Fig. 23).

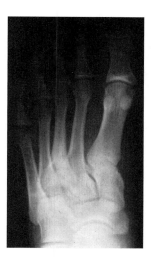

Figure 24 Sclerosing osteomyelitis of Garre. The third metatarsal is noted to be thickened and dense and although this was thought to be a stress phenomena, at biopsy it was found to be due to chronic osteomyelitis.

On biopsy, evidence of a chronic osteomyelitis is found, but usually, no organisms are present, nor can they be found in the bloodstream or adjacent to the involved bone. This was first described over 100 years ago and has remained a mystery until fairly recently, when another form of recurrent chronic osteomyelitis in adolescent children has been described, and this is discussed below. Radiologically, the differential diagnosis of this appearance would be of a stress phenomenon of some type (Fig. 24). The treatment of sclerosing osteomyelitis of Garre is uncertain at this time.

Chronic Multifocal Recurrent Osteomyelitis

A few years ago, we began to see a number of children who presented with one thickened, sclerotic bone, suggesting osteomyelitis of Garre, which would subside over time, and then the patient would develop another and then another. Chronic multifocal recurrent osteomyelitis (CMRO) was first described as recently as 1972, but I have seen four cases of the condition in the past 10 years. It is said to predominantly affect females, although three of my cases were male. The majority of the patients are adolescents or younger, and it affects long bones primarily, although involvement of the spine and mandible have also been described. The patient will complain of months, or even years, of arthralgias, and will often have one of the pustulotic forms of acne, such as pustulosis palmoplantaris. The drug cultures are invariably negative. Its etiology is unknown, although some form of autoimmune disease associated with a very slow-growing bacterium has been suggested.

Radiographically, CMRO may look like any form of chronic or subacute osteomyelitis, from a Brodie's abscess to sclerosing osteomyelitis of Garre (Figs. 25A–F and 26A–D) to the more characteristic appearance of a chronic osteomyelitis with a fluffy periosteal reaction (involucrum) and central sclerotic area (sequestrum) (Fig. 27).

Bone scans will show mildly increased activity. Histologically, there is an appearance of chronic osteomyelitis with inflammatory cells, plasma cells, lymphocytes, and a periosteal reaction. Although the course of the disease is long, the condition is benign and self-limiting, and the patient grows out of it. This is almost certainly the same disease described by Ribbing as a forme frust of Engelmann's disease.

A recent article by Mortenssen et al. (3) described CMRO in 31 children: 12 boys and 19 girls, who presented with pain in one or more limbs or joints and decreased range of motion. Their age range was from 3 years up to 14.5 years, with a mean of 10 years. The X-ray appearances were as described above, and there were 89 lesions in the 31 patients occurring distally in 33, proximally in 12, in the foot 12, and in the vertebrae 11. Histologically, the findings were of chronic osteomyelitis without bacteria, fungi, or tuberculosis. These and other authors have also noted that antibiotics appear to have no effect on the course or the outcome of the condition.

Vanishing Epiphyseal Ossification Center

Although this should probably be under the heading of septic arthritis, there is an entity in infants where an epiphyseal ossification center, such as a femoral head or humeral head, will disappear as a result of a septic joint. Initially, a large effusion will be present, displacing the femoral head outward and presumably damaging the blood supply to the growth plate (Fig. 28A, B).

The underlying infection is invariably *S. aureus,* and the children are aged between six months and two years. Once the diagnosis has been made and the infection treated, most of the ossification centers reappear and the joint returns to a relatively normal state (Fig. 29A–C).

Primary Subacute Epiphyseal Osteomyelitis

Although the vast majority of skeletal abscesses are of the Brodie's type, occurring in the metaphyses of adolescent children, there is one form of osteomyelitis that occurs within the epiphysis. Although very rare, some young children, aged between two and six, will present with a painful limp and swelling and develop a well-defined lytic area in their epiphysis. The majority are caused by *S. aureus,* although some may be sterile. The distal femoral epiphysis is the most frequently involved, and, radiologically, these abscesses look like an epiphyseal

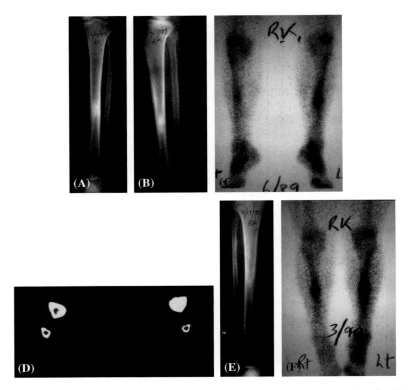

Figure 25 (**A, B**) Chronic multifocal recurrent osteomyelitis. The initial films show involvement primarily of the midshaft of the left tibia with possible some involvement on the right. (**C**) Chronic multifocal recurrent osteomyelitis. Bone scan shows involvement primarily of the midshaft of the left tibia with possibly some involvement on the right. (**D**) Chronic multifocal recurrent osteomyelitis. CT scan confirms these findings. (**E**) Plain film of the right tibia taken eight months later shows further involvement of the right tibia. (**F**) Bone scan of both lower legs shows further involvement of the right tibia and left ankle.

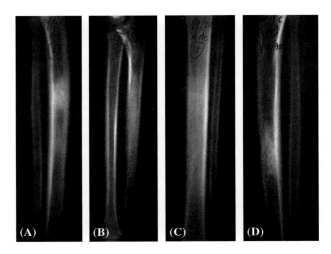

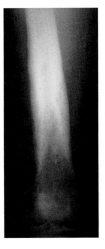

Figure 26 (**A, B**) Chronic multifocal recurrent osteomyelitis. Another patient with a similar picture. Plain films show involvement of the left mid tibia in October 1989. (**C**) Chronic multifocal recurrent osteomyelitis. Plain film of left tibia two years later when the osteomyelitis had recurred. (**D**) Chronic multifocal recurrent osteomyelitis. Plain film taken two years later when the osteomyelitis first presented in the right tibia.

Figure 27 Classic chronic osteomyelitis with marked cortical thickening as well as involvement of the intramedullary canal.

form of Brodie's abscess. In fact, some of these epiphyseal lesions can be contiguous with a metaphyseal abscess. CT, and particularly MRI, can be very helpful in the diagnosis. The differential diagnosis of a purely epiphyseal lesion in a

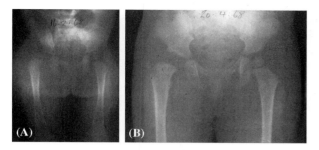

Figure 28 (**A**) Vanishing epiphyseal ossificiation center. On the initial film there is soft tissue swelling of the right hip. (**B**) Vanishing epiphyseal ossificiation center. On a film taken two months later the right femoral head has vanished.

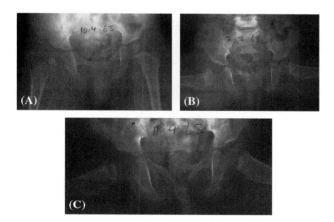

Figure 29 (**A**) Vanishing epiphyseal ossificiation center. On the initial film there is a large right-side joint effusion with subluxation of the hip joint. (**B**) Vanishing epiphyseal ossificiation center. Five months later the right femoral head has vanished. (**C**) Vanishing epiphyseal ossificiation center. Six months later it has reappeared although smaller than its original size.

child is eosinophilic granuloma, chondroblastoma, osteoid osteoma, and infection. A review article on 21 children by Sorensen et al. (4) reported that 20 lesions were at the knee, 16 in the femur, and 4 in the tibia. The children presented with pain and a limp, and the white blood cell count and sedimentation rate were normal. Usually, a bone scan was positive. The bacteria involved were *S. aureus* in 15 cases and *Streptococcus* in 2 cases. Four of these cases had sterile abscesses. The treatment was antibiotics and curettage.

Septic Arthritis

It may seem strange to separate out septic arthritis from bacterial osteomyelitis, yet it behaves somewhat differently, and it forces us to think of a number of causes of a somewhat hot, swollen joint other than juvenile chronic arthritis in children and gout or pseudogout in older

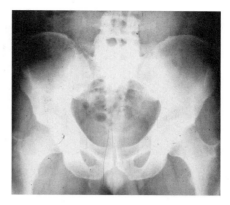

Figure 30 Septic arthritis left hip. Apart from soft tissue swelling, no specific abnormality can be seen on the plain film.

patients. This is exactly the problem that we have with septic arthritis; many radiologists seem to have forgotten that it exists. Septic arthritis is often difficult to diagnose; for example, a patient presents with a painful, swollen joint, and an X ray shows no obvious abnormality except perhaps a minor effusion (Fig. 30).

Your differential diagnosis would depend on the age of the patient, so let us assume that the joint involved is the knee and the patient is a child of five or so; thus, juvenile chronic arthritis would be your first thought. Please put a needle in the joint, aspirate some fluid, and send it to the laboratory to exclude a septic arthritis. Septic arthritis may affect any joint in the body, but bacterial infections seem to have a predilection for the larger joints including the hip, shoulder, wrist, and sacroiliac joint (Fig. 31A–C), although the symphysis pubis can be fairly often involved in male patients who have chronic prostatitis and female patients with chronic cystitis (Fig. 32).

Radiographically, the bones may initially appear normal, although juxta-articular osteoporosis will occur in 10 to 14 days. If not diagnosed at this stage, then erosions and loss of joint cartilage will ensue over the course of the next three to four weeks (Fig. 33A, B).

The way to differentiate a bacterial septic arthritis from a tuberculous arthritis is by the time course: two to three weeks for a staphylococcal infection, and the patient is usually febrile with an increased white count and sedimentation rate; three to six months for tuberculosis, and the patient has few signs and symptoms and is not febrile. One of the problems with the diagnosis of septic arthritis is its insidious onset, although joint aspiration will give you an early diagnosis and allow you to treat the patient with the correct antibiotic. In majority of cases, septic arthritis is still caused by *S. aureus,* and the newer, broad-spectrum antibiotics are often effective. One final comment is that in most of the cases, septic arthritis cause only juxta-articular synovial erosions and do not really involve the subchondral bone. However, a continuing septic

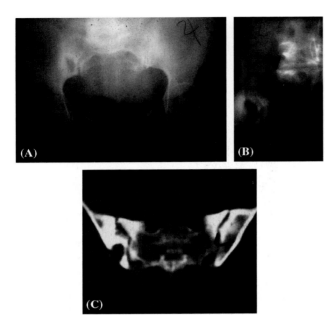

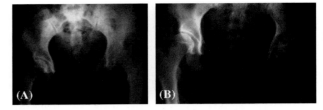

Figure 33 (A) Septic arthritis in the left hip of a mentally retarded adult. Initial film shows a relatively normal pelvis and hip. (B) Plain film taken three months later shows destruction of the cartilage with subchondral cysts extending both into the femoral head and acetabulum.

Figure 31 (A, B) Septic arthritis right sacroiliac joint. On the initial films, irregularity of the right sacroiliac joint can be seen with an abscess cavity adjacent to and connecting to the joint. (C) A CT scan shows the characteristic appearance of septic arthritis in the anterior synovial part of the joint. The defect posteriorly was caused by an ill-informed orthopedic surgeon trying to get into the infection!

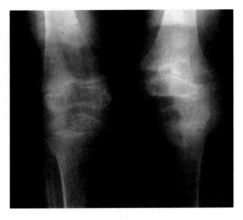

Figure 34 Meningococcemia. Note the irregularity of the growth plates and surrounding bone in both knees although much more advanced on the left.

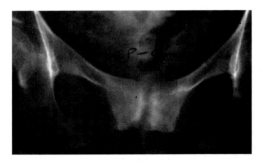

Figure 32 Septic arthritis in the symphysis pubis secondary to chronic cystitis in a 51-year-old female patient.

arthritis will obviously produce an underlying osteomyelitis, and this occurs in approximately 10% of cases of septic arthritis.

Epiphyseo-Metaphyseal Changes in Children Following Meningococcemia

Many young children die from meningococcal septicemia, but the few that survive develop a number of problems, including intravascular coagulation, which leads to a

combination of osteomyelitis and infarction in the skeleton. This appears to primarily involve the epiphysis, although secondary metaphyseal changes are apparent (Fig. 34).

The age of the children is classically two to five years. Once recovered from the infection, the prognosis is of increasingly severe orthopedic problems, with premature fusion of the growth plate, angular deformities at the ends of the long bones, as well as premature arthritis.

Sepsis After Orthopedic Instrumentation

Inherently, any orthopedic procedure can lead to infection, and the presence of an orthopedic device, plate, or screw in the skeleton can lead to an increasing risk of sepsis (Figs. 35 and 36).

Conventional wisdom says that the infection rate is 2% following any orthopedic procedure, but this varies depending on the procedure, and this will be discussed in much greater detail in chapter 8.

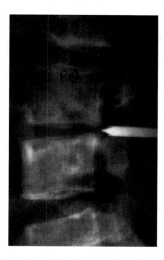

Figure 35 Infection following orthopedic instrumentation. Single lateral view of the lumbar spine following a laminectomy. Note the irregularity of both end plates with patchy areas of destruction and sclerosis. Note also the biopsy needle poised to make the correct diagnosis, which was an *S. aureus* disc space infection.

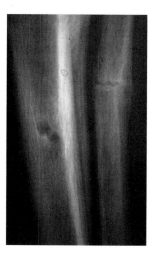

Figure 36 Infection following orthopedic instrumentation: pin-track infection in the mid tibia in this young male patient whose external fixator was removed because of continuing sepsis. Note that the pin-track hole instead of having clean-cut margins is rather blurred, which is a typical sign of early infection.

Spinal Infection

It may seem somewhat arbitrary to separate out spinal infections from the rest, but the discs, being relatively avascular, respond to infection differently than, say a bone or a joint. In fact, because of the avascular nature of the disc, the older literature made great play of the fact that bacterial infections affected the bones (i.e., they were really osteomyelitis); whereas tuberculosis affected Sharpey's fibers at the front of the disc, which were

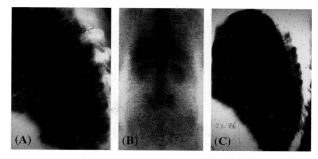

Figure 37 (**A**) Disc space infection. On the initial lateral film of the thorax spine no major abnormality was seen. (**B**) The early nuclear medicine scan shows increase uptake in the mid thorax region. (**C**) On a repeat lateral film taken two months later, there is vertebral end plate loss at T8/9 typical of an early disc infection.

relatively vascular (i.e., the equivalent of a synovial infection) and hence, one could tell them apart. This is really not true any longer, even if it were true then. The only way bacterial and tuberculous spinal infections can be separated is the time course: 6 to 8 weeks for bacterial infections and 6 to 12 months for tuberculous infections. Also, on the whole, the longer the time course, the more chance of reactive sclerosis, but this is not entirely true either, and surrounding sclerosis is frequently seen in association with bacterial infections as well as tuberculous ones. In either situation, the majority of patients get infections of their lumbar spine, although spinal infections can be seen from C2 (cervical) down to S1 (sacral) in both bacterial and tuberculous diseases.

Spinal infection starts anteriorly probably because of the good blood supply around the anterior longitudinal ligament. The reason for the preponderance of lumbar infections is almost certainly the relationship between the spine and the abdomen where renal infections, along with retroperitoneal node inflammation, can spread directly into the spine. Often the initial radiograph is normal and the patient has a mildly elevated sedimentation rate and white blood count and fevers and night sweats (Fig. 37A–C).

If infection is considered a possibility, a radionuclide study, either a gallium scan or indium-111 white cell scan, will be positive. A CT scan will show a soft-tissue abscess and, possibly, early bone destruction, but an MRI will definitely confirm the diagnosis, demonstrating both abscess and early bone destruction. However, if the diagnosis is not made at this early stage, the patient is told to go home, probably on analgesics, and unfortunately, probably on an inadequate course of antibiotics.

In bacterial infections, the patients usually present at six to eight weeks with destruction and erosion of the vertebral end plates adjacent to the involved discs (Fig. 38A, B).

Often there is bony sclerosis, demonstrating an attempt to wall off the infection (similar to the periosteal new bone

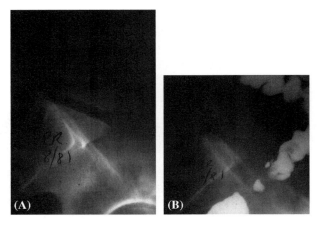

Figure 38 (**A**) Disc space infection in a drug addict. Initial film is normal. (**B**) Disc space infection in a drug addict. Follow-up film two months later shows marked destruction of the lower end plate of L5 vertebral body due to an *S. aureus* infection.

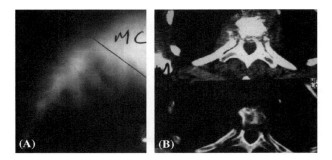

Figure 39 (**A**) Disc space infection. This 40-year-old man had received radiation to his mediastinum for lymphoma. The tomogram of the upper thoracic spine shows marked destruction of several of the vertebral bodies and end plates. (**B**) The CT scan confirms the tomogram findings and shows a large soft tissue abscess, which was aspirated to reveal an *S. aureus* infection.

and involucrum seen in infections of long bones). The disc space is usually involved throughout its whole width so that if the infection is allowed to continue untreated, the two vertebral bodies will ultimately collapse into each other symmetrically, and usually vertically, so that there is no subsequent angulation. At this late stage, one can differentiate an old, burnt-out bacterial infection from a tuberculous infection: in the former, the spine is straight; and in tuberculous, there is marked angulation.

Once the infection has been seen on plain films, there is no real need to image it any further, although a CT-guided aspiration, usually from the soft-tissue abscess rather than the involved disc, should be performed to identify the actual organism (Fig. 39A, B).

In otherwise normal patients, *S. aureus* is still the cause of over 95% of spinal infections. In drug addicts and in

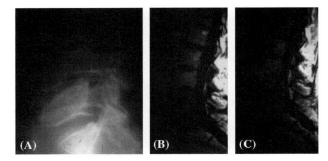

Figure 40 (**A**) Disc space infection at L4/5. The plain film shows the characteristic appearance of an infection. This is confirmed by the MR scan. (**B**) T1-weighted sagittal image. (**C**) T2-weighted sagittal image showing both the bony destruction and a large anterior and posterior soft tissue extension.

patients who are immunosuppressed, *Staphylococcus* accounts for 75% of infections, with a variety of other common, or even strange, organisms causing the other 25%. These include *Pseudomonas, Klebsiella,* and some forms of anaerobic streptococci. However, the radiographic appearance is the same regardless of the underlying cause. Obviously, the infection will be hot on indium-111 and gallium scanning, although it may be cold on Tc99m bone scanning. A CT scan will show the destruction of both the disc and the adjacent bone, as well as the extent of the soft-tissue abscess (Fig. 39B). An MRI is probably the investigation of choice today because it will also show if there are any other disc infections, higher or lower (Fig. 40A–C).

Once again, if an aspiration biopsy is being planned, CT is the technique of choice, although, of course, at this stage of the disease, blood cultures will probably be positive and make the diagnosis easy. Treatment is done by giving the appropriate antibiotic, intravenously at first for three to four weeks and then orally. The end result is usually spontaneous fusion without angulation between the adjacent vertebral bodies.

Although tuberculosis will be discussed in further detail shortly, spinal tuberculosis is very similar to bacterial spinal infections except for two things, and both have already been mentioned: the time course of spinal tuberculosis is 9 to 12 months, and tuberculosis of the spine erodes the anterior parts of the vertebral bodies, particularly, thus producing a wedge-shaped area of destruction, so that once the spine collapses, a marked angulation occurs, and this is referred to as a "Gibbus" (or hump) (Fig. 41).

Tuberculosis and spinal tuberculosis will be dealt with in more detail in the next section.

Finally, we need to discuss an entity described by the pediatric community called "discitis." In reality, this

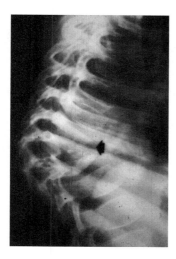

Figure 41 Typical Gibbus deformity seen following tuberculosis. Note the V-shaped vertebral body with two sets of pedicles posteriorly.

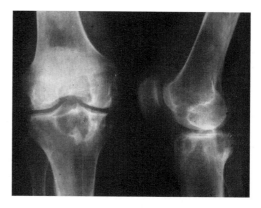

Figure 42 Typical tuberculosis (or other chronic synovial infection) in a knee. Note the large synovially based erosions mainly in the intracondylar notch (where the cruciate ligaments originate and insert) but also medial and laterally on the tibial plateau where the lateral and medial collateral ligaments run. This case of tuberculosis came from Nigeria. *Source*: Courtesy of Stanley Bohrer, MD.

refers to a spinal infection almost invariably due to *S. aureus* but occasionally due to *Streptococcus* in a child who presents with low-grade fever, back pain, and normal X rays. A recent review article confirms my bias, and radionuclide studies will confirm the disc space infection, even if not visible on plain radiographs.

The treatment is broad-spectrum antibiotics with some form of immobilization. I believe that discitis is simply a bacterial spine infection seen in children rather than in adults before radiographic changes occur.

Tuberculosis

Radiologists seem to forget that tuberculosis is still prevailing, even in the United States and Europe. In 1998, the World Health Organization reported on an incidence of 1.2 per 100,000 population in the United States, and estimated 10 million new cases worldwide with approximately 3 million deaths. As I write this section, I saw two new cases of tuberculosis (one pulmonary and one in the sacroiliac joint) in my department in the last month. Before we begin the description of osteoarticular tuberculosis, three things should be kept in mind, first, osteoarticular tuberculosis is a secondary manifestation of the disease, with the primary site being either the lungs or the kidneys. Second, tuberculosis of the musculoskeletal system should be considered primarily a joint or disc infection, not an osteomyelitis. Finally, tuberculosis in a joint or disc resembles a bacterial infection radiologically, except for its time course. Initially, the patient will complain of pain and swelling for six to eight weeks, although the radiographs are often normal at this stage. Joint effusions and soft-tissue swelling become apparent at

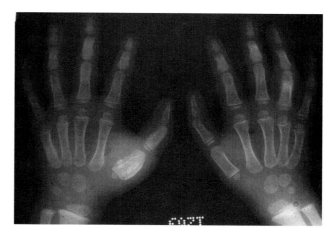

Figure 43 Tuberculous dacylitis. There is a characteristic appearance of osteomyelitis in the first left metacarpal and the fourth right proximal phalanx as well as more discrete changes seen elsewhere.

about three months, and if the diagnosis is not made at this stage, juxta-articular osteoporosis and discrete erosions will be seen at about six months. Loss of joint cartilage and increasingly obvious osteopenia with larger erosions will occur at about nine months (Fig. 42).

In adults, the spine, knee, wrist, and sacroiliac joints are quite commonly involved. However, children can get two forms of true osseous involvement, a dactylitis in the hands (Fig. 43) and a very rare condition known as spina ventosa (Fig. 44).

Dactylitis occurs mainly in young children aged four to nine, and primarily affects the small bones of the hands and feet, with an appearance typical of a bacterial

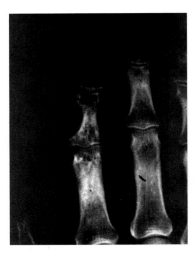

Figure 44 Spina ventosa in tuberculosis. Note the appearance of lucencies in the distal phalanx and distal end of the middle phalanx of the index finger of the right hand. This appearance is almost identical to that seen in sarcoidosis and in fact may actually be related to that condition.

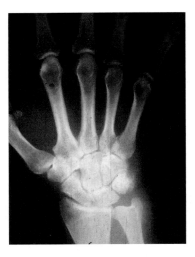

Figure 45 *Microbacterium marinum*. This patient was fishing and got his hook caught in the soft tissues of his right hand adjacent to the hamate. Note the soft tissue swelling and discrete erosions of several of the carpal bones on their ulnar aspect.

osteomyelitis with a fluffy periosteal reaction, cortical thickening, and some patchy loss of cancellous bone. In bacterial infections, dactylitis usually affects only one bone, whereas in tuberculous dactylitis, three or four bones, phalanges, and/or metacarpals will be involved (Fig. 43).

The differential diagnosis of tuberculous dactylitis is a curious syndrome seen in infants with sickle cell anemia called the "hand-foot" syndrome where they develop widespread dactylitis throughout their hands and feet. In tuberculosis, it is usually only one hand or one foot that is involved. Spina ventosa means "holey" bones and refers to a type of primary osseous tuberculosis that resembles sarcoidosis in the phalanges of one or more fingers (Fig. 44).

I believe that it is, in fact, another manifestation of sarcoidosis, which will be discussed elsewhere in this book.

Getting back to the more usual articular form of tuberculosis, an article from Kuala Lumpur in Malaysia (5) discusses 71 patients with osteoarticular tuberculosis. Apparently, the author had over 7000 patients with pulmonary tuberculosis and 1% of them developed bone changes. They were mainly aged between 20 and 50, and the spine was involved in 56 patients (cervical spine, 13; thoracic spine, 20; and lumbar spine, 23). There was only one sacroiliac-joint infection, although the hips were involved in six patients. The metaphyseal ends of long bones were involved in four patients, three of whom had an adjacent septic arthritis. Fifteen of the patients had multiple sites of involvement. The radiographic findings were the same as I outlined above, soft-tissue swelling, juxta-articular osteoporosis, synovial erosions, and finally,

loss of cartilage and/or disc height. Before we leave osteoarticular tuberculosis, one final comment is that the *Mycobacterium* is ubiquitous, and some strange presentations can occur as a result of local inoculation of an atypical mycobacterium. For instance, *Mycobacterium marinum* occurs in large game fish and can be transmitted to fishermen if they get the hook caught in their soft tissues (Fig. 45).

Although it is said that a picture is worth a thousand words and the text is accompanied by a number of good illustrations, a verbal description of tuberculosis will also be useful. In the wrist, initially some soft-tissue swelling will be seen, and then discrete, synovially based erosions will occur, and these can be most easily seen in the line of the collateral ligaments, with erosions at the tip of the ulnar styloid, at the base of the fifth metacarpal, on the ulnar aspect of the distal hamate, and the lateral aspect of the triquetrum and pisiform (Fig. 46A–C).

On the radial aspect of the wrist, the erosions are somewhat more difficult to find, but can usually be seen at the tip of the radial styloid, in the region of the styloid of the scaphoid (the outermost radial aspect of the distal scaphoid), and at the base of the trapezium. In tuberculosis of the wrist, juxta-articular osteoporosis is a late occurrence and will not be seen at this stage (3–6 months). However, as the disease progresses, the erosions enlarge and become more obvious, as well as becoming more widespread, involving many of the intercarpal spaces such as the triscaphe joint, the scaphocapitate space, and the capitohamate joint. Now, juxta-articular osteoporosis as well as obvious soft-tissue swelling and early loss of joint cartilage space will occur (6–9 months). If the disease

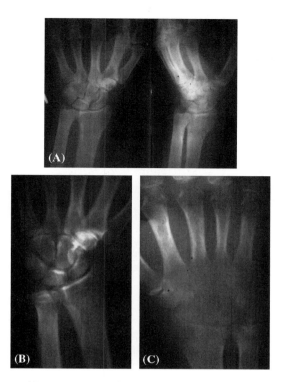

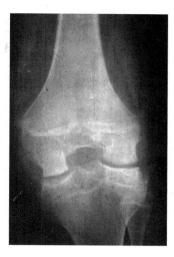

Figure 47 Typical tuberculosis of the knee: another classical case with synovial erosions at the origin and insertion of both the MCL and the femoral fibular ligament as well as within the intercondylar notch.

Figure 46 Progressive tuberculosis of the left wrist. (**A**) The initial film was read as normal. (**B**) A film three months later was also read as normal, but in retrospect there are large erosions of the distal scaphoid. (**C**) Another three months later and there are now marked widespread destruction of many of the carpal bones with juxta-articular osteoporosis.

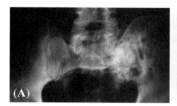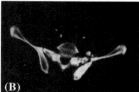

Figure 48 Tuberculosis of the left sacroiliac joint. (**A**) Plain film showing the destruction and sclerosis of the left sacroiliac joint. Note all the small ossific loose bodies (which are known as psammatous loose bodies). (**B**) A CT scan confirms these findings.

continues untreated, then complete destruction of the joints will occur, culminating in bony fusion of the wrist.

In the knee, similar changes take place, with a joint effusion and some soft-tissue swelling in the first instance (3 months), and then slowly progressive synovial erosions occur from three to six months, culminating at six to nine months with the characteristic widening of the intercondylar notch, erosions of the lateral margins of the lateral femoral condyle, and the medial margin of the medial femoral condyle as well as the lateral and medial margins of the tibia (Fig. 47).

On the lateral view, large erosions in the region of the tibial spines can be clearly seen. If one remembers one's anatomy, the central erosions occur because of synovial overgrowth surrounding the cruciate ligaments, and the peripheral erosions occur because of synovial overgrowth around the collateral ligaments. Although theoretically in the knee, loss of joint cartilage can also occur, as can fusion of the joint, this is a relatively rare complication of the condition since most patients will seek medical care before this happens because of the decrease in range of motion in the joint. Incidentally, the other causes of

widening of the intercondylar notch are all synovially based diseases: juvenile chronic arthritis, fungal infections, hemophilia, and synovial tumors such as pigmented villonodular synovitis.

In the sacroiliac joint, tuberculosis is usually unilateral and produces changes similar to that seen in bacterial infections of the joint; erosions, sclerosis, and often an actual abscess, will occur (Fig. 48A, B).

However, once again it is the time course of the disease that separates bacterial infections from tuberculous infections of the sacroiliac joint: four to six weeks for bacterial infections and six to nine months for tuberculosis. Also, the tuberculous infections are more inclined to be associated with a large, cold abscess containing calcified granulation bodies known as psammomatous bodies. If the abscess is anterior, it can run down the iliopsoas muscle and point just below the inguinal ligament (Fig. 49A, B).

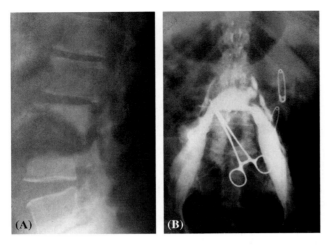

(A)   (B)

Figure 49 (**A**) Lateral lumbar spine showing extensive destruction of a disc space with sclerosis of the adjoining vertebral bodies suggestive of tuberculosis. (**B**) Contrast was injected into a cold abscess in the groin where it ran up large, bilateral abscess cavities lying superior to the psoas muscles.

Classically, tuberculosis is said to affect the right sacroiliac joint rather than the left because of the mesenteric drainage from the kidneys when they act as the primary site of infection. However, tuberculous sacroiliitis can be seen in either the left or the right sacroiliac joint. To complete this discussion, unilateral sacroiliitis can also be seen in psoriatic arthritis, in degenerative arthritis (most commonly), and with gout.

Tuberculosis in the spine also has a fairly characteristic appearance. It involves the anterior part of the two vertebral bodies adjacent to the disc. Initially, there are only discrete erosions without any reactive sclerosis or collapse, but about four to six months into the infection, angulation through the disc space will occur. This is because tuberculous involvement of the disc space and vertebral body is primarily the anterior part of the discovertebral segment. This produces an acute angulation at this level, which is known as a Gibbus (from the Latin for hump) (Fig. 50A, B).

Although the bone changes are what we see on the plain X rays, spinal tuberculosis is almost invariably associated with a large, soft-tissue mass lying anteriorly and laterally to the involved discs. Because it is a chronic disease, these abscesses are often called "cold abscesses" because they contain no organisms. In the chest, they appear as a posterior mediastinal mass, and may even calcify. They are often associated with psammomatous bodies. If aspirated, pus is withdrawn, but it frequently fails to contain any organisms. In the lumbar region, these abscesses will often connect with the fascia running over the iliopsoas muscle, and classically run down the muscle to present as a cold abscess in the groin. Once again, psammomatous bodies and calcifications can be seen in association with this abscess.

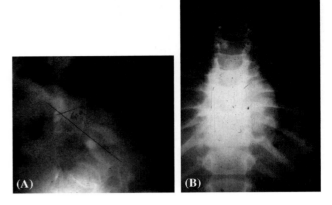

(A)   (B)

Figure 50 Gibbus with a large cold abscess. (**A**) Lateral thorax spine film shows a typical 60° wedge-shaped vertebral body with two sets of pedicles entering posteriorly. (**B**) An AP view shows the large cold abscess.

Old tuberculosis of the spine is easy to diagnose because this somewhat triangular, apparently single vertebral body has two sets of pedicles entering it posteriorly, one set from the remains of the upper vertebral body and the second from below (Fig. 50A).

Nowadays, tuberculosis of the spine is often diagnosed before this occurs, and the patient is given antituberculous drugs and placed in a brace so that the fusion of the spine is more vertically oriented. One final comment is that tuberculosis of the spine may, in fact, involve the whole disc space and resemble a bacterial infection, and this is particularly true in drug addicts and in those patients who are markedly immune suppressed, such as AIDS patients. Another paper reviewed the findings in 123 patients with tuberculosis of the spine in Riyadh, Saudi Arabia (6). The average age was 41, and 118 patients had no less than 284 vertebrae involved; 50% had two adjacent vertebral bodies involved, 25% had three or more, and 25% had only a single vertebral body. Nineteen cases were in the cervical spine, 76 cases in the thoracic spine, and 36 patients had lumbar involvement. In 14 patients, the involvement was multiple. Radiologically, the infection was associated with a soft-tissue mass, loss of the end plates, disc-space narrowing, and erosions of the vertebral bodies. The main area of infection appeared to be the anterior, inferior segment of the bone, and the adjacent paravertebral soft tissue. This study also examined the use of bone scanning in the diagnosis of spinal tuberculosis, and of 56 patients who had Tc99m bone scans, 35 were positive, 20 were normal, and 1 was "cold." Gallium scans were performed in 10 patients, 3 of whom were positive and 7 were read as normal. Thus, neither gallium nor Tc99m is particularly useful in the diagnosis of spinal tuberculosis, presumably because of the chronicity of the infection. One final comment about tuberculosis of the

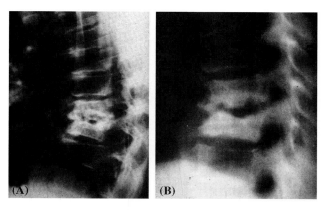

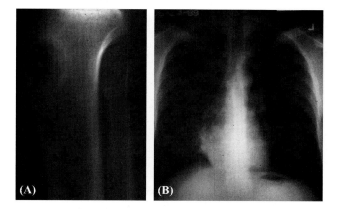

Figure 51 (**A, B**) Two cases of Brucellosis involving the spine in different patients with sclerosis of two adjacent vertebral bodies and destruction of the disc space.

Figure 52 (**A**) Brucellosis. Chronic abscess in the anterior tibia in a park ranger who also had pulmonary involvement. (**B**) Brucellosis in a park ranger who had pulmonary involvement with scarring and collapse of part of the right middle lobe.

spine to remember is that tuberculosis can be reactivated by radiation, and in the past three years, we have seen two patients with tuberculosis of the mid-thoracic spine reactivated as a result of radiation for previous lymphoma who presented with serious neurological complications as a result of collapse of two adjacent vertebral bodies (Fig. 39A, B).

Fungal Infections

Although rarer than tuberculosis, fungal infections of the musculoskeletal system are still fairly frequently seen, particularly in the Third World and in the more rural areas of the United States. Each different fungus has a different mode of entering the human body; some are airborne, some by direct inoculation, and some by hematogenous spread. They can cause abscesses in the lungs and soft tissues and can afflict the bones, joints, and discs in the musculoskeletal system. In the bones, a fungal infection most resembles either a chronic osteomyelitis or, more likely, appears like a Brodie's abscess, but occurring in the wrong age group and in the wrong place. In the joints, fungal infections are synovially based, and so resemble tuberculosis of a joint, with soft-tissue swelling, synovial erosions, and ultimately, loss of joint cartilage space. In the spine, fungal infections are usually chronic, and once again, are likely to resemble tuberculosis rather than bacterial disc infection. At this point, I will briefly discuss the musculoskeletal findings in a number of specific fungal infections, namely, brucellosis, blastomycosis, coccidiomycosis, and sporotrichosis.

Brucellosis

Brucellosis usually occurs in the spine. It has an appearance similar to a chronic bacterial infection, but it also can produce dense vertebral bodies in its healing phase (Fig. 51A, B).

Thus, brucellosis and unusual infections should be included in the differential diagnosis of an ivory vertebra. Outside the spine, brucellosis is similar to chronic osteomyelitis, although it can produce large abscesses (Fig. 52A, B).

In joints, it will lead to intense, reactive sclerosis, hypertrophic changes, and bony fusions.

Blastomycosis

Hematogenous spread from skin or from the lungs. This is a very destructive infection that produces many soft-tissue and bone abscesses with draining sinuses (Fig. 53A–C).

Coccidioidomycosis

This is spread hematogenously from the chest into the soft tissues and the skeleton. It can involve the spine, pelvis, ribs, and long bones. The appearances resemble infection, either acute or chronic, although, in the chronic phase, the lesions can be somewhat destructive (Fig. 54).

There is often reactive bone sclerosis with draining sinuses.

Sporotrichosis

This is another fungal infection involving people who work in horticulture or farming, or who are gardeners. It can occur at any age, but is commoner in middle-aged patients, many of whom remember a specific injury (Fig. 55A–C).

Lymphocutaneous spread is common and occurs in the majority of patients, although some may have intra-articular infections or soft-tissue infections as a result of deep cuts (Fig. 56).

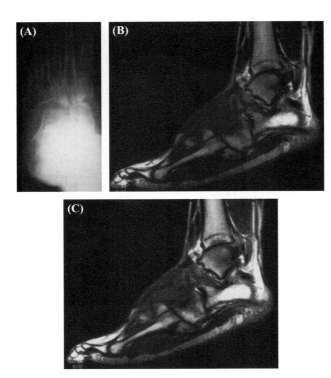

Figure 53 (**A**) Blastomycosis. Plain film showing marked destruction of many of the mid tarsal bones and joints. (**B**) MR sagittal sequence confirms these findings. (**C**) MR sagittal sequence confirms these findings.

Rowe et al. (7) described 48 patients with sporotrichosis, 12 of whom had joint infections that presented with decreased range of motion. There was usually a delay in diagnosis since many of these infections were thought to be due to another form of arthritis, internal derangement of the joint, pigmented villonodular synovitis, or even sarcoidosis. Once the diagnosis had been established, the treatment is with potassium iodide amphocerotin-B and arthrodesis.

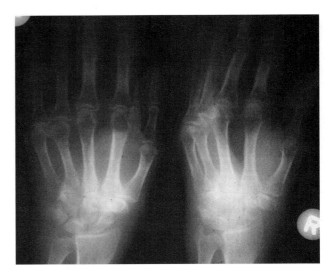

Figure 54 Coccidiodomycosis in the right wrist. There is soft tissue swelling and loss of joint cartilage space. This again resembles tuberculosis (Fig. 46)

Nocardiasis

Nocardiasis is spread directly from pulmonary involvement to the chest wall. It usually spreads locally rather than by hematogenous spread, leading to osteomyelitis in the chest wall. However, hematogenous spread may occur as can be seen from this patient's films (Fig. 57A–C).

Madura Foot

Madura foot is general term for a fungal infection of the foot, mycetoma pedis. It may be caused by actinomycosis, nocardiasis, *Streptomyces,* or *Madurella.* In Mexico, 90% of cases of Madura foot are due to *Nocardia.* It occurs in the tropics where people walk around barefoot, and the fungus is in the soil, where it enters the foot through a cut

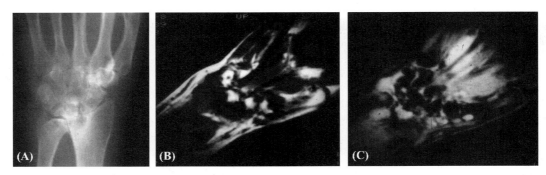

Figure 55 (**A**) Sporotrichosis. This 52-year-old vicars wife was gardening and sustained an open wound. Three months later she developed a swollen painful wrist. The plain film shows marked destruction of many of the carpal joints with erosions. (**B**) Sporotrichosis. MR coronal T1 sequence shows the marked synovial proliferation with erosion of many of the carpal bones. (**C**) Sporotrichosis. MR coronal fat-saturated T2 sequence shows the marked synovial proliferation with erosion of many of the carpal bones. This appearance can be seen in any chronic infection including tuberculosis.

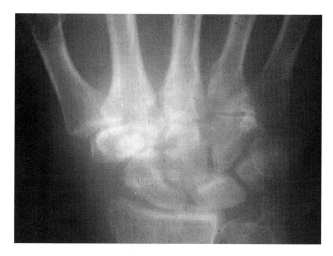

Figure 56 Sporotrichosis in the wrist of a different patient with similar findings although more localized to the radial side of the wrist.

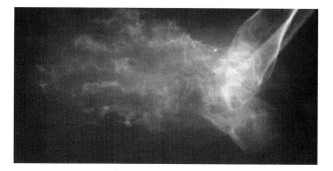

Figure 58 Madura foot. Note the marked soft tissue swelling and destruction of all the tarsal bones, metatarsals, and phalanges. In this patient, this appearance was caused by *Nocardia*.

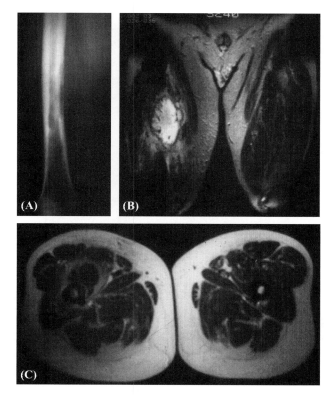

Figure 57 (**A**) Nocardiasis. Plain film. Demonstrates this large abscess with bony destruction of the midshaft of the right femur. The patient managed a large wildlife ranch. (**B**) Nocardiasis. MRI coronal delayed T2 sequence confirms these findings. (**C**) Nocardiasis. MRI axial T1 sequence confirms these findings.

and involves the soft tissues, the muscles, and finally, the bones, causing a chronic infection with granulomas and sinus tracts (Fig. 58).

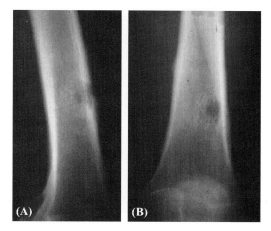

Figure 59 (**A**) Lateral and (**B**) AP plain films. Atypical mycobacterium. Plain film of the distal femur showing indolent chronic periostitis with an underlying abscess cavity. The differential diagnosis would include almost any form of chronic osteomyelitis. On biopsy this proved to be a case of atypical mycobacterium.

There is extensive destruction of the bones of the foot, with multiple lytic defects, but without sequestration or periosteal reaction.

Unusual Infections

Atypical Mycobacterium

Atypical mycobacterium can cause an appearance similar to that of tuberculosis or of a chronic bacterial osteomyelitis (Fig. 59A, B).

Gonorrhea

Gonorrhea causes a septic arthritis rather than an osteomyelitis in most cases. It is characterized by a generalized loss of joint cartilage without juxta-articular osteoporosis in the first instance (Fig. 60A–C).

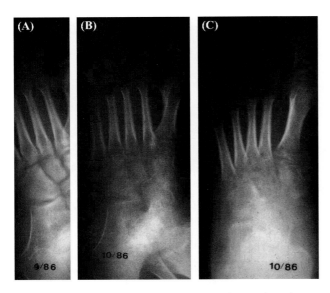

Figure 60 (**A**) Gonococcus. Progressive destructive changes are seen in the foot of a prostitute. The initial film shows early destructive changes around the lateral cuneiform. (**B**) Three weeks later there is further destruction with increasing juxta-articular osteoporosis on the lateral aspect of the foot. (**C**) Three weeks after this, the infection has progressed to involve the whole of the mid-foot.

However, as the disease progresses, there will be increasing reactive osteopenia surrounding the infection.

Histoplasmosis

Histoplasmosis, in the North American type, can produce an appearance similar to that of a chronic osteomyelitis or similar to that seen in tuberculosis. In the African type of histoplasmosis, there are diffuse irregular areas of bone destruction with periosteal reaction resembling more chronic infection (Fig. 61A, B).

Hydatid Disease

Hydatid disease (echinococcus) is relatively common in certain parts of the world, although it only rarely involves the skeleton. Seventy-five percent of cases of hydatid are in the liver, 15% are in the lungs, and only 2% in the bones. The definitive host is the dog with an intermediate host being the sheep, from whom man gets the disease. In the pelvic or long bones, hydatid looks like a bone cyst, with sharply demarginated edges and some surrounding sclerosis (Figs. 62 and 63).

Typhoid

When typhoid was common, some patients developed a chronic osteomyelitis, which was unusual in that it

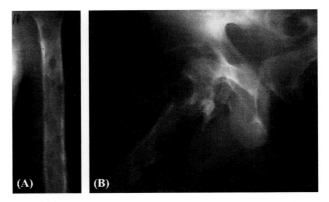

Figure 61 (**A**) Histoplasmosis. AP humerus showing patchy areas of bone destruction in the shaft of the bone in an adolescent. (**B**) Histoplasmosis. Lateral view of the right hip in a different younger patient shows large erosions suggesting soft tissue lesions encroaching on the bone from outside, perhaps synovially based. *Source:* Courtesy of Stanley Bohrer, MD.

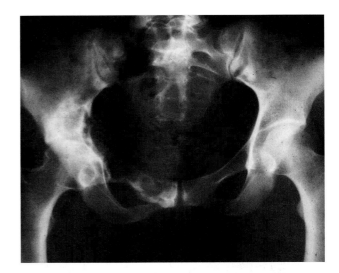

Figure 62 Hydatid. There is a large expansatile lucency involving the right pubic ramus and medial wall of the right acetabulum. The normal differential diagnosis would include fibrous dysplasia, aneurysmal bone cyst, giant cell tumor, and plasmacytoma.

involved long bones symmetrically, such as both femurs and both tibias (Fig. 64).

It has the appearance typical of any form of chronic osteomyelitis.

Ainhum

Although this may not be due to an infection, but may be developmental, it involves the fifth toe in black patients in

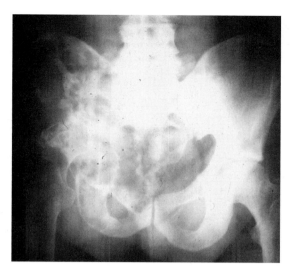

Figure 63 Hydatid. Another patient. The patient is from Greece with a large destructive lesion of the roof of the right acetabulum where the femoral head has subluxed upward into the cyst.

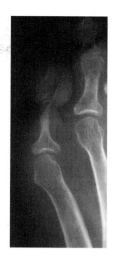

Figure 65 Ainhum. There is a fibrous tissue band around the PIP joint of the little toe with soft tissue swelling and decreasing bone mineral distally.

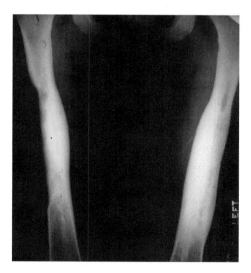

Figure 64 Typhoid. Both femurs show typical findings of a chronic osteomyelitis of whatever cause.

their fourth or fifth decade. It is commoner in women. There is soft-tissue swelling with loss of the outer diameter of the phalanx, ultimately leading to resorption and dissolution of the whole bone (Fig. 65).

Pathologically, a fibrous band can be found crossing the fifth metatarsophalangeal joint that causes the loss of the little toe.

Treponemal Infections

Syphilis

Syphilis could be seen at any age. However, the appearances are somewhat different, depending on if the disease is transmitted through the placenta or acquired.

Congenital syphilis occurs under two years of age and is associated with generalized periostitis running along the length of all the long bones (Fig. 66A–C).

There are also metaphyseal lucent bands that can be seen, particularly in the distal radius, distal femur, and proximal tibia. These can be associated with erosions. There is in fact, a Wimberger sign, which is medial tibial metaphyseal lesions with symmetrical cortical erosions (Fig. 67).

Some children with congenital syphilis are stillborn, however, the classical radiological finding in a living child is of widespread periosteal reaction.

Juvenile syphilis usually has only an appearance of a dactylitis similar to the one that can be seen in tuberculosis.

Adult syphilis has a number of different presentations, including gummas, which are large, destructive lesions of both bone and soft tissue (Fig. 68A, B).

The patient may also have Hutchinson's teeth, which are curious, pointed teeth, and there are some skin and nerve changes including eighth nerve deafness. Several of the patients develop saber shins, which is an anterior curvature of the tibias bilaterally (Fig. 69A, B).

A form of neuropathic joint has been described in some of these patients, which has been referred to as

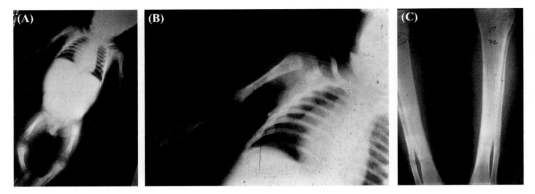

Figure 66 (**A**) Congenital syphilis. Neonate with widespread periostitis. (**B**) Congenital syphilis. Right arm of the same child in **A**. (**C**) Congenital syphilis. Periostitis seen along both tibias in an older patient.

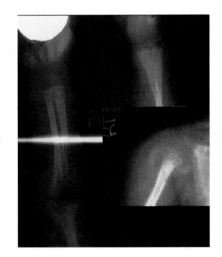

Figure 67 Congenital syphilis. Three views of the skeleton in a young child with metaphyseal lucent bands and discrete erosions.

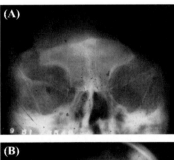

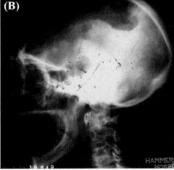

Figure 68 (**A**) Gumma of the skull. AP view. (**B**) Gumma of the skull. Lateral view shows a large destructive lesion involving the calvarium typical of a gumma.

Cluttons joints, but, in reality, these are simply neuropathic joints.

Yaws

Yaws is caused by *Treponema pertenue*. It resembles syphilis in all its different stages. The secondary and tertiary stages of yaws are very similar to syphilis, and the appearance of the skeleton is that of a chronic osteomyelitis and is somewhat nonspecific (Fig. 70A, B).

The primary stage of yaws has a widespread periosteal reaction similar to syphilis, which is often exuberant. This can be mainly seen in the tibias, ulnas, and phalanges (Fig. 71).

Destructive metaphyseal lesions (Wimberger's sign) have also been described.

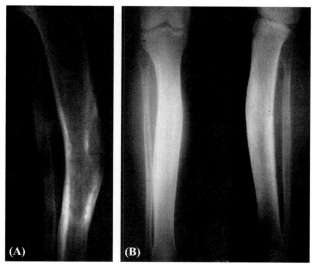

Figure 69 (A) Sabre shins. Lateral view of a tibia showing bowing and deformity of the anterior tibial cortex with periostitis and thickening. (B) Sabre shins. AP and lateral views in a different patient showing similar changes.

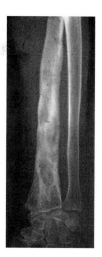

Figure 71 Yaws. Close-up AP view of the left ulna in a patient with primary yaws.

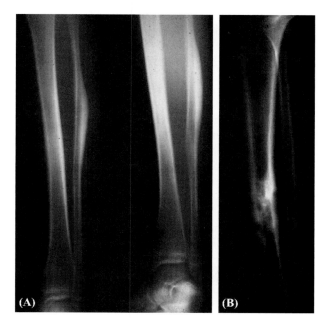

Figure 70 (A) Yaws. AP and oblique view of the left leg in a young patient with yaws and periosteal thickening. (B) Yaws. More aggressive changes seen in a different patient with yaws.

Leprosy

There appear to be two types of bone involvement in leprosy, an osteitis, which involves 15% of the patients with bone destruction, and dissolution of the phalanges "twisted fingers" (Fig. 72).

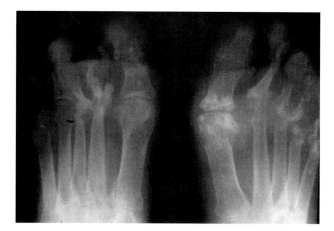

Figure 72 Leprosy. This is the appearance of "twisted toes" with central destruction and sclerosis of many of the MTP joints and toes.

The bone destruction is inclined to be central, with collapse of the fingers (Fig. 73A, B).

Nonspecific changes are more typical of leprosy and have been described in 50% of patients, and this includes neuropathic changes. Sometime ago, over 2000 patients with longstanding leprosy were reviewed, of whom 200 had bone changes. Resorption of the tufts occurred in 40%, resorption of the metatarsals in 50%, bone destruction in the toes in 14%, and bone destruction of the metatarsals in 17%. Twenty percent of the 200 patients had neuropathic arthropathy.

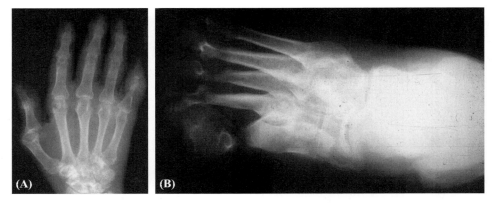

Figure 73 (**A, B**) Leprosy. Similar findings in the hand and foot of a different patient with leprosy.

Infections in Relationship to Specific Conditions

There are at least two situations where infection plays a major role in the patient's welfare, and although each of these are dealt with elsewhere in this text, I feel that these conditions should be dealt with separately here. The two conditions are diabetes and sickle-cell anemia.

Infection in Patients with Diabetes

The problem with the diagnosis of infection in a patient with diabetes is the complexity of the late stage of this condition. In a diabetic patient with essentially normal feet, the diagnosis of acute osteomyelitis is relatively easy, but, as the patients develop a polyneuropathy with loss of proprioception and pain sensation, the diabetic patient will have five radiological features, which when put together make the diagnosis of "diabetic foot." These are vascular calcification (medial wall); periosteal reaction running along the shafts of several metatarsals; patchy osteopenia, particularly in the metatarsal heads; a neuropathic joint, usually at the chopart (calcaneocuboid and talonavicular) or lisfranc level (tarsometatarsal); and finally, infection both in the soft tissues and in the underlying bones and joints. Thus, to find an acute osteomyelitis in a diabetic foot is often extremely difficult, plain films would show all the chronic changes and the disordered anatomic appearance of the bones. Most radionuclide studies would be hot due to the neuropathic changes in any case, and CT scanning is useless. On the other hand, ultrasound can be useful in finding soft-tissue abscesses, but is not particularly helpful in demonstrating acute osteomyelitis.

With the advent of MRI, a better way of assessing the osseous structures of the foot became available. In acute osteomyelitis, there is decreased bone marrow signal on the T1-weighted images of the involved bone, and on the fat-saturated T1 images, the same region becomes very high signal. So, in a patient who is otherwise normal, the MR diagnosis of acute osteomyelitis is relatively easy. In patients with all of the other conditions present, the diagnosis can be much more difficult, particularly if there is widespread cellulitis (low signal on T1, high signal on fat-saturated T1) or a complex neuropathic joint (Fig. 74A–D).

Neuropathic joints lead to stress phenomena in the surrounding bones (low signal on T1, and intermediate signal on fat-saturated T1); thus, the correct way to assess an MRI of the diabetic foot is to have the plain film beside you and compare the lateral plain film with the sagittal T1 images, compare bone for bone and joint for joint. Then compare both of these with the fat-saturated T1 sagittal images, looking for any areas of particularly high signal: fluid in a neuropathic or other joint, fluid around tendons, moderate high signal in bones adjacent to a neuropathic joint, and very high signal anywhere in any bone of the foot (Fig. 75A, B).

Once an area of very high signal is found on the sagittal view, confirm it on the axial and coronal views, and you have almost certainly found an area of acute osteomyelitis.

Unfortunately, it is not always this easy, since reactive bone marrow edema is commonly seen in association with both cellulitis and disordered joints, so secondary signs of osteomyelitis need to be looked for: a sinus tract, an actual break in the cortex, and the presence of an abscess (Figs. 76A–C and 77A–C).

As our experience with MR imaging in diabetic feet has increased, we are getting better at differentiating cellulitis, reactive bone edema, and osteomyelitis from

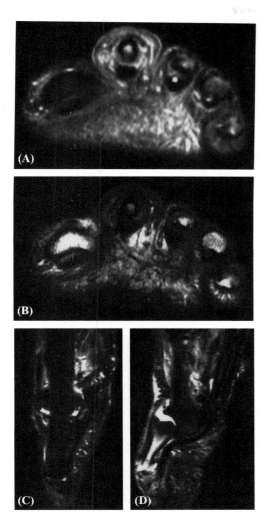

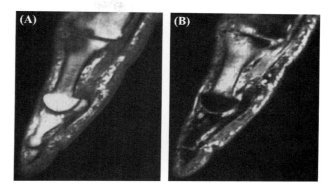

Figure 75 (**A**) Two sagittal images through the foot. The image shows normal marrow with high signal on PD. Note the discordant signal in the proximal end of the 1st metatarsal. (**B**) On this fat-saturated image, the 1st metatarsal signal has become high, signifying osteomyelitis.

Figure 74 (**A**) MRI in a foot of a diabetic patient with known infection. Axial fat-saturated sequence shows the patchy high signal in the soft tissue produced by cellulitis and the high signal in the shaft of the proximal phalanx of the 2nd toe typical of osteomyelitis. (**B**) MRI in a foot of a diabetic patient with known infection. Delayed T2 axial image shows the normal bone marrow signal in the 1st, 3rd, 4th, and 5th toes and the low signal in the 2nd toe typical of osteomyelitis. (**C**) MRI in a foot of a diabetic patient with known infection. Coronal fat-saturated image of the 1st toe that is normal. (**D**) MRI in a foot of a diabetic patient with known infection. Coronal fat-saturated image of the 2nd toe proximal phalanx that shows osteomyelitis. This was confirmed at biopsy.

each other. Plain X rays are about 40% sensitive, clinical examination 50% sensitive, bone scanning about 80% sensitive, and MR about 90% sensitive. If gadolinium is given, reactive edema shows little change in signal, whereas there is increased high signal in osteomyelitis, which increases MR sensitivity and accuracy up to about 95%. Secondary signs can also be very useful and if an ulcer, an abscess, or definitive cortical break is detected, osteomyelitis is more likely to occur. Remember that a "discordant" bone marrow signal is also a very useful MR sign of osteomyelitis.

Infection in Patients with Sickle-Cell Anemia

As has been eluded earlier, patients with sickle-cell anemia have a two to three times higher incidence of infection than people without it. This is partly because of the nature of the disease, partly due to the multiple infarcts that occur, and partly due to the recurrent bacteremia that these patients get from pulmonary, genitourinary tract, gastrointestinal tract, and other primary sites. Although it is well known that patients with sickle-cell anemia have a high incidence of *Salmonella* infections, in fact these only comprise 23% of the whole, 70% are still due to *Staphylococcus,* and the remaining 7% to other, more unusual organisms. Patients with sickle-cell anemia can get infections anywhere in their bodies, although disc-space infections and sacroiliac-joint infections appear to be particularly prevalent. However, long-bone infections are not uncommon, and this is probably because a young or, adolescent patient develops penetrating arteries through the cortex of their long bones secondary to the endosteal and periosteal infarctions. The diagnosis of infection in patients with sickle-cell anemia is mainly based on plain films and MRI, since Tc99m bone scans will be positive in any case because of the infarct. However, indium-111 white blood cell scanning or gallium may also be useful.

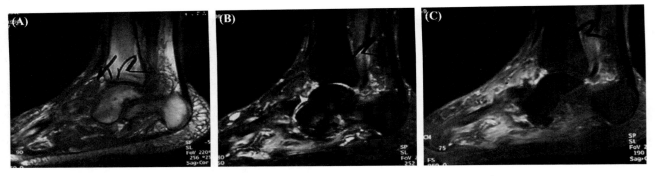

Figure 76 (**A**) Three sagittal MR images of the left foot of a young diabetic with a known Charcot joint. This is a PD image: note the patchy bone marrow abnormality in the talus and calcaneus. (**B**) Fat-saturated T2 image shows patchy high signal in the same bones. This represents reactive bone edema and not osteomyelitis. (**C**) A sagittal MR image of the left foot of a young diabetic with a known Charcot joint. Delayed T2 shows normal bone marrow signal in the bone but cellulitis in the soft tissues.

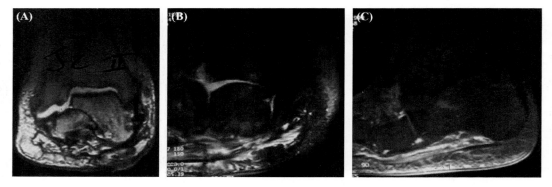

Figure 77 (**A**) Diabetic patient with suspected osteomyelitis but with a neuropathic ankle joint. Coronal PD image shows a large joint effusion but no MR evidence of osteomyelitis. (**B**) Diabetic patient with suspected osteomyelitis but with a Charcot ankle joint. Sagittal fat-saturated image shows a large joint effusion but no MR evidence of osteomyelitis. (**C**) Diabetic patient with suspected osteomyelitis but with a Charcot ankle joint. Sagittal delayed T2 image shows a large joint effusion as well as cellulitis but no MR evidence of osteomyelitis.

REFERENCES

1. Green NE, Beauchamp RD, Griffin PP. Primary subacute epiphyseal osteomyelitis. J Bone Joint Surg Am 1981; 63-A: 107–114.
2. Poyhia T, Azouz EM. MR imaging evaluation of subacute and chronic bone abscesses in children. Pediatr Radiol 2000; 30(11):763–768.
3. Mortensson W, Edeburn G, Fries M. Chronic recurrent multifocal osteomyelitis in children. A roentgenologic and scintigraphic investigation. Acta Radiol 1988; 29(5):565–570.
4. Sorensen TS, Hedeboe J, Christensen ER. Primary epiphyseal osteomyelitis in children. Report of three cases and review of literature. J Bone Joint Surg Br 1988; 70(5): 818–820.
5. Rathakrishnan V, Mohd TH. Osteo-articular tuberculosis. Skeletal Radiol 1989; 18(4):267–272.
6. Weaver P, Lifeso RM. The radiological diagnosis of tuberculosis of the adult spine. Skeletal Radiol 1984; 12(3): 178–186.
7. Rowe JG, Amadio PC, Edson RS. Sporotrichosis. Orthopedics 1989; 12(7):981–985.

4

Metabolic and Hematological Bone Disease

BASIC BONE METABOLISM

Inherently there are only three metabolic bone disorders, although of course there are in actuality many others. Osteoporosis, osteomalacia, and hyperparathyroidism (both primary and secondary) are the three major disorders that are usually discussed under the heading of metabolic bone disease. To understand these disorders more fully, some knowledge of basic bone metabolism is needed. When one sees a patient with thin bones, the correct term is "osteopenia," rather than osteoporosis. Osteopenia is a radiological finding, and osteoporosis is a disease (Fig. 1).

During metabolic adult life (from approximately 20 to 45 years in women and from 20 to 65 years in men) bone formation keeps up with bone resorption, and thus the skeleton is stable. However, in older people and in certain other metabolic situations, bone formation becomes less, whereas bone resorption remains normal. This is thought to be the primary problem in patients with osteoporosis.

Bone is formed on a collagen matrix. There are several disorders that can affect the matrix, and these are osteogenesis imperfecta, scurvy, and steroid therapy. Obviously, Cushing's disease will have the same effect as steroid therapy and diabetics can develop disorders of their collagen matrix. Each of these conditions has been associated with a situation described as exuberant callus formation. This can be seen following a fracture and is fairly characteristic of this group of diseases: i.e., osteogenesis imperfecta, scurvy, steroid therapy, Cushing's disease, and diabetes. Osteoblasts enter the collagen

matrix and start laying down osteoid. It is at this biochemical stage that it is thought that the osteoblasts stop forming bone in postmenopausal women, leading to postmenopausal osteoporosis, in some men (so-called senile or involutional osteoporosis), and in patients with severe calcium or protein deficiency. Osteoid itself can be affected by steroids and in some unusual forms of secondary osteomalacia as well as in some of the renal tubular disorders. At this stage the osteoid needs to be mineralized, and apart from some trace metals (such as zinc and magnesium), the body needs adequate supplies of both vitamin D and calcium to form mineralized bone from unmineralized osteoid. Thus, disorders of bone mineralization are caused primarily by lack of vitamin D, and this is known as osteomalacia in adults and rickets in children. The metabolic pathway of vitamin D will be discussed later. Once bone matures, it will eventually be resorbed by osteoclasts. An exaggeration of osteoclastic activity occurs both in primary and secondary hyperparathyroidism, as well as in disuse osteoporosis, thyrotoxicosis, and possibly in relationship to calcitonin.

OSTEOPOROSIS

Osteoporosis is a major health problem affecting over 20 million patients in the United States alone. There are 1.5 million fractures a year, and the estimated health care costs are over $3.8 billion a year (figures from 1998). In adult life, bone formation equals bone resorption; however, as we get older, bone formation decreases, whereas bone resorption remains the same, and this produces

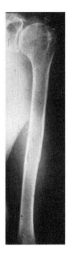

Figure 1 Osteopenia. This 99-year-old lady fell in her bath but did not sustain a fracture. This is her humerus that is osteopenic but probably normal for her age.

osteoporosis. Bone mineral, or bone density, increases up to age 25 or so in both sexes and then remains stable in men up to age 55 or 60, before it starts dropping at a rate of 0.3% to 0.5% a year. In women, bone mineral only remains stable up to age 40 or 45 (i.e., in the premenopausal or perimenopausal period), and then also starts dropping. However, it drops at a rate of 2% to 3% per year in postmenopausal women, finally flattening out at about age 60 to the same rate of decrease as is seen in men. It has been estimated that women lose 35% of their cortical bone and 50% of their trabecular bone over their lifetime. This compares to an estimated 22% loss of cortical bone and 35% of trabecular bone in men. Thus, the menopause seems to accelerate this bone loss at a rate of 10% to 15% for the appendicular skeleton and 15% to 20% for the axial skeleton. Various activities and mechanical conditions can also affect bone mineral. Hence, good nutrition with a daily calcium intake of over 800 mg a day is the recommended dose to maintain bone equilibrium in normal women, increasing up to 1500 mg/day in postmenopausal women. Exercise (particularly weight-bearing exercises) is important to maintain or increase bone mineral, whereas smoking and heavy drinking decrease bone mineral. However, other factors also contribute to this loss of bone. In a recent study of 180 patients with osteoporosis, 14% had a history of corticosteroid use, 9% of early menopause, 10% of vitamin D deficiency, 4% of chemotherapy, 4% malabsorption syndrome, and 4% hyperparathyroidism. It is also known that there is a familial tendency toward osteoporosis, with the short, slight, fairhaired English women being more predisposed to develop it. There are also at least two primary types of osteoporosis: the postmenopausal type and what is now being called the involutional type. In postmenopausal women, there is increased bone turnover with increasing resorption, but there is also some increased formation, but not enough to sustain bone mineral. On the other hand, in the involutional type, which is mainly seen in men, there is normal resorption, but decreased formation.

Before we get onto the treatment, it is also necessary to consider a relatively new concept: the fracture threshold. This is the absolute level of bone mineral below which there is an increasing risk of fracture, and it appears to be 1 g/cm^2 of bone mineral at any age. Thus, prevention of osteoporosis is much more important than treatment, since once the fracture threshold has been reached, it is much more difficult to increase the bone mineral to more than this absolute level rather than to slow or stop the loss of bone. Preventive measures include adequate weight-bearing exercise, adequate calcium, and a good diet. To this can be added estrogen, in postmenopausal women. Theoretically, it would also be useful in population groups to be able to increase the total bone mineral in young people by giving them adequate milk and exercise in adolescence, but few studies have addressed this side of the equation.

Treatment includes not only the use of calcium and estrogen but also other therapies. For actual stimulation of new bone, sodium fluoride, some of the new synthetic parathyroid hormones, and various growth factors have been used. For slowing the resorption, calcium, estrogen, calcitonin, some of the new biphosphonates (particularly editronate), anabolic steroids, calcitriol, and the newer vitamin D analogues can also be used. Some, if not all, of these drugs have adverse side effects, and certainly fluoride, calcitonin, and the biphosphonates need to be given in a cyclical fashion, i.e., three months on and three months off. All should be given with calcium supplementation, and fluoride also should have vitamin D supplementation. Prolonged estrogen therapy is associated with a mildly increased risk of both breast and cervical cancer. However, if given cyclically or in association with progesterone, there seems to be no adverse side effects other than the patient restarting her periods, which many older women find difficult. However, more information on the actual management of osteoporosis can be found elsewhere.

Radiographically, osteoporosis does not become apparent until at least 30% of bone mineral in a specific bone has been lost. The secondary trabeculae get resorbed first, so that the metaphyseal ends of long bones and the vertebral bodies are often the first areas to appear osteopenic. It is often difficult to assess osteopenia radiologically in fat or large patients because of the overlying soft-tissue bulk, but even in short, thin people, it can also be difficult to see early osteoporosis. However, once it has become established, osteoporosis is easier to diagnose. In the metaphyseal ends of long bones, there is a decrease in trabecular bone, with increasing osteopenia. In the vertebral bodies, the end plates become more obvious because of the loss of the internal vertebral trabecular bone. It is as though one has taken a sharp, white pencil and drawn a box representing the end plates surrounding the black vertebral body that is devoid of trabeculae. This is in comparison to both osteomalacia and hyperparathyroidism (primary or secondary) where the end plates become blurred as osteoporosis progresses. The vertebral trabeculae often become blurred and indistinct as well as increased in density.

As the disease progresses, vertebral compression fractures may occur, and these can involve the anterior aspect of the vertebral body, particularly in the thoracic spine, where osteoporosis produces "wedging," or may involve the horizontal upper and lower end plates of the vertebral body, producing a more central collapse with curved end plates and loss of height in the middle of the body. I usually refer to these as end-plate compression fractures (Fig. 2).

This can occur anywhere in the spine but is usually seen initially at the thoracolumbar junction and in the lumbar region rather than in the thoracic spine (Fig. 3).

There is a purely mechanical explanation for both of these appearances: The anterior wedging occurs because the weight-bearing aspect of the thoracic spine is situated more anteriorly than posteriorly, and as the kyphosis increases with age, so does the vertebral wedging. The central wedging occurs because the lumbar disc becomes relatively stronger than the vertebral body itself and encroaches on the end plates, slowly pushing then

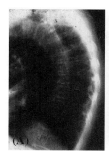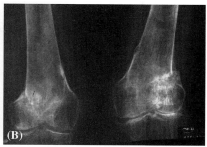

Figure 3   (A) Thoracic spine: Severe osteoporosis in a 52-year-old woman who had a surgical menopause at age 30 and received no replacement therapy. Note all the compression fractures with increased kyphosis. (B) Knees. Note there are fractures of both distal femurs, almost complete loss of trabecular bone, and marked thinning of the cortical bone.

inward. This has been called a "fish-mouth" or "codfish" vertebra.

To digress for a moment: Osteoporosis produces central wedging with the end plates gently collapsing, leaving a uniform curve from one corner of the vertebral body to the other. Sickle cell anemia produces a localized, rather straighter central collapse in a patient who has normal, or even increased bone mineral; this is known as an H-shaped vertebra. Multiple myeloma and metastases usually produce a more localized, jagged collapse, with the margins of the end plates remaining horizontal, although multiple myeloma can present with generalized osteoporosis rather than focal punched-out lesions, and so, in fact, may be indistinguishable from primary osteoporosis. Thus, if one sees a youngish male patient with quite severe osteopenia, multiple myeloma needs to be excluded. Finally, Schmörl's nodes represent a localized herniation of disc material through the vertebral end plate. These have clear-cut, sclerotic margins with an otherwise normal end plate and are fairly characteristic (see page 278).

Measurements of Bone Density

In the olden days, attempts to measure bone mineral density using X-rays were common. However, let me state again that it requires over 30% of the bone mineral to be lost before any evidence of osteoporosis becomes apparent on a radiograph. On the other hand, once established, it is possible to use a hand X-ray to follow the course of the disease by utilizing the metacarpal index. This is a measurement taken at the midpoint of the second or third metacarpal. A horizontal line is drawn across the bone from side to side. In a normal person, 40% of the bone is cortical and 55% is trabecular. Once osteoporosis is established, since the metacarpal is a tubular cortical

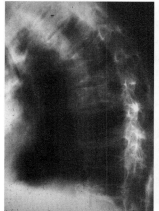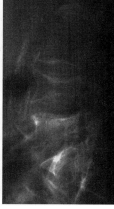

Figure 2   Thoracic spine. Osteoporosis in a 64-year-old postmenopausal woman with severe osteoporosis. Note all the compression fractures with wedging and end-plate fractures. Note the increased lordosis as well as some vertebral bodies that are sclerotic, indicating healing.

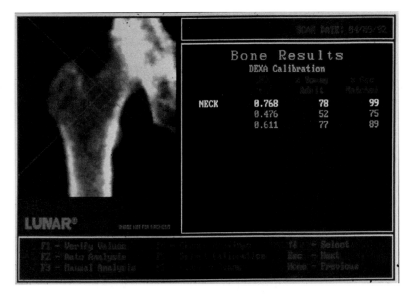

Figure 4 Bone mineral analysis of the proximal femur. Note that the computer gives you readouts of the femoral neck, Ward's triangle, and trochanteric region. *Source*: Courtesy of Lunar.

bone, there is loss of cortex, and thus the metacarpal index starts decreasing slowly as a result of endosteal resorption. Thus, it is possible to chart the course of osteoporosis and the patient's response to therapy using this index, although dual-energy X-ray photon absorptiometry (DEXA) scanning is more accurate and is now readily available. On the other hand, there have recently been a number of articles stating that there is no relationship between the metacarpal index and the presence of fractures of either the vertebral bodies or the proximal femur, and today most investigators would recommend DEXA scanning for the measurement of bone mineral.

Various attempts to measure the bone mineral density using physical methods have come and gone, although single-photon absorptiometry devices remain in widespread use in renal dialysis centers. These machines are inexpensive and easy to use; however, they really only measure the cortical bone mineral in the peripheral arm bones, so are of no use in the diagnosis and follow-up of patients with early osteoporosis. They are useful in following patients with hyperparathyroidism who may have marked subperiosteal resorption of bone. Double-photon absorptiometry is now obsolete. Some people are still using CT bone mineral measurement, which is very accurate and reproducible, and one is able to measure the bone mineral where one needs to, i.e., the central part of the vertebral body and proximal femur, for example, both of which are purely trabecular bone. However, I believe that the radiation dose is too high, being about 1 rad for a conventional CT scanner. There are some dedicated bone mineral CT scanners where the dose is said to have been reduced to about 400 milligray. This compares to a radi-

ation dose of less than 10 milligray in DEXA scanning. Finally, ultrasound is being increasingly used to assess bone mineral; the machines use sound waves and bounce these across the calcaneus. Early results appear promising, and this technique, of course, uses no x-radiation.

DEXA scanning, or DEXA, is the technique that is in widespread use today. It has a low radiation dose, is reliable and reproducible, and since it is basically a small, low-resolution X-ray machine, can measure the bone mineral where you want it to measure: vertebral body [anteroposterior (AP), lateral, cortical and trabecular, or just trabecular], upper femur (intertrochanteric, transcervical, or Ward's triangle), arm (cortical, midshaft, or trabecular at the distal metaphysis of the radius), or whole body (Figs. 4 and 5).

The precision for DEXA scanning also varies depending on the body part: AP vertebral body, 1%; lateral vertebral body, 2%; femur, 1% to 2%; and total body, less than 1% in accuracy. Most scans take less than 15 minutes, and they are easy for the patient to tolerate. The highest radiation dose is for the lateral lumbar region, and even this is only 8 milligray. The scan that takes the longest time is for the whole body, and with the new generation of scanners, this only takes about 10 minutes. DEXA scanners have been placed in most radiology departments but also are often found in screening clinics where a woman can have her mammogram and a bone mineral estimation done at the same time.

The definitions of normal bone mineral, osteopenia, and osteoporosis are based on populations of patients who have been studied by DEXA scanning. By definition, a normal bone mineral value is considered to be not more

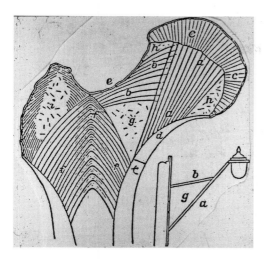

Figure 5 Diagram of Ward's triangle. In 1882, Ward used the analogy of a London street lamp to explain the triangular area of pure trabecular bone seen in the femoral neck lying between the femoral calcar (weight-bearing trabeculi) and the supporting trabeculi arching over the femoral neck.

than one standard deviation below the mean value of peak bone mass in young normal women. Osteopenia is where the bone mineral is between 1 and 2.5 standard deviations below the mean value of peak bone mass in young normal women. Osteoporosis is where the bone mineral is below 2.5 standard deviations mean value of peak bone mass in young normal women. Established osteoporosis is similar but occurs in the presence of fractures. People with this area of interest use two other definitions: T-scores and Z-scores. The T-score is the relationship to normal, young, adult females with mean scores given in standard deviations. The Z-score is the relationship to normal age- and sex-matched control subjects given in standard deviations. Finally, it is of interest to note that for each 10% decrease of bone mineral density, the fracture rate apparently doubles.

The next questions are—who should be scanned and how often? Most authorities suggest that bone mineral scans should be performed at the same time as routine, screening mammograms. Certainly, all women should have a screening bone mineral at or near the menopause. Women considered at high risk should also be scanned, i.e., those with positive family history, those having slight or slim build, those with a poor diet or malabsorption, those on steroids, and particularly those who had an early menopause. Follow-up scans should be performed semi-annually on those women who are being treated for osteoporosis and yearly for the rest of the population. If the bone mineral is normal at menopause, the recommended follow-up time for the bone mineral scan to be repeated is every two years.

PRIMARY CUSHING'S DISEASE AND STEROID THERAPY

Although the precise action of steroids on bone is still not fully understood, it is thought that they affect all the processes required for bone metabolism. It is known that they uncouple resorption formation rates. They also elevate parathyroid hormone levels due to decreased intestinal absorption of calcium. Steroids also affect osteoblast function directly, producing decreased bone formation, no doubt producing the osteoporosis that is seen in steroid therapy. There also appears to be a decrease in osteoid production. Thus, prolonged therapy with steroids produces generalized osteoporosis, and if this becomes severe, as can be seen in patients with rheumatoid arthritis or collagen vascular diseases who are on long-term steroid therapy, then increasing vertebral biconcavity and wedge fractures of the thoracic and lumbar vertebral bodies occur (Fig. 6).

However, steroids also affect the bone matrix, and thus one can see exuberant callus (Fig. 7) following fractures in these patients. Steroids also affect small vessels and can produce both infarcts, which are usually intramedullary and metaphyseal, as well as avascular necrosis, classically of the femoral head but also in the shoulder and knee, as well as elsewhere. This will be discussed further under "Avascular Necrosis." Prolonged steroid therapy can also lead to such clinical side effects as obesity, cardiomegaly and hypertension, premature vascular calcification, and an increased susceptibility to infection.

Primary Cushing's syndrome is quite rare. In fact, I have only seen three overt cases of the condition in the past 30 years. It usually occurs as a result of adrenal hyperplasia but may also be seen in association with

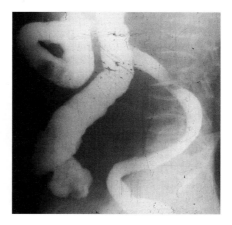

Figure 6 Effects of long-term steroid therapy. This 24-year-old man with ulcerative colitis had received corticosteroid enemas as well as steroids by mouth and has now developed severe osteoporosis.

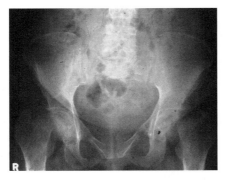

Figure 7 Primary Cushing's disease. This pelvis shows the classical radiological findings in this condition with obesity, osteoporosis, avascular necrosis of the right femoral head, and exuberant callus surrounding the ramal fractures also on the right.

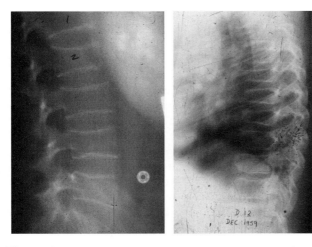

Figure 8 Primary Cushing's disease in two young patients. Both of these young female patients developed severe osteoporosis as a result of adrenal hyperplasia. Note the compression fractures that resolved once the adrenals had been removed.

adrenal adenomas, adrenal carcinomas, and with a number of pituitary tumors. Radiologically, patients with primary Cushing's syndrome have osteopenia with vertebral compression fractures and increased biconcavity, avascular necrosis, and exuberant callus. Anterior vertebral wedging can also be seen in children with primary Cushing's syndrome (Fig. 8).

As a footnote, local steroids also have some other side effects. If a patient has repeated injections of steroids into a joint, then joint destruction may result. This is due to the fact that corticosteroids destroy the hyaline cartilage by releasing hyaluronidase, which destroys the articular cartilage. Thus, the excess use of intra-articular steroids will affect the relevant joint and produce a neuropathic-type appearance on X-ray.

OSTEOMALACIA

To understand the radiographical appearance of osteomalacia, it is necessary to understand the metabolic pathway of vitamin D. Vitamin D is needed to mineralize the osteoid into mature bone. Thus, without an adequate supply of vitamin D, the osteoid fails to mineralize and osteomalacia occurs. We assimilate vitamin D from two chief sources—sunlight and our diets. Sunlight releases the precursor of vitamin D in the skin and this travels to the liver via the lymphatics, where it is stored as 25 hydroxycholecalciferol. Most green vegetables, milk, and dairy products contain vitamin D, and this gets absorbed from the small intestine (primarily the proximal part) and is transported to the liver via the lymphatics, where it also is stored as 25 hydroxycholecalciferol. When mature vitamin D is required, this travels to the kidneys, where it receives a second hydroxylation into vitamin D_3, i.e., 1.25 dihydroxycholecalciferol. There are complex feedback mechanisms between the kidneys, the liver, and the small intestine to ensure that an adequate supply of vitamin D_3 is on hand (usually about 18 months' supply) (Fig. 9).

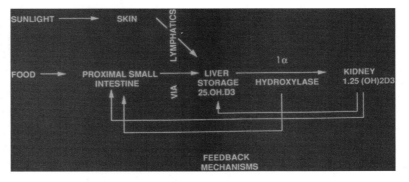

Figure 9 Metabolic pathways of vitamin D.

Table 1 Etiology of Osteomalacia

Dietary
  1. Vitamin D lack
Intestinal malabsorption
  1. Celiac disease
  2. Idiopathic steatorrhea
  3. Postgastrectomy
  4. Chronic cirrhosis
  5. Biliary rickets (congenital biliary obstruction)
  6. Inflammatory bowel disease
Renal diseases
  1. Fanconi syndrome
  2. Familial vitamin D-resistant osteomalacia
  3. Hyperchloremic renal acidosis
  4. Chronic acetozemic renal failure
Other
  1. Hypophosphatasemia
  2. Anticonvulsant therapy
  3. Hemangioendotheliomas

Osteomalacia can occur because of any number of causes (Table 1); however, the commonest cause of osteomalacia is seen histologically in association with renal bone disease. Probably the commonest cause of osteomalacia that we see radiologically is from profound liver disease such as primary biliary atresia, although one can occasionally see osteomalacia or rickets in patients on long-term anticonvulsant therapy and even more rarely in association with hemangioendotheliomas and other rare tumors.

The bone mineral in osteomalacia is decreased, but because of all the unmineralized osteoid, the trabecular pattern becomes disorganized, with the trabeculae themselves appearing blurred and indistinct, and the overall radiological density may actually appear increased rather than decreased. Thus, the bone mineral in osteomalacia may be decreased, increased, or mixed.

The radiological hallmark of osteomalacia is the presence of pseudofractures. These are usually bilateral and symmetrical and occur at right angles to the weight-bearing cortex of various bones, particularly the pubic and ischial rami, the femoral neck, the humeral neck, the scapuli, ribs, and clavicles, and more rarely the long bones (Figs. 10 and 11).

Initially there is a lucent line that looks like a true fracture but is, in fact, due to localized resorption of bone mineral, presumably along a stressline, hence the term "pseudofracture." Obviously these areas act as a point of weakness, and so true fractures can occur through the pseudofractures. Thus, obvious deformities of the pelvis and slippage of the femoral heads can occur, for example (Fig. 12).

Sometimes an attempt at healing will occur, and the margins of the pseudofracture become sclerotic. These were first described by a Viennese physician called Looser in 1910 and are primarily seen in long bones. They are now known as Looser zones (Fig. 10). The whole, full-blown appearance of osteomalacia, which one never sees today, was also described by Milkman and has been termed "Milkman's syndrome." This is not after the dairyman, but after a physician in the 1920s. The few cases of primary osteomalacia that one sees today are usually associated with somewhat dense bones with a blurred trabecular pattern and discrete pseudofractures often seen in the femoral necks running horizontally from the medial cortical margin.

RICKETS

When osteomalacia occurs in children, it is called rickets. Since mineralization of osteoid is an essential part of the growth of long bones, rickets manifests itself primarily in the growing ends of long bones with painful swelling of the knees and wrists particularly. Ultimately, the ends of the ribs will also swell (i.e., a rickety rosary), and the long bones will bow, particularly the femur and tibias.

Radiographically, the growth plate widens and becomes cup-shaped and frayed. The metaphysis itself expands (hence, the swelling that is seen clinically) (Fig. 13).

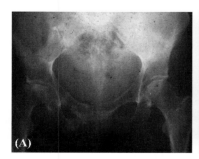
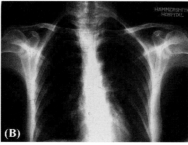
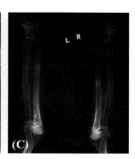

Figure 10 (**A**) Pelvis. Classical osteomalacia in a 45-year-old female missionary who did not take her vitamin D supplementation while in Africa. Note the pseudofractures of all four rami, the severe osteopenia, and irregular trabecular pattern as well as true fractures of both femoral necks. (**B**) Rib cage. Note the osteoporosis and pseudofractures of the upper ribs. (**C**) Looser zones with pseudofractures of both ulnars now with sclerotic margins, indicating healing.

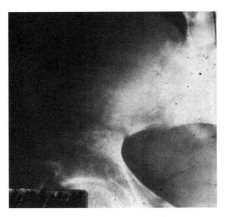

Figure 11 Pseudofractures with osteomalacia. This was a young female patient, with end-stage renal failure, who developed severe secondary osteomalacia.

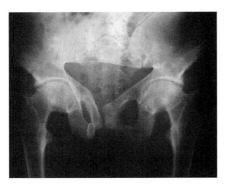

Figure 12 End result of pseudofractures following therapy. The patient has developed bilateral protrusio acetabuli with a "champagne glass" deformity of the pelvis typical of this condition. Bilateral protrusio only occurs as a result of osteomalacia or rheumatoid arthritis and occasionally in Paget's disease if this involves both sides of the pelvis.

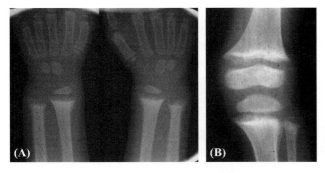

Figure 13 (A) Wrists. Classical Rickets. Note the osteopenia, the fraying and cupping of the metaphyseal ends of the long bone, and the widening of the growth plate and the metaphysis itself. The epiphysis is relatively spared. (B) Knee. Classical rickets in the same patient. Note the osteopenia, the fraying and cupping of the metaphyseal ends of the long bone, and the widening of the growth plate and the metaphysis itself. The epiphysis is relatively spared.

The overall skeletal appearance is of osteopenia, with blurred, irregular trabeculae, which conversely can produce both osteopenia or osteosclerosis in the skeleton. Treatment with vitamin D reverses and corrects all these deformities.

SCURVY

A lack of vitamin C results in scurvy, and this was well known to the 17th century sailors who would get petechiae and lose their teeth because of excessive bleeding. This was treated by providing them with limes, hence the term, "limey," for the British sailor. Vitamin C is needed for the integrity of the underlying collagen matrix of both blood vessels and the skeleton, and lack of vitamin C leads to increased capillary fragility, which produces the bleeding. Hence, exuberant callus can be seen following fractures. However, similar to a lack of vitamin D, scurvy manifests itself primarily at the growing ends of long bones in children, with a disorganized and fragmented growth plate. Although enough vitamin D and calcium is present, the matrix is weak and collapses. Thus, the radiological appearance of scurvy is quite characteristic, although very rare today (Fig. 14).

The growth plate is of normal width: there is a sclerotic line on the metaphyseal side (Frankels white line). Under this the bone fragments, and so a lucent line can be seen (the Trummerfeld zone of increased fragmentation, which is in reality a fracture). The white metaphyseal line is not firmly attached to either the epiphysis or to the metaphysis and frequently subluxes outward (Pelken's sign) and may carry a lucent area under it (corner sign) (Fig. 15).

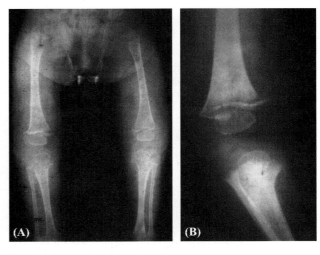

Figure 14 (A) Classical Scurvy. Knees in a nine-year-old. (B) Classical Scurvy. Right knee in a different and somewhat older patient. Note that the growth plate is of normal width and that the changes involve primarily the metaphyseal ends of the long bones as well as the epiphysis (contrast to Fig. 13).

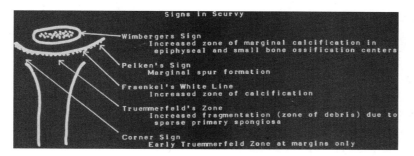

Figure 15 Diagram of the terminology associated with scurvy.

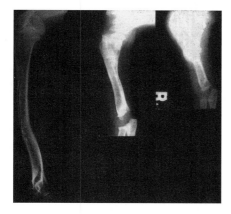

Figure 16 Scurvy. Series of X-rays of a child with treated scurvy who calcified a subperiosteal hematoma (right-hand image) that slowly resolved over time (middle and left-hand image).

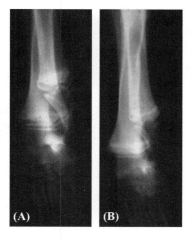

Figure 17 Great Dane with scurvy. (**A**) Note the Trummerfeld zone. (**B**) The Trummerfeld zone disappears following three weeks of therapy with vitamin C.

Similar rings of sclerotic bone with an underlying ring of lucency in the epiphysis are known as Wimberger's sign. Once vitamin C has been given, the growth plate will heal and the mineralization will return to normal.

However, not only do patients with scurvy have cutaneous petechiae, but they can also get large internal bleeds, including periosteal hematomas, which, following treatment, will also mineralize and heal and slowly regress over the course of several years (Fig. 16).

Recently we saw a Great Dane who was only fed dry dog food and not allowed outside to eat grass. He developed scurvy, which was treated with vitamin C, and his metaphyseals healed rapidly (Fig. 17).

PHOSPHATE ABNORMALITIES

There are basically two abnormalities of phosphate metabolism: namely, hyperphosphatasia and hypophosphatasia. Hyperphosphatasia is a familial condition with a high-to-very high alkaline phosphatase and has been called juvenile Paget's disease. It is extremely rare. On the other hand, hypophosphatasia has several forms, most of which are familial, and is associated with low alkaline phosphate, hypercalcemia, and radiologically with osteoporosis, rickets, or a mixture of the two. Hypophosphatemic rickets is one of these disorders and probably the commonest. This is a familial renal tubular disorder in which radiologically we see rickets.

Hypophosphatemic rickets is the commonest form of renal rickets and occurs as a sex-linked dominant in male patients only. Biochemically, there is hypophosphatemia, a decreased renal tubular resorption of phosphate, a low alkaline phosphate, and hypercalcemia. The X-rays are basically similar to those seen in rickets, with short stature, but there is also premature fusion of the epiphyses and, often, the bones have apparently increased bone density. The treatment for hypophosphatemic rickets is the use of vitamin D and oral phosphate (Fig. 18).

Hypophosphatasia, in general, comes in four forms: the infantile or congenital form, which is lethal and in which the baby is stillborn, apparently with no visualized ossified skeleton (Fig. 19).

There is a neonatal form in which the bones are short and bowed and have club-shaped ends (Fig. 20).

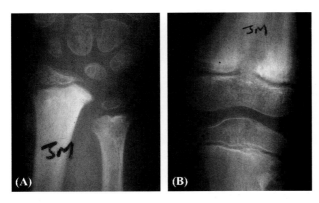

Figure 18 Wrist. Hypophosphatasia, adolescent type in a 12-year-old boy. (**A**) The growth plate is somewhat widened with irregular erosions reminiscent of rickets. (**B**) Knee. The growth plate is somewhat widened with irregular erosions reminiscent of rickets.

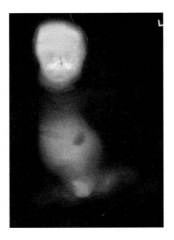

Figure 19 Hypophosphatasia neonatal type in a stillborn infant. Note the almost total lack of ossification in the skeleton and the opaque lungs.

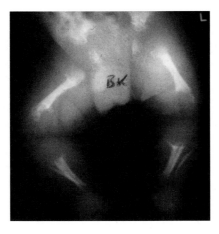

Figure 20 Hypophosphatasia infantile type. Note the irregular and widened ends of the long bones with soft tissue swelling around the knees, again reminiscent of rickets.

They are also of increased density, and this appears radiologically like a very severe case of rickets. The tarda adolescent form, which is the commonest form seen in hypophosphatemic rickets, is equivalent to mild rickets with curious "bites" taken out of the metaphyseal ends of the long bones (Fig. 18). Overall, the skeleton is usually osteopenic and fractures occur. The final form is a tarda form which occurs in adults and is equivalent to a mild type of osteomalacia with blurred, indistinct trabecular pattern, osteopenia, and, very rarely, pseudofractures.

On the other hand, primary hyperphosphatasia is a familial condition in which the radiographical appearance is equivalent to that seen in Paget's disease, hence its name, "juvenile Paget's disease," although it is not associated with the adult disease in anyway. Biochemically, there is an elevated alkaline phosphatase, and hyperphosphatasia occurs in the blood. The bones appear thick and expanded. They are often sclerotic but with large lytic areas. The long bones are bowed, and there is patchy osteoporosis (Fig. 21).

There is often loss of definition between the cancellous and the cortical bone. However, this condition is extremely rare and will not be seen by the average radiologist in practice.

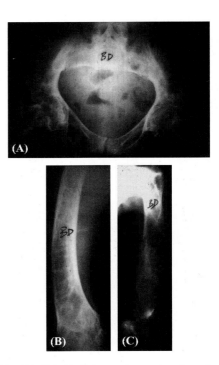

Figure 21 (**A**) Pelvis: Primary hyperphosphatasia (Juvenile Paget's disease). The bowing and widening of the long bones with mixed sclerosis and lucency of both flat and long bones are similar to that seen in adult Paget's disease except that this patient is only 21. (**B**) Femur. (**C**) Humerus.

Hyperparathyroidism

Although primary hyperparathyroidism is very rare, particularly in its later, well-developed stages, secondary hyperparathyroidism is actually quite common and occurs, as it does, fairly frequently in patients with end-stage renal disease. Von Recklinghausen was the first well-known person to describe the effects of hyperparathyroidism, and he named the condition "osteitis fibrosa et cystica." He was also the person to describe the localized cystic areas of resorption, which he called "brown tumors" because of their color. The radiological features of primary and secondary hyperparathyroidism are identical albeit occurring with a somewhat different frequency in the two conditions. Renal bone disease is a rather complex condition made up of osteoporosis, osteomalacia, as well as secondary hyperparathyroidism and will be considered separately after discussion of the classical findings seen in primary hyperparathyroidism. Elevation of the parathyroid hormone occurs as a result of a tumor or hyperplasia in one or more of the four parathyroid glands at the base of the neck (Figs. 22 and 23).

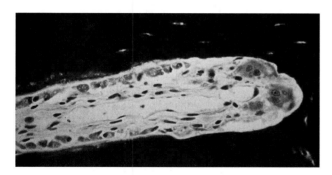

Figure 22 Normal cutting cone. There are multinucleate osteoclasts at the leading edge of this cutting cone trailing uninucleate osteoblasts along the edge of the cone laying down osteoid and new bone.

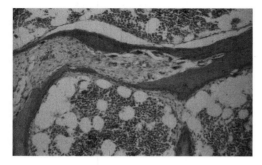

Figure 23 Cutting cone in hyperparathyroidism. There are multiple multinucleate osteoclasts but few osteoblasts. Fibrous tissue is laid down in lieu of osteoid, hence the term "osteoitis fibrosis et cystica."

This leads to bone resorption, predicated by the biochemical effect of the parathyroid hormone on the osteoclast. In a normal person, there is a balance between the calcium and phosphate levels in the blood. As the level of parathyroid hormone increases, the osteoclasts resorb more and more bone to elevate the calcium level. Thus, the phosphate level drops, and the bone resorption continues in an attempt to keep the calcium/phosphate balance intact. This bone resorption occurs both generally, where it will produce osteoporosis, as well as locally, at some very specific sites. In normal patients, as the osteoclasts resorb bone, osteoblasts will lay down new bone in what is called a "cutting cone," in which the two processes of resorption and new bone formation are closely integrated. In hyperparathyroidism, this process is disturbed, and osteoclastic resorption is followed by fibroblasts and not osteoblasts so that the bone is replaced by fibrous tissue, and hence, the old name of osteitis fibrosa et cystica. Tertiary hyperparathyroidism occurs when a patient with severe secondary hyperparathyroidism develops parathyroid adenomas that are often refractory to treatment.

Generalized loss of the secondary trabeculae caused by increasing levels of parathyroid hormone leads to generalized osteopenia. Interestingly, the trabecular pattern becomes blurred and even appears to have a somewhat increased density in hyperparathyroidism, so that it is often possible to separate pure osteoporosis (which presents with a clear-cut loss of bone, with the remaining trabeculae being clearly defined) from the osteopenia of hyperparathyroidism, where the trabeculae are blurred and the bone density can be greater than normal. However, the generalized osteopenia still leads to vertebral compression fractures as well as insufficiency fractures and ultimately to true fractures.

Localized loss of bone occurs at a number of specific sites, of which the best known is the so-called subperiosteal erosion seen in the fingers. In its early stages, this is best seen with high-resolution X-ray film, such as mammography film, and occurs characteristically on the radial aspect of the middle phalanx of the index and long fingers (Fig. 24).

It is also said that the tufts of the fingers show similar changes, but I find this area more difficult to assess (Fig. 25).

Once established, subperiosteal erosions can be seen all over the phalanges of the hands and the feet, and this is a pathognomonic sign of hyperparathyroidism, be it primary or secondary. No one understands why it is the radial aspect of the phalanges that get involved first, although many theories have been put forward.

Other characteristic sites for resorption are the ends of the clavicles, both distal (which is very characteristic) and proximal (which is much more difficult to see) (Figs. 26 and 27).

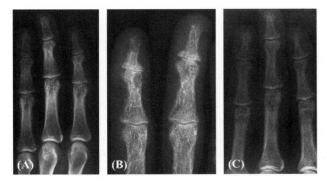

Figure 24 Subperiosteal erosions in the hands of three patients. (**A**) Secondary hyperparathyroidism due to renal failure. There are erosions of the radial aspect of the middle phalanx of the index and long fingers in all three patients. (**B**) Primary hyperparathyroidism in a 36-year-old female patient who also has small localized lucencies in a number of phalanges representing "brown tumors." (**C**) Another patient with renal failure and secondary hyperparathyroidism. Marked subperiosteal erosions throughout all the small bones of the hands as well as the tufts.

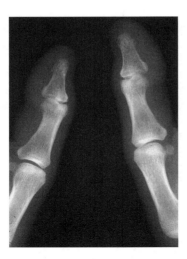

Figure 25 Subperiosteal erosions of the tufts of the thumbs seen in an advanced case of secondary hyperparathyroidism.

The differential diagnosis of resorption of the distal clavicle includes rheumatoid arthritis (where both the acromion and the clavicle become eroded) and recurrent subluxation as a result of trauma. However, it is only in hyperparathyroidism where the distal clavicle is resorbed alone, and there is no evidence of acromioclavicular separation, and there is no history of trauma. Similarly, erosions can be seen in the sacroiliac joints, (Fig. 28) usually bilaterally and symmetrically, involving both sides of the joint. The differential diagnosis here lies with the seronegative spondyloarthropathies, and the clinical history should be able to differentiate these conditions. In

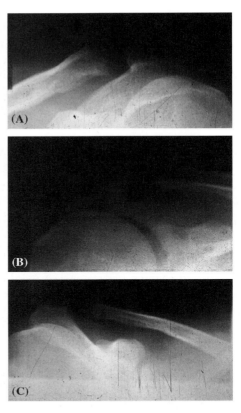

Figure 26 Erosions of the distal clavicle seen in three different patients with hyperparathyroidism. (**A**) Secondary to renal failure. Note the loss of the distal clavicle with sparing of the acromion in each case unlike in patients with rheumatoid arthritis who develop erosions of both acromion and clavicle. (**B**) Primary hyperparathyroidism. Note the loss of the distal clavicle with sparing of the acromion. (**C**) Another patient with secondary hyperparathyroidism due to renal failure. Note the loss of the distal clavicle with sparing of the acromion.

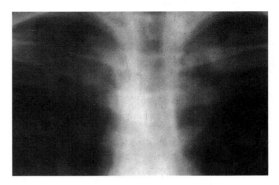

Figure 27 Erosions of the sternoclavicular joints: these are more difficult to see than those at the outer end of the clavicle although they occur in most patients with secondary hyperparathyroidism.

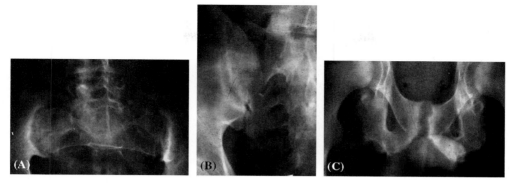

Figure 28 (**A**) Secondary hyperparathyroidism due to renal failure. Erosions of the sacroiliac joints and pelvis in three different patients. Both sides of the sacroiliac joints are involved with widening, erosions, irregularity, and some sclerosis. (**B**) Another patient with secondary hyperparathyroidism. Both sides of the sacroiliac joints are involved with widening, erosions, irregularity, and some sclerosis. (**C**) Patient with primary hyperparathyroidism. With erosions of the symphysis and rami.

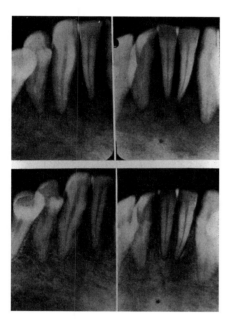

Figure 29 Loss of the lamina dura. Lower images show a normal lamina dura surrounding all the teeth; the upper images show loss of the lamina dura in a patient with primary hyperparathyroidism. *Source*: Courtesy of Jack Edeiken.

the skull, there is said to be erosion of the lamina dura around the pituitary fossa and around the roots of the teeth, so that hyperparathyroidism is actually a condition that a dentist might be able to pick up from X-ray (Fig. 29).

Once established, periosteal resorption can be seen anywhere in the skeleton, such as the rami of the pelvis and the metaphyseal ends of long bones (Fig. 30).

An unusual finding in hyperparathyroidism is increasing bone density or osteosclerosis rather than osteopenia, and this is seen in 3% to 5% of patients with primary hyperparathyroidism and in up to 30% of patients with secondary hyperparathyroidism (Figs. 31 and 32).

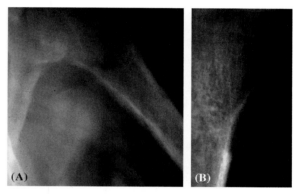

Figure 30 (**A**) Shoulder. Erosions elsewhere. This patient had severe tertiary hyperparathyroidism that was resistant to treatment and developed erosions all over her skeleton including her proximal tibia and proximal humerus. (**B**) Proximal tibia in the same patient.

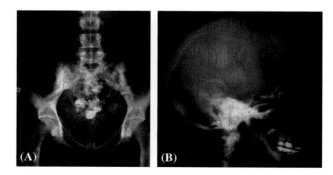

Figure 31 (**A**) Osteosclerosis in a 55-year-old female patient with primary hyperparathyroidism. Note that all the bones show increased density as well as a few punched out lucencies representing small "brown tumors." (**B**) Skull in the same patient with primary hyperparathyroidism showing generalized increase in bone density.

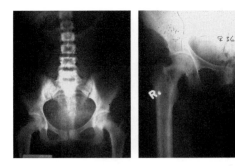

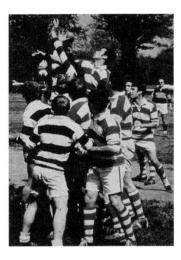

Figure 34 Rugger jerseys in action.

Figure 32 Osteosclerosis in two different patients with secondary hyperparathyroidism and renal failure. There is generalized increased density in the spine, pelvis, and proximal femurs of both patients. Note also the involvement of the sacroiliac joints, which is typical of hyperparathyroidism.

Once again, a number of theories have been advanced, but none seem to make much sense in a condition that is usually primarily destructive. This increased density can be seen in a generalized fashion or in local areas such as the skull, where a mixture of increased density and increased resorption leads to a patchy appearance of the calvarium, which is known as "salt-and-pepper" skull (Fig. 33).

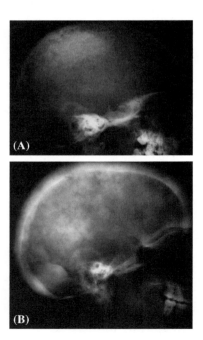

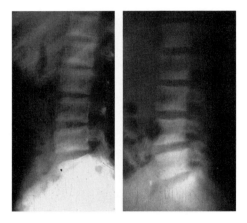

Figure 35 (**A**) Rugger jersey spine seen in two patients with secondary hyperparathyroidism. Note the sclerotic margins adjacent to both the upper and lower end plates of each vertebral body.

This is found almost equally in patients with primary and secondary hyperparathyroidism. On the other hand, the increased density seen adjacent to the vertebral end plates in the lower thoracic and the lumbar spine known as "rugger jersey" spine occurs almost exclusively in secondary hyperparathyroidism and renal bone disease, where it affects upward of 20% of patients who have osteosclerosis of any degree (Figs. 34 and 35).

In patients with renal failure, this localized increased density has been explained by the fact that many of these patients have osteomalacia and disordered bone metabolism, so that osteosclerosis is thought to represent increasing mineralization of otherwise abnormal osteoid. However, such an explanation for osteosclerosis in primary hyperparathyroidism does not hold true. Localized areas of resorption, which Von Recklinghausen described as "brown tumors" (because they were brown histologically),

Figure 33 (**A**) Primary hyperparathyroidism. The classical "salt-and-pepper" appearance is easier to see in this patient with primary hyperparathyroidism although both patients show areas resorption and new bone formation. (**B**) Secondary hyperparathyroidism. The classical "salt-and-pepper" appearance is easier to see in the patient with primary hyperparathyroidism although both patients show areas of resorption and new bone formation.

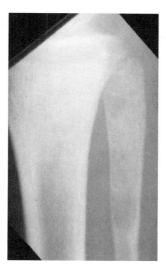

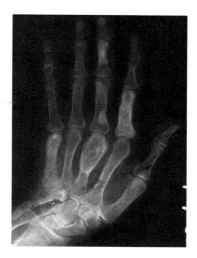

Figure 36 Brown tumor in primary hyperparathyroidism. There is a long well circumscribed lucency with a "ground-glass" appearance in the proximal fibula. It has a thin cortical margin and appears benign. This is a typical brown tumor but the differential diagnosis would include fibrous dysplasia and other benign tumors.

Figure 38 Brown tumor. Multiple brown tumors of different ages in a patient with long-standing primary hyperparathyroidism.

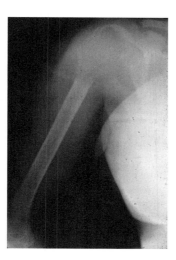

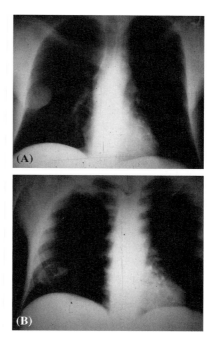

Figure 37 Brown tumor. This expansile destructive lesion of the proximal humerus appears almost malignant except that the patient had severe renal bone disease and this was a brown tumor.

occur in both primary and secondary hyperparathyroidism (Figs. 36 and 37).

They are common in the former, and can occur anywhere, but are most often seen in the metaphyseal ends of long bones and in the phalanges of the hands and feet (Fig. 38).

They can vary from being quite small to being 5 or 6 cm across. Brown tumors usually appear benign and are usually poorly marginated. They may even be expansile and so present an interesting differential diagnosis: if they are metaphyseal and central—unicameral bone cysts and

Figure 39 Brown tumor in a 32-year-old patient with generalized bone pain and fatigue. (**A**) Routine chest X-ray. (**B**) More penetrated film of the ribs show a well-circumscribed expansile lesion of the right eighth rib with some internal calcification. The generalized osteoporosis was initially not noted. However, at work-up the patient was found to have primary hyperparathyroidism.

fibrous dysplasia; if they are eccentric—giant-cell tumor and even osteogenic sarcoma; if they are marginated—fibrous dysplasia; if they are small and adjacent to a joint—geodes or subchondral cysts. Thus, it behooves one to keep the diagnosis of brown tumors in mind as part of the differential diagnosis of a solitary cystic lesion in bone in many differing situations (Fig. 39).

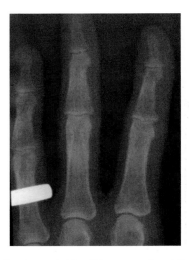

Figure 40 Erosive arthritis of hyperparathyroidism. There are marginal erosions of many of the interphalangeal joints. This was a young female patient with renal failure. In an older patient, the differential diagnosis would include erosive osteoarthritis.

Hyperparathyroidism also can be associated with a number of different types of arthritis. In fact, there is a specific form of erosive arthritis associated directly with hyperparathyroidism known as "erosive arthritis of hyperparathyroidism" (Fig. 40).

This involves the interphalangeal joints of the fingers and is seen in association with obvious subperiosteal resorption. The erosions are presumably due to synovial overgrowth. This is much more common in secondary than in primary hyperparathyroidism and is seen predominantly in females. Occasionally one will see larger erosions at the ends of long bones, such as the humeral head and femoral head, for example, but these are often caused by amyloidosis, which will be dealt with later on in this chapter. Other forms of arthritis seen in association with secondary hyperparathyroidism include gout and calcium pyrophosphate disease (or pseudogout). Obviously, patients with renal failure are unable to remove uric acid from the body, so an elevated serum uric acid level is to be expected. But, in fact, the incidence of gout in dialysis patients is only slightly above that of the normal population because of careful dialysis. The disease looks identical to that seen in patients with primary gout. Similarly, the calcium pyrophosphate disease (pseudogout) that occurs in renal dialysis patients resembles that seen in normal people, although the patients will be younger and their joints are frequently smaller, i.e., the hands and feet rather than the knees and shoulders.

Finally, with all the profound metabolic changes seen in hyperparathyroidism, soft-tissue calcification can occur, probably as a result of the elevated serum phosphate. Patients with primary hyperparathyroidism and

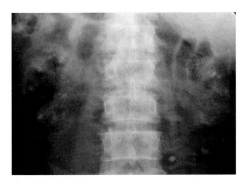

Figure 41 Nephrocalcinosis with multiple renal stones in a patient with primary hyperparathyroidism.

normal renal function will also develop renal stones (Fig. 41).

On the other hand, nephrocalcinosis can be seen in both primary and secondary hyperparathyroidism. Although both cortical and medullary nephrocalcinosis have been described, medullary nephrocalcinosis is probably the commonest form of interrenal calcification seen in association with primary hyperparathyroidism. Soft-tissue calcifications elsewhere have also been well described in both primary and secondary disease but are more common in secondary hyperparathyroidism. These calcifications appear almost tumoral, are usually rounded in shape, and I believe that they represent calcifying hematomas following trauma, since they usually appear adjacent to the hips and pelvis or to the shoulder girdle (Fig. 42).

They appear mainly in people on long-term dialysis in whom there are either low vitamin D levels or the calcium/phosphate balance has not been properly maintained. Finally, vascular calcification is also common but mainly occurs in secondary hyperparathyroidism frequently in association with diabetic renal failure (Fig. 43).

RENAL BONE DISEASE

All three of the primary metabolic bone abnormalities occur in renal bone disease: osteoporosis caused by low serum calcium, osteomalacia caused by vitamin D deficiency (brought on by the failure of the secondary stage of hydroxylation into 1.25 dihydroxycholecalciferol), and hyperparathyroidism due to increasing secretion of parathyroid hormone brought on by the decreasing serum calcium. Metabolically, the kidneys fail, so that phosphate excretion drops, and thus, the serum phosphate increases, causing the serum calcium to decrease. This will stimulate the parathyroid glands to secrete more parathyroid hormone and, ultimately, to undergo hyperplasia (this has been termed "tertiary hyperparathyroidism"). Occasionally a parathyroid adenoma will actually occur as a result of this condition, and this has been called quaternary

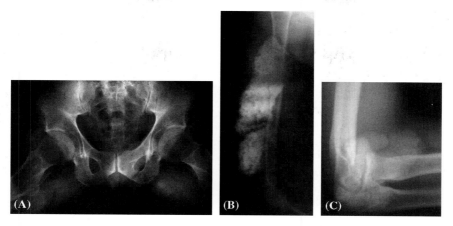

Figure 42 Tumoral calcinosis in three different patients. (**A**) This is a young female patient with tumoral calcinosis around both hip joints following minor trauma. (**B**) and (**C**) Tumoral calcinosis in two different patients around the distal humerus and around the elbow.

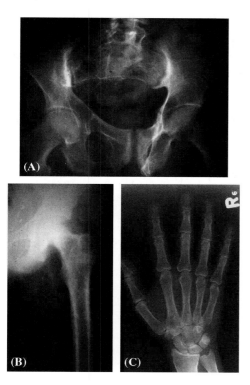

Figure 43 (**A**) Vascular calcification in three different patients. There is widespread vascular calcification in this young female patient with severe secondary hyperparathyroidism. Note the erosions of the sacroiliac joints and the symphysis pubis. (**B**) The upper leg in a young male patient with severe secondary hyperparathyroidism and marked vascular calcifications. (**C**) The hand in another young 25-year-old male patient with terminal renal failure secondary to diabetes with marked vascular calcification.

hyperparathyroidism. Of the three metabolic conditions seen in renal bone disease, osteomalacia is the most common, histologically affecting at least 80% of patients on

dialysis. On the other hand, secondary hyperparathyroidism is the one most commonly seen radiographically. To be honest, it is often difficult to ascertain how much of the osteopenia that one sees in these patients is due to osteoporosis, osteomalacia, or secondary hyperparathyroidism.

All the features of primary hyperparathyroidism occur in renal bone disease: subperiosteal erosion of the radial aspect of the middle phalanges of the index and middle fingers, of the tufts of the fingers, of the distal clavicles, of the sacroiliac joints, of the symphysis pubis, of the sternoclavicular joint, and elsewhere, if the disease is not managed properly. Nowadays, less than 5% of patients on chronic dialysis show any major changes of hyperparathyroidism, although, with the use of high-resolution radiographs (mammographic film, for example), discrete subperiosteal resorption in the phalanges can be seen in about 20%. The skull and jaw changes can also be seen in renal bone disease, and, in fact, the incidence of the so-called salt-and-pepper skull is probably higher than in primary hyperparathyroidism. This is almost certainly because the incidence of osteosclerosis is much higher in secondary hyperparathyroidism than in primary.

Osteosclerosis in renal bone disease occurs in 10% to 30% of patients, depending on the dialysis technique used. In fact, it may be the only manifestation of secondary hyperparathyroidism in young patients. Osteosclerosis may be generalized, with increased trabecular bone in the metaphyses and increasing cortical thickness in the long bones. However, more commonly, it affects the lumbar spine in a linear fashion, producing increased new bone adjacent to the vertebral end plates and an appearance known as a "rugger jersey" spine. There is sparing of the central part of the vertebral body, presumably because the nutrient canal (of Hahn) enters centrally and posteriorly. If the parathyroid glands are surgically removed, the osteosclerosis gradually disappears, suggesting that osteosclerosis is a manifestation of hyperparathyroidism. However, the truth is that we do not know what causes the osteosclerosis in renal bone disease and why it is relatively common.

Osteopenia does occur in a significant number of patients with renal failure, particularly in the elderly. It may be the result of osteoporosis, osteomalacia, or hyperparathyroidism, or various combinations of the three. Thus, there is an increasing incidence of fractures in these patients; both true fractures (caused by trauma on an already weakened bone) and insufficiency fractures. True fractures will occur at the usual sites: distal radius, proximal femur, and vertebral bodies. Insufficiency fractures will occur at the distal ends of the tibia and fibula, the pelvic rami, the sacrum, and in the ribs, causing distortion of the rib cage.

There are some other, rarer manifestations of renal bone disease, and one of these is periosteal new bone formation, which can be seen in the fingers and in the pelvis adjacent to the iliopectineal line. A possible cause of this could be scurvy, since dialysis successfully removes most of the serum ascorbic acid. Another finding in patients who have been on dialysis longer than eight years is amyloid deposition or amyloidosis. Primary amyloidosis is very rare, only occasionally involving the skeleton. However, secondary amyloidosis can be seen in renal failure and is becoming increasingly common because more and more patients are now surviving on long-term dialysis. In the olden days, secondary amyloidosis could be seen in patients with long-standing rheumatoid arthritis and other chronic diseases. Amyloidosis is a group of disorders, which are characterized by the deposition of amyloid proteins in various organs such as the heart and kidneys. In long-term dialysis patients, musculoskeletal involvement is usually associated with the deposition of β-2 macroglobulin in the synovium. In renal failure, amyloid deposition appears to occur either around large joints, i.e., the shoulders, knees, and wrists, or in the spine, where it produces a destructive spondyloarthropathy, particularly seen in the cervical region. Many patients will present with carpal tunnel syndrome, but what we see radiologically is large, synovially based cysts and erosions destroying the bone adjacent to the joint (Fig. 44).

We have recently seen a number of patients with involvement primarily of their shoulders, where the fact that the condition is bilateral and often fairly symmetrical excludes the other causes of synovial overgrowth, such as pigmented villonodular synovitis, hemophilia, and juvenile chronic arthritis, for example (Fig. 45).

The MR characteristics of amyloid are fairly unique: amyloid is characterized by a long T1 and a short T2 relaxation time giving a low signal on all sequences—T1W, T2W, and fat suppression, although there can be some mixed higher signal on the latter.

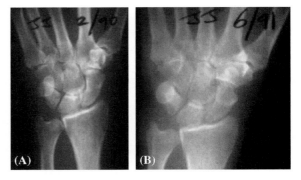

Figure 44 Progressive amyloidosis in a patient with renal failure on long term dialysis. (**A**) Initial Film. (**B**) Film taken 5 years later showing synovially based erosions involving many of the carpal bones.

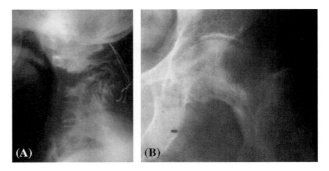

Figure 45 (**A**) Destructive spondyloarthropathy at C2/3/4 in another patient with amyloidosis secondary to renal failure. (**B**) Amyloid deposits of the hip in a different patient with a large lateral erosion involving the lateral side of the femoral neck.

One interesting historical aside is probably appropriate at this stage of the discussion on renal bone disease. As dialysis came into more widespread clinical use, we became aware of a very strange form of vitamin D-resistant rickets, which many patients developed.

In spite of the use of high doses of vitamin D, even of the newer, synthetic analogues, unmineralized osteoid built up on the margins of the bone, and histologically, there was a curious, green-colored layer between the osteoid and the bone. This was found to be due to aluminum, and after years of speculation and controversy, it was discovered that this came from both the water used in the dialysate and from the pipes of the dialysis machine itself. Once this was realized, dialysis machines were changed, and only purified water used for dialysis, so that the incidence of aluminum toxicity dropped to almost zero.

Hyperparathyroidism in Children

It is rare for primary hyperparathyroidism to appear in those aged less than 20, but there are many children who develop renal failure as a result of congenital disease. Although the classical subperiosteal erosions and other findings described above do occur in children, most of the damage is seen at the growth plates, where a mixture of rickets, scurvy, and hyperparathyroidism can be seen. Thus, the growth plate will be widened and frayed, the metaphyseal ends of the long bones will also widen and appear somewhat sclerotic, and the trabecular pattern will become blurred.

Children also have a higher incidence of generalized osteosclerosis. The skull in children with renal failure frequently has a "salt-and-pepper" appearance, with areas of sclerosis and areas of resorption. If the secondary hyperparathyroidism is not managed properly, the bones remain shorter than normal, the bone age is retarded, and the joints become clinically enlarged, similar to those seen in rickets.

Another complication of renal failure that can be seen in older children is slipped capital femoral epiphyses. For that matter, any major epiphysis can slip, and I have seen a child whose humeral epiphyses slipped. The slip occurs, presumably, as a result of the combination of rickets and hyperparathyroidism and is usually posteromedially in the hips. Slipped capital femoral epiphysis (SCFE) occurs in a number of other conditions including following trauma, postradiation, and in rickets and heavy metal poisoning. For a fuller explanation and description of SCFE, please see chapter 5. Other problems that have been described in children in renal failure include coxa vara, epiphysiolitis, and Legg-Calvé-Perthes disease, which is equivalent to avascular necrosis of the hip in children. As the child grows older, long-bone bowing becomes more apparent. However, nowadays, those dialysis centers that deal with children are well aware of these complex biochemical abnormalities and will manage the child's biochemical needs accordingly.

Hypoparathyroidism

Although this condition is not rare clinically, it has few radiographic changes. In congenital hypoparathyroidism, short metacarpals and metatarsals can be seen, and in fact premature closure of the epiphyses can occur. In adolescents and young adults, hyperostosis of the calvarium and the acetabular roof has been described. A curious dense line around the femoral condyles has also been described associated with dense, sclerotic bands at the growth plates and surrounding the margins of the vertebral body. However, all these are rare findings and difficult to confirm radiographically (Fig. 46).

The most common radiographic finding in hypoparathyroidism is intracranial calcifications, classically involving the basal ganglia, but soft-tissue calcifications have also been described involving the intraspinous ligaments (Fig. 47).

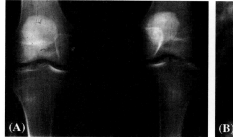
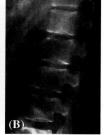

Figure 46 (**A**) Knee. Idiopathic hypoparathyroidism. These films purport to show increased density of the articular margins and growth plate remnants typical of this condition. (**B**) Lumbar Spine. Idiopathic hypoparathyroidism. These films purport to show increased density of the vertebral end plates typical of this condition.

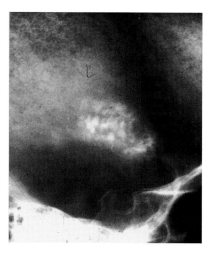

Figure 47 Hypoparathyroidism. Basal ganglia calcifications in another patient.

THYROID BONE DISEASE

Both hyperthyroidism and hypothyroidism cause bone changes. In hyperthyroidism, with the increased metabolic rate, the patients can develop osteoporosis, but this is only rarely seen radiographically.

On the other hand, hypothyroidism will often produce specific bone changes. In neonates and young children, cretinism, as it is also known, presents with a combination of retarded bone age, increasing density of long bones, and fragmentation of the femoral heads. The main findings are a delay in skeletal maturation associated with what appears to be an epiphyseal dysplasia, although there are often secondary metaphyseal changes also (Fig. 48).

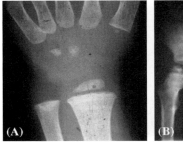
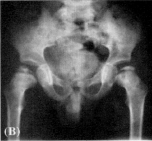

Figure 48 (**A**) Hand. Hypothyroidism (cretinism). The hand shows osteopenia, evidence of retarded bone age, and failure of maturation. The bone age is about two. (**B**) Pelvis. Hypothyroidism (cretinism) in the same five-year-old boy. AP view of the pelvis in the same child shows retarded bone age, sclerosis, and fragmentation of both femoral heads reminiscent of an epiphyseal dysplasia. *Abbreviation*: AP, anteroposterior.

It is said that there is a characteristic appearance to the pelvis, with squaring off of the iliac wings, as well as quite marked osteosclerosis. If the condition progresses, the vertebral bodies become somewhat longer and denser than usual. Platybasia of the base of the skull has also been described. Occasionally, children with hypothyroidism will develop abnormal calcifications in their vessels, soft tissues, and kidneys. Incidentally, the fragmentation of the femoral heads can easily be misdiagnosed as an epiphyseal dysplasia. So in children who have this finding, thyroid hormone levels need to be assessed. (See also the chapter "Congenital and Developmental Abnormalities.")

There is an extremely rare condition called thyroid acropachy. This occurs in patients who have been severely hyperthyroid but have had either a radionuclide ablation of the thyroid gland or the gland removed surgically and who are now profoundly hypothyroid. These patients develop pretibial myxedema on their anterior shins but may also develop a curious perpendicular periosteal reaction along the distal shaft of the first, second, and third metacarpals (Fig. 49).

This is fairly characteristic but is so rare that one will probably only find it in the books!

ACROMEGALY

If an excess of growth hormone occurs in a child, then gigantism occurs. This is extreme overgrowth of all the long bones, with delayed epiphyseal fusion, leading to a giant. This is a relatively rare situation. However, increased growth hormone in middle-aged patients is not uncommon, and this is known as acromegaly. Basically, anything that can overgrow, does. Thus, in the hand, there is increased thickness of both the bones and the soft

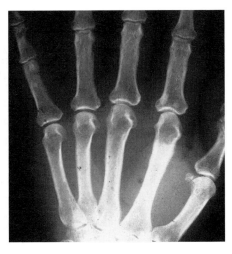

Figure 49 Thyroid acropachy. This hand X-ray shows the characteristic, but very rare finding of discrete perpendicular periosteal reaction along the distal shafts of the second and third metacarpals.

tissues. There is increased size of exostoses, and there is an overall increase in the thickness of the joint cartilage. The hand has been described as "spade-like" (Fig. 50).

The acromegalic hand has new bone laid down at the medial and lateral edges of the radius and ulna as well as at both ends of all the metacarpals and phalanges. The tufts widen and square off, and there is increase in the width of the joints, which is best seen at the metacarpophalangeal joint. There is also obvious increase in the thickness of the soft tissues, hence the term spade-like. Similarly, in the heel pads, there is increased thickness of the soft tissues. In a normal person, the heel pad measures

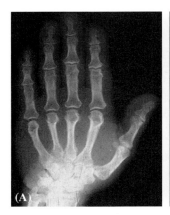
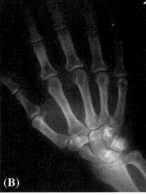

Figure 50 Acromegaly. (**A**) "Spade-like" hand in two different patients. Note the enlarged soft tissue and joint spaces as well as the overgrowth of the distal radius and ulna and tufts of the fingers. (**B**) Similar changes are present in this hand, but there is also "beaking" of the metacarpal heads.

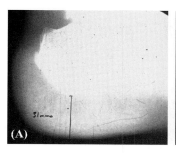
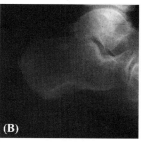

Figure 51 Acromegaly: Heel pads in two different patients. (**A**) There is marked thickening of the soft tissues of the heel pad. The width of the heel pad measured from the undersurface of the calcaneus down to the skin measures 31 mm (normal is under 21 mm in most adults. (**B**) This shows marked thickening of all the soft tissues, widening of the heel pad, and overgrowth at the insertion of the Achilles tendon and origin of the plantar fascia. Thus, acromegalics are considered to be "bone formers" and this is another example of an enthesopathy.

no more than 22 mm in a vertical line drawn from the most dependent part of the calcaneus down to the skin. In the majority of acromegalic patients, the heel pad usually measures over 25 mm (Fig. 51).

In the skull, there is increased thickness of the calvarium, as well as elongation and widening of the angle of the mandible, which in turn produces loss of the teeth. There is enlargement of the sinuses, particularly the frontal sinuses, which causes frontal "bossing." There is also often hyperostosis of the occipital protuberance (Fig. 52).

As a result of the pituitary adenoma, there is enlargement of the sella turcica. In the vertebral bodies, there is increased concavity of the posterior end plates, particularly in the lumbar region, due to overgrowth of the theca, which causes a characteristic appearance (Fig. 53).

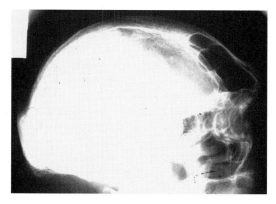

Figure 52 Acromegaly: Skull. There is thickening of the calvarium, marked enlargement of the frontal sinus, widening of the angle of the jaw, enlargement of the tongue, and overgrowth of the occipital protuburance. Note the enlargement of the sella turcica produced by the adenoma, which caused the patients acromegaly. This is the same patient as shown in Figure 50(**A**) and 51(**A**).

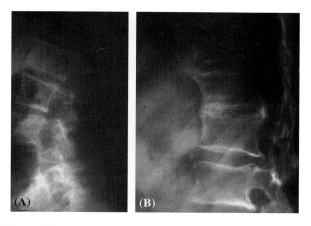

Figure 53 Acromegalic spine. Thoracolumbar spine in two different patients. (**A**) Shows the typical anterior overgrowth of the thoracic vertebral bodies as well as the increasing concavity of the posterior end-plates of the lumbar vertebral bodies caused by overgrowth of the theca. (**B**) Shows similar changes although with large overgrown anterior syndesmophytes again evidence of an enthesopathy.

The increased growth hormone also induces new bone formation anteriorly on the front of many of the vertebral bodies, particularly in the lower thoracic spine.

Finally, in acromegaly there is significant overgrowth of joint cartilage. Once we have reached maturity, there is as much hyaline cartilage as there is ever going to be. What occurs in acromegaly is that the elevated growth hormone promotes formation of fibrocartilage, which grows into the hyaline cartilage and causes actual widening of the joint space. In fact, the only cause of true widening of a joint cartilage space is acromegaly. Unfortunately, fibrocartilage is not as strong as hyaline cartilage and often patients with acromegaly will present with loss of joint cartilage and early degenerative arthritis (Figs. 54 and 55).

A recent study looked at 18 pelvic X-rays in acromegalics aged between 20 and 77 and compared them with 75 age- and sex-matched normal controls. They found that the normal width of the hip joint is from 3 to 5 mm, with a mean of 4 mm. In the acromegalic patients, the width varied from 4 to 10 mm, with a mean of 7.3 mm. However, actual widening of the joint space is not particularly common radiographically, since most patients go on to damage their articular cartilage and develop premature degenerative arthritis, particularly in weight-bearing joints.

DENSE BONES

There are two congenital causes of generalized dense bones, namely, osteopetrosis and Engelmann's disease, which are discussed in the chapter "Congenital and

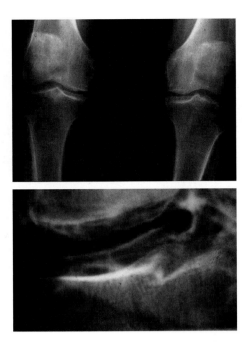

Figure 54 Plain films. Acromegalic knees. There is genuine thickening of the articular cartilage seen in both films. The plain film is taken standing and the widening of the joint cartilage space is only seen in acromegaly.

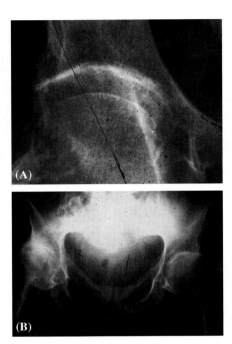

Figure 55 Acromegaly. Hips in two different patients. (**A**) Shows genuine widening of the right hip joint in a patient with well-established acromegaly who has not yet developed secondary degenerative arthritis. (**B**) AP Pelvis. This film was taken in a 44-year-old male with marked acromegaly and advanced degenerative change in his right hip with severe bony overgrowth. The left hip shows similar but not such advanced changes. Note the huge "acromegalic" osteophytes on the undersurface of both hip joints. *Abbreviation*: AP, anteroposterior.

Developmental Abnormalities." There are at least six other causes of generalized dense bones, of which two have already been discussed: hyperparathyroidism (mainly secondary and due to renal bone disease) and hypothyroidism. The other causes are primarily either hematological disorders (myelosclerosis, sickle cell anemia, thalassemia, and mastocytosis) or due to "poisons," such as fluoride, overdoses of vitamins A and D, heavy-metal poisoning, or due to congenital enzyme abnormalities, such as Gaucher's disease. There are three congenital causes of patchy, increased bone density: osteopathia striata, osteopoikilosis, and melorheostosis, which are also discussed in the chapter "Congenital and Developmental Abnormalities." There are at least five other causes of patchy, dense bones, including metastases, Paget's disease, sickle cell anemia, Gaucher's disease, and mastocytosis.

Let us begin with those hematological disorders, which produce skeletal manifestations.

Myelofibrosis and Myelosclerosis

Myelofibrosis is a not an uncommon disorder of older patients, usually male, which has an insidious onset. The bone marrow slowly undergoes fibrosis leading to a chronic iron-deficiency anemia. The condition progresses inexorably, and approximately 20% of the patients develop dense bones, which is usually generalized, involving primarily the axial skeleton, although it may be somewhat patchy in appearance. The dense bones are caused by osteoblasts migrating into the fibrosing marrow and laying down new bone, hence the term "myelosclerosis." It is seen primarily in those bones in which there is active bone marrow, i.e., the ribs and spine (Fig. 56).

The cortices become thickened, and there is loss of the intramedullary cavity. In the spine this can be generalized or localized to the vertebral end plates, producing a rugger-jersey spine appearance similar to that seen in secondary hyperparathyroidism. The calvarium of the skull becomes thickened and sclerotic. As the disease progresses, the patients develop an enlarged liver and spleen (Fig. 57).

Occasionally extramedullary hematopoiesis can be seen in the most severe cases, and this presents as large, paraspinal masses of metastatic bone marrow adjacent to the lower thoracic spine as well as in the lumbar region. Patients also develop cardiomegaly and congestive heart

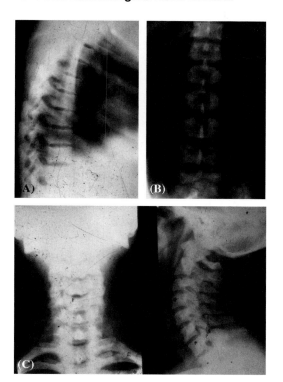

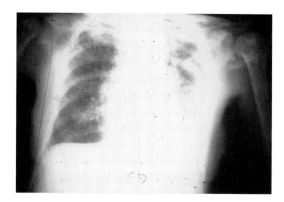

Figure 58 Myelofibrosis. Extramedullary hematopoiesis. Note the dense bones, enlarged heart, and soft tissue masses in the left hemithorax representing metastatic bone marrow deposits.

Figure 56 Myelofibrosis. (**A**) Spine in a 60-year-old male patient. Lateral thoracic spine showing marked increased bone mineral in all the visualized bones including the rib cage. (**B**) Myelofibrosis: AP lumbar spine in the same patient. (**C**) Cervical spine in the same patient. Note the generalized increased density in all the visualized bones. *Abbreviation*: AP, anteroposterior.

THALASSEMIA

There are at least three forms of thalassemia: (1) thalassemia major (Cooley's anemia); (2) thalassemia minor; and (3) thalassemia intermedia. Thalassemia major is the most severe example of marrow hyperplasia, associated with widened marrow cavities and coarse, linear trabeculae, as well as with osteopenia. In the skull there is a characteristic "hair-on-end" appearance, with thickening of the calvarium, but with loss of the outer diploic space (Fig. 59).

This can also be seen in other forms of hyperplastic anemia. Thalassemia in children will lead to growth retardation and premature fusion of epiphyses, often involving the outer half, leading to a tilt or angulation of the growth plate. Also in children with thalassemia, the sinuses fail to aerate, and the facial bones appear thickened. In the rib cage, there can be thickening of the ribs, as well as a "bone-within-a-bone" appearance. Finally, if the disease progresses far enough, hepatosplenomegaly occurs and extramedullary hematopoiesis can be seen.

OTHER ANEMIAS

Many severe anemias can lead to a hair-on-end appearance in the skull, including congenital nonspherocytic hemolytic anemia and severe, long-standing iron deficiency anemia. On the other hand, hereditary spherocytosis leads to generalized osteopenia in the skull and spine as well as thickening of the diploic space. Patients with hypoplastic anemia have few skeletal changes because they die young, although a triphalangeal thumb can be seen in carriers of the condition as well as in some of the patients. Thrombocytopenia with absent radii syndrome (TAR syndrome) presents with absent radii bilaterally, although the thumb is always present. They also have

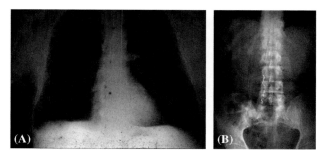

Figure 57 Myelofibrosis in a 74-year-old male patient. (**A**) Chest PA shows increased density in all of the visualized bones. (**B**) Myelofibrosis in a 74-year-old male patient. KUB showing dense bones and enlarged liver and spleen. *Abbreviations*: PA, posteroanterior; KUB, kidney, ureter, bladder.

failure, and often the chest X-ray is pathognomonic, with dense bones, an enlarged heart, extramedullary hematopoiesis, and evidence of cardiac failure (Fig. 58).

There are two forms of myelosclerosis: a benign one, which is commoner, and the malignant form, which is a precursor to a group of myeloleukemic disorders.

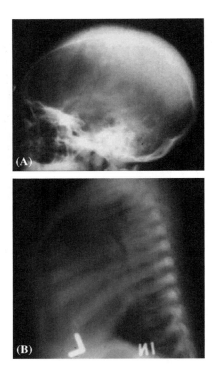

Figure 59 Thalassemia and other anemias. (**A**) Skull. The skull shows the characteristic "hair-on-end" appearance with marked thickening of the calvarium. (**B**) Lateral chest X-ray. Showing the expanded ribs and abnormal trabecular pattern.

a severe anemia, which is present from birth, although it rarely kills the patient. Finally, Fanconi's aplastic anemia is associated with pancytopenia and multiple congenital anomalies, including radial club hand and hypoplastic phalanges on the radial side of the arm. These changes may be bilateral or unilateral, and the children usually die of the anemia within the first three years of life (Fig. 60).

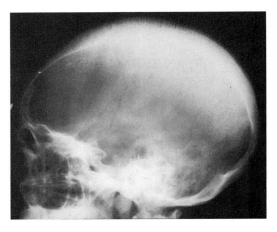

Figure 60 Hemolytic anemia with generalized thickening of the calvarium.

SYSTEMIC MASTOCYTOSIS

Systemic mastocytosis is a disease of unknown etiology characterized by the abnormal accumulation of mast cells in the skin and other organs—gastrointestinal tract, liver, spleen, lymph nodes, and bones. The age range is 30–90 (median 60), and it has an equal sex incidence. The signs and symptoms include fatigue, night sweats, and weakness (60%), diarrhea (40%), arthralgias and bone pain (20%), enlarged spleen and liver (60%), and skin lesions (60%). The patient suffers systemic effects due to the release of vasoactive substances (probably histamine), leading to flushing, headaches, bronchospasm, and diarrhea. In the skeleton, 50% to 70% of the patients have bone changes, of whom half have generalized and one-third have patchy osteosclerosis (Fig. 61).

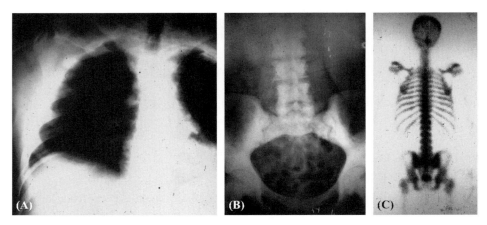

Figure 61 Mastocystosis in a 46 year-old-male patient. (**A**) Chest X-ray shows patchy increased density of many of the bones, particularly of the ribs. (**B**) KUB shows generalized increased bone density and enlarged liver and spleen. (**C**) Mastocystosis in a 46-year-old male patient. Bone scan: "super scan" with no obvious excretion in the kidneys or the bladder. *Abbreviation*: KUB, kidney, ureter, bladder.

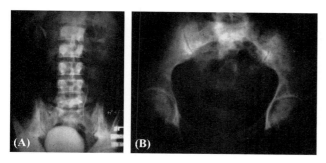

Figure 62 Mastocytosis in another patient showing patchy increased uptake in the skeleton. (**A**) KUB during an IVP. (**B**) Pelvis in the same patient with changes similar to those seen in Paget's disease. *Abbreviations*: KUB, kidney, ureter, bladder; IVP, intravenous pyelogram.

The remainder has mixed sclerotic and lytic areas. Bone scans may be normal, with patchy uptake of isotope or appear as a superscan, i.e., all the technetium is taken up by the skeleton and is not excreted, so that the kidneys and bladder are not visible on the bone scan (Fig. 61).

Systemic mastocytosis is associated with urticaria pigmentosum, and there are at least five syndromes associated with the combination. If a patient presents with urticaria pigmentosum, but no other manifestations of systemic mastocytosis, there is a 10% risk of systemic involvement. Of the patients with systemic disease, the five-year survival rate is 70%, with 30% who die of some malignant complication, such as leukemia, lymphoma, or neoplasms elsewhere. Once the systemic manifestations occur, the treatment varies from antihistamines, steroids, and chemotherapy. As has been mentioned, the bone changes may be generalized or patchy. If generalized, they resemble those seen in myelosclerosis. If patchy, they resemble those seen with blastic metastases or in Paget's disease (Fig. 62).

The bone scan will usually be helpful, but a normal, alkaline phosphatase will exclude Paget's disease, and an enlarged liver and spleen will usually tip the diagnosis toward mastocytosis.

SICKLE CELL ANEMIA

Sickle cell anemia originated in Africa and occurs almost exclusively in the black population. There are a number of forms, of which sickle cell S disease is the commonest, but there is also sickle cell C disease, sickle cell E disease, sickle cell trait, and sickle cell thalassemia. The main defect in sickle cell disease is with the red blood cell, which tends to become "S" shaped when hypoxic, and hence, block small blood vessels and cause infarcts. These can occur almost anywhere in the body but tend to be in the lungs, abdomen, and skeleton.

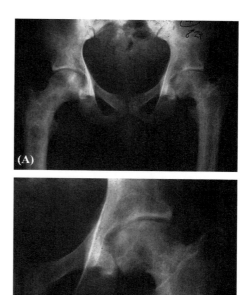

Figure 63 Sickle cell anemia. Two views of the pelvis in the same 25-year-old male patient. (**A**) Pelvis shows patchy increased density typical of widespread infarcts as well as avascular necrosis of the left femoral head with collapse. (**B**) Close-up of the left hip, which also shows intramedullary endosteal new bone formation in the femoral shaft as well as collapse of the femoral head secondary to avascular necrosis.

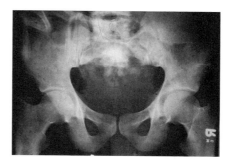

Figure 64 Sickle cell anemia in another young male patient with patchy but widespread increased bone density due to multiple infarcts.

In the skeleton, the infarcts produce increased density, mainly due to the reparative influence of osteoblastic activity. However, impaction and collapse also lead to increased density. Thus, the bones may become dense, either in a generalized or in a localized fashion. Bone infarcts, bone-within-a-bone, as well as endosteal new bone formation may all be seen (Figs. 63 and 64).

Many of these patients develop a hair-on-end appearance of the skull. Endosteal new bone formation is a very useful sign of increased intramedullary bone marrow

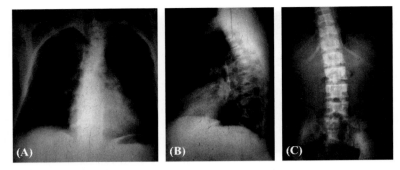

Figure 65 Sickle cell anemia. (A) Chest PA showing cardiomegaly, basilar pulmonary infarcts, and patchy increased density in the bones. (B) Lateral X-ray shows the typical "H"-shaped vertebral bodies with classical central defects. (C) KUB in the same patient showing the typical "H"-shaped end-plate defects as well as patchy increased density of all the bones and hepatosplenomegaly. *Abbreviation*: KUB, kidney, ureter, bladder.

activity and can be seen particularly in diseases that cause intramedullary infarcts, for example, sickle cell anemia, Gaucher's disease, and decompression disease but can also be in association with primary bone marrow diseases, such as eosinophilic granuloma, leukemia, lymphoma and in chronic infection. Patients with sickle cell anemia have a high incidence of avascular necrosis, particularly of their femoral heads, and this is discussed in more detail on pages 24 and 57. The incidence of avascular necrosis in patients with sickle cell anemia is about 10% overall and is seen more commonly in those patients with sickle cell S disease. In the spine, central infarcts lead to the characteristic, so-called "H"-shaped vertebra, with localized central collapse of many of the vertebral end plates, which appear sclerotic (Fig. 65).

Often the defects look more like Schmörl's nodes, except that the infarcts in sickle cell anemia are central and have sclerotic margins, whereas the defects seen in Schmörl's nodes are more peripheral, usually smaller, less sclerotic, and less well defined. In the ankle and shoulder of a child, infarcts can lead to premature fusion of part of the end plate, leading to a slant or tilt. In the ankle, this is known as a tibiotalar tilt. Because of the widespread nature of the disease, there is a high incidence of musculoskeletal infections, including septic arthritis (occasionally seen in the sacroiliac joints) and osteomyelitis. Although every medical student knows that patients with sickle cell anemia have a high incidence of salmonella infection, the commonest organism found in these patients is still staphylococcus, accounting for over 70% of all musculoskeletal infections, whereas salmonella accounts for only 20% to 25%. Finally, in neonates with sickle cell anemia, a curious syndrome can be seen in the extremities known as the "hand-foot" syndrome (Fig. 66).

This represents a widespread dactylitis and is due to a combination of infarcts and infection. Although rare, this is important to remember because the differential diagnosis includes tuberculous dactylitis and congenital syphilis.

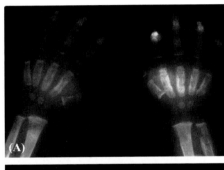
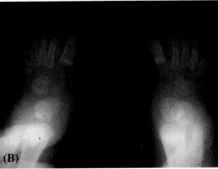

Figure 66 Sickle cell anemia. Hand foot syndrome. (A) Hands showing widespread dactylitis. (B) Feet in the same infant showing widespread dactylitis.

PATCHY DENSE BONE DISEASE

This heading is perhaps better than "others," but there are always a number of conditions, which do not readily fit anywhere else. Incidentally, I have always found it intriguing that two of the more common diseases seen in the skeleton, Paget's disease and diffuse idiopathic skeletal hyperostosis (DISH), usually get classified under "others."

Paget's Disease

Sir James Paget described a man with a bowed tibia, an enlarging skull, and "arthritis" in his hip in 1876, and the disease was named after him shortly thereafter. In fact, it was quite common in England at the time and, for that matter, it still is. It is also seen in those member states of the old British Commonwealth where the British went or were sent to, like the convicts who were sent to Australia, where Paget's disease is very common. Similarly, Paget's disease is not uncommon in Scandinavia and is also seen in places where Scandinavian immigrants came over to the United States, including the midwest and Canada. Europeans also populated the east coast of the United States, so Paget's disease is quite common there as well. The majority of patients who develop certain complications of Paget's disease such as soft-tissue granulomas and malignant bone tumors can be traced to one family who originated from Avelino in Italy. But as one goes toward the equator, Paget's disease becomes increasingly rare, so that it is only rarely seen in southern Europe, Africa, or in Central and South America. Although the etiology is unknown, it is once again being postulated that Paget's disease is due to a slow virus. In those places where it does occur, Paget's disease is seen in approximately 5% of the population over 50. It has an equal sex ratio and is extremely rare below the age of 45. The so-called juvenile Paget's disease is, in fact, hyperphosphatasia, which is now known to be caused by a renal tubular disorder and is not related to adult Paget's disease.

The train of histological events in Paget's disease is disorganized osteoclasis, causing bone resorption, followed eventually by disordered osteoblastic changes. Histologists refer to this as "metabolic madness," and the characteristic histological finding is of a "mosaic pattern," which represents the disordered nature of the condition. Radiologically, one sees a lucent area preceding a disorganized blastic or sclerotic area, with disorderly trabeculae running this way and that. The bone becomes extensively remodeled, enlarges in width, and develops thickened, but disorganized, cortices. This is associated with the hallmark of Paget's disease, which is a high-to-very high alkaline phosphatase—300 to 3000 international units (normal: <100).

The bones involved in Paget's disease, in order of frequency, are the pelvis (and proximal femur), the spine, and the skull. However, Paget's disease has been described in every bone in the body, including the ossicles of the ear. Incidentally, it is inclined to be purely blastic in the peripheral skeleton. In long bones, Paget's disease characteristically starts in the epiphysis and spreads down through the metaphysis into the shaft of the bone. However, there is one rather common and well-known exception, and that is the tibia, where Paget's disease seems to start in the middiaphysis and spreads proximally (Fig. 67).

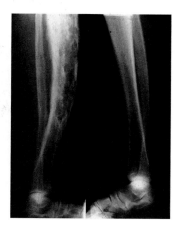

Figure 67   Paget's disease: tibia. This film shows the bowing and widening as well as the classical "candle-flame" in the midshaft of the right tibia. The left tibia is normal and shown for comparison.

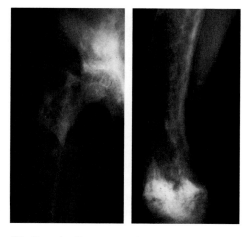

Figure 68   Paget's disease: the femur. These two films show the characteristic disorganization of both trabacular and cortical bone caused by Paget's disease. Note the anterior bowing as well as the widening of the distal femur extending down into the epiphysis, which is sclerotic.

As I stated earlier, in long bones we initially see a lytic area that can have a triangular configuration, starting just under the cortex and leading to a "candle-flame" appearance. Once established, patchy and disorganized new bone formation occurs, leading to a mixed sclerotic and lytic pattern, with widening of the bone, thickening of the cortices, bowing of the bone, and a disorganized trabecular pattern. Increased cortical striations may be seen in the cortex of long bones (Fig. 68).

In the pelvis, Paget's disease is usually mainly blastic, with increased bone density and cortical thickening as well as having a disorganized trabecular pattern (Fig. 69).

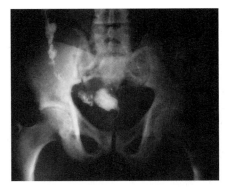

Figure 69 Paget's disease: pelvis. This shows the marked sclerosis of the right hemipelvis with cortical thickening particularly well seen in the ramal region and in the iliopectineal line. However, although the proximal femurs are not involved, the left hemipelvis also shows early Pagetoid changes.

The margins of the iliac bone become involved first, with increasing sclerosis adjacent to the sacroiliac joint and running along the iliopectineal line, which become thickened in 75% of patients with pelvic Paget's disease. Then the ischial and pubic bones become dense and widened (compare them to the uninvolved side), and the disease spreads up the outer edges of the iliac bone with thickening and increasing density of the iliac crest, anterior/superior iliac spine, anterior/inferior iliac spine, and roof of the acetabulum. Characteristically, Paget's disease of the pelvis involves only one side, but obviously both sides may become involved, either together or at separate times. Frequently, one or the other femoral head becomes involved, usually in the blastic phase, and with the disorganized bone matrix, the patient will often develop a distorted acetabulum, leading to the arthritis that Sir James Paget described (Fig. 70).

In reality, Paget's disease is a bone disorder and not a form of arthritis. Incidentally, total hip replacements in patients with Paget's disease do not do well and frequently loosen because of the progressive nature of the condition.

In the spine, the involvement is usually in the lumbar region, although Paget's disease may involve any part of the spine from the atlas and odontoid down to the coccyx. Classically, Paget's disease involves the body and the pedicles as well as the posterior elements. On a lateral view of the involved vertebral body, there is often a "bone-within-a-bone" appearance, which is known as a "picture frame" vertebral body. The differential diagnosis of a solitary, dense vertebral body (or "ivory" vertebra) includes Paget's disease, hemangioma, lymphoma, metastases, and infection. Of these, involvement of the posterior elements is unique to Paget's disease (Fig. 71).

In the skull, Paget's disease has two distinct appearances: in the initial osteoclastic stage a lucent band

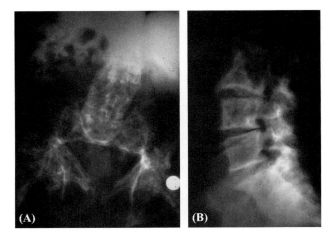

Figure 70 Paget's disease: lumbar spine and pelvis. There is marked involvement of all visualized bones. (**A**) AP view shows the deformity of the pelvis with bilateral protrusio as well as involvement of the left femoral head and neck, causing arthritis in both hip joints. (**B**) Lateral view of the lumbar spine. All the vertebral bodies are involved including L2/3, which was surgically fused years before. L4 shows the characteristic "window frame" or "picture frame" appearance. *Abbreviation*: AP, anteroposterior.

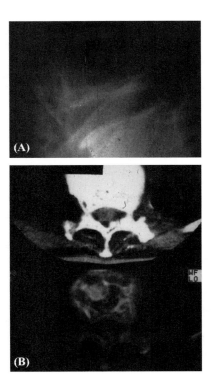

Figure 71 Paget's disease: lumbar spine. (**A**) Lateral view shows the typical "picture frame" appearance. (**B**) CT scan through L5 shows the remarkable disorganization of the trabeculae pattern with both lytic and sclerotic areas, overall enlargement of the bone, cortical thickening, and involvement of the posterior elements that is characteristic of Paget's disease.

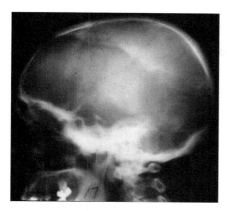

Figure 72 Paget's disease. Lateral skull with osteoporosis circumscripta. There is a lucent band apparently running across the lower half of the calavrium.

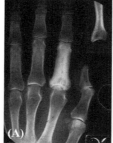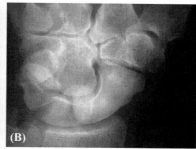

Figure 74 (**A**) Paget's disease of two peripheral bones in two different patients. The proximal phalanx of the index finger is noted to be sclerotic and widened as well as thickened. This was picked up serendipitously on a bone scan. (**B**) Paget's disease in another patient, the scaphoid is somewhat enlarged and sclerotic. This occurred in a patient with widespread polyostotic Paget's disease.

appears around the calvarium, which is known as osteoporosis circumscripta (Fig. 72).

However, this is nearly always associated with blastic changes in the base of the skull and occasionally with platybasia and basilar invagination. Hence, osteoporosis circumscripta is fairly characteristic of early Paget's disease. In the later osteoblastic stage, the metabolic madness has taken over and the calvarium becomes thickened with a mixed and disorganized blastic and lytic pattern. Usually the base of the skull is also involved in these patients, so that the differential diagnosis between Paget's disease and metastatic disease from breast carcinoma, for example, is easy, since metastases will not usually involve the base of the skull (Fig. 73).

Incidentally, patients with Paget's disease of the skull are prone to many complications, and apart from platybasia and basilar invagination, the slow encroachment on the eighth cranial nerve leads to deafness. The marked thickening of the skull is equivalent to an arteriovenous

shunt, and the constant rushing sound leads some patients with untreated Paget's disease of the skull to commit suicide. Other nerve roots may also get involved.

In the peripheral skeleton, Paget's disease is usually found serendipitously when a hot spot is discovered coincidentally on a bone scan. Paget's disease usually involves the whole bone, which seems dense and somewhat enlarged when compared with the opposite side (Fig. 74).

We have already discussed some of the complications of Paget's disease, but only about 10% of patients with Paget's disease have any symptoms at all, and, for example, Paget's disease is often picked up serendipitously during an intravenous pyelogram or upper gastrointestinal series, for example. The commonest complication is bone pain, which occurs in 5% to 10% of patients with Paget's disease and is usually manageable with calcitonin therapy or the use of some of the milder chemotherapeutic drugs. Obviously, with all of the remodeling, bowing occurs and fractures are not uncommon. These may be incremental, involving only the outer cortex of bone such as the femur and are known as "banana fractures," but are more usually true fractures, requiring internal fixation (Fig. 75A, B).

Incidentally, fractures in Paget's disease heal well and rapidly. As has been mentioned, Paget's disease acts as a left-to-right shunt because of the marked increase in metabolic bone activity, and thus, patients in borderline congestive cardiac failure may be thrown into true heart failure. If both sides of a joint are involved, the distortion of the adjacent bones leads to arthritis (Figs. 68, 70A and 75A). Total joint replacement does not work well because of the increased metabolic activity, and many of the prostheses loosen within the first year of implant.

Finally, a number of tumors have been described in association with Paget's disease: in spite of popular wisdom, giant-cell tumors of bone do not occur in Paget's

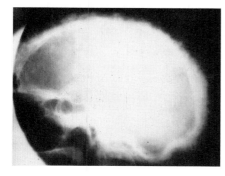

Figure 73 Paget's disease. Lateral skull with more characteristic and advanced Pagetoid changes. Note the cortical thickening, fluffy new bone formation, and sclerosis at the base of the skull.

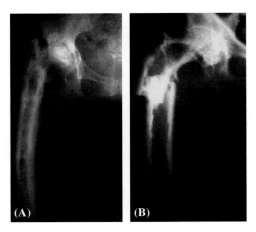

Figure 75 (**A**) Paget's disease. Incremental fractures or "banana" fractures of the proximal femur. These are horizontal sclerotic lines starting on the outer aspect of the bowed bone and running across the bone at irregular intervals. (**B**) True fractures in a different patient with Paget's of the left femur. The fracture is horizontal and probably started as an incremental fracture.

disease, but, on the other hand, giant-cell granulomas of soft tissues have been described in the disease. These can be related back to one family in East Anglia in Britain. They are thought to be reactive granulomas, which can be seen in association with a number of other disorders. However, the worst complication is malignant change in Paget's disease, and all the classical textbooks state that the incidence of this malignant change is 2% of all cases of Paget's disease, in which case all the hospital beds in the United Kingdom and Australia would be full of patients with terminal sarcomas associated with the condition. The true incidence of malignant change is probably between 1 in 10,000 and 1 in 100,000 patients. Malignant change occurs more typically in patients with long-standing polyostotic Paget's disease, and it can be seen in almost any involved bone, but appears to be rare in the spine, and occurs most frequently in the pelvis, proximal femur, proximal humerus, and skull (Figs. 76–78).

The tumor is usually very anaplastic and consists of a mixture of osteosarcoma, chondrosarcoma, and malignant fibrous histiocytoma, but may be predominantly of one cell type. The prognosis is dreadful, with most patients dying within six months of diagnosis.

Gaucher's Disease

This is an exceedingly rare, inherited condition, where failure of an enzyme leads to a buildup of glucocerebrosides in various organs, including the liver, spleen, and bone marrow. The gene can be traced back to a group of Ashkenazi Jews in Poland, and the disease is autosomal recessive in pattern. There are three subtypes of Gaucher's

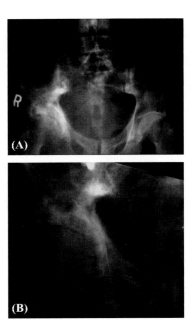

Figure 76 (**A**) Pelvis. Malignant change. There are definite Pagetoid changes seen in the right hemipelvis (also in L3). However, there is a huge soft tissue mass centered on the medial wall of the right acetabulum with a perpendicular periosteal reaction extending into the mass which is well seen in part (**B**). (**B**) Close-up of the right acetabulum. These are typical findings of malignant transfiguration of Paget's disease: this was found to be an undifferentiated pleomorphic sarcoma (Malignant fibrous histocytoma—see chapter 6).

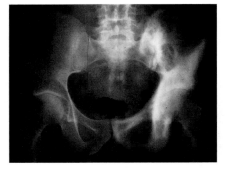

Figure 77 Paget's disease: Pelvis. Malignant changes. There are Pagetoid changes throughout the left pelvis with a poorly circumscribed lucency adjacent to the left sacroiliac joint. This was an osteosarcoma and the patient died within three months.

disease. Type I is the most common form and is described below. Type II occurs in infancy and is fatal. Type III presents in the first year of life with progressive hepatosplenomegaly.

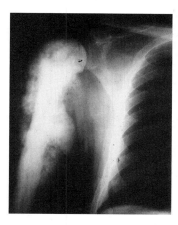

Figure 78 Paget's disease. Malignant change in the humerus in a 78-year-old male patient, with long-standing Paget's disease, whose ancestory came from Avelino in Italy.

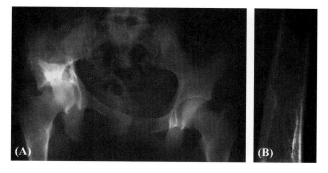

Figure 80 Gaucher's disease. Two films of a different patient with Gaucher's disease. (A) Pelvis shows patchy sclerotic areas with a pathological fracture of the right acetabulum. (B) Close-up of a distal femur showing the endosteal new bone formation as well as the widening of the whole shaft, again characteristic of Gaucher's disease.

Gaucher's disease is an inborn error of glycosphingolipid metabolism, which is a lysosomal storage disorder. There is decreased glucocerebrosidase activity, with accumulation of glucocerebrosides within the lysosomes of macrophages. This leads to progressive visceral enlargement and gradual replacement of bone marrow with lipid-laden macrophages. Anemia, coagulation abnormalities, and enlarging liver and spleen occur in most patients. Skeletal involvement occurs in 75%.

The skeletal findings include bone infarcts, avascular necrosis, localized sclerotic and lytic areas with an increased risk of fractures (Figs. 79 and 80).

Similar to sickle cell anemia, endosteal new bone formation may also be seen in Gaucher's disease because of intramedullary infarction. However, the hallmark of

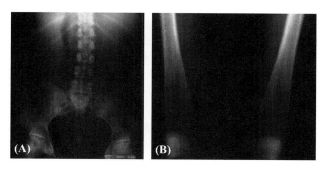

Figure 79 Gaucher's disease. (A) KUB showing the patchy dense bones secondary to infarcts as well as bilateral avascular necrosis. Note the large liver and extremely enlarged spleen. (B) Gaucher's disease. Distal femur in the same 24-year-old girl shows the characteristic flaring of the distal femur, the Erlenmeyer flask deformity characteristic of Gaucher's disease. *Abbreviation*: KUB, kidney, ureter, bladder.

Gaucher's disease is the presence of Erlenmeyer flask deformities, which occur as a result of marrow packing, so that tubulation (or remodeling) of the distal femoral metaphysis does not occur (Figs. 79 and 80). The appearance is that of an Erlenmeyer flask that used to be employed in chemistry, and can be seen, not only in Gaucher's disease but also in Ollier's disease (enchondromatosis, which is also a marrow-packing disorder), thalassemia, osteopetrosis, and Engelmann's disease, where periosteal resorption, as well as endosteal resorption, fails in childhood. Erlenmeyer flask deformities can also be seen in association with multiple osteochondromatosis.

POISONS THAT AFFECT THE MUSCULOSKELETAL SYSTEM

Very few poisons affect the musculoskeletal system in a visible manner, but fluorosis, although rare, does produce characteristic skeletal changes. Overdose with either vitamin A or vitamin D leads to enthesopathy, and poisoning with heavy metal, such as lead, affects the growth plates in children.

Fluorosis

Fluoride is a poison that affects the central nervous system, the cardiovascular system, and the lungs, as well as the skeleton. It occurs in certain endemic areas in the world, including north India and some Native American Indian reservations in the United States (Fig. 81).

To my knowledge, there are no reported cases of fluorosis that have occurred as a result of eating too

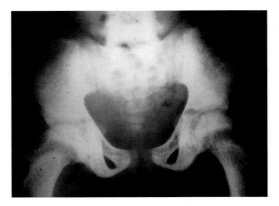

Figure 81 Fluorosis: American Indian child born on an Indian Reservation in North Dakota where endemic fluorosis is a problem. Note the generalized increased density of all the bones with a dislocated irregular trabecular pattern.

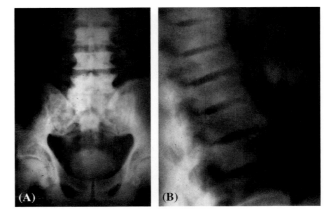

Figure 83 Fluorosis in a different patient with fluoride poisoning. (**A**) KUB with generalized increase in bone density secondary to fluoride poisoning. Note the ossification of the sacrotuberal ligament typical of fluorosis. (**B**) Lateral spine in the same patient shows the ossification of the anterior longitudinal ligament. *Abbreviation*: KUB, kidney, ureter, bladder.

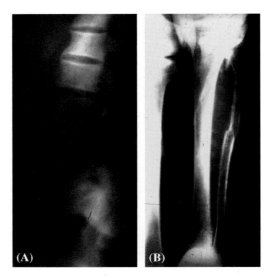

Figure 82 Fluorosis. (**A**) Lateral spine. This film shows ossification of the paraspinal ligaments in the lower thoracic and upper lumbar spine similar to that seen in one of the enthesopathies. However, there are also patchy areas of increased density in various other bones and the patient is only 35-years old. (**B**) Fluorosis. Lower leg in the same patient. There is ossification of the intraosseous membrane. The bones are brittle secondary to osteomalacia, and there are insufficiency fractures of both fibulas.

much toothpaste, in spite of, or because of, the warning on the packet! Fluorosis produces dense bones associated with an enthesopathy, with ossification of various ligaments (Fig. 82).

It is this finding that distinguishes fluorosis from all the other forms of dense bones (Fig. 83).

Usually in adults, the skeleton becomes fairly uniformly dense, with an abnormal, indistinct trabecular pattern. Although any bone may be involved, it is often easier to see the increase in density in the spine and pelvis. Once the ligamentous ossification has been identified, the diagnosis is easy. Any ligament may ossify, but the paraspinal ligaments and the sacroiliac and sacrotuberous ligaments are most commonly involved.

At a histological level, fluoride alters the configuration of the hydroxyapatite crystal and changes its shape from rhomboid to oblong, thus altering the structural integrity of the skeleton and making it prone to fracture. The situation of multiple fractures in a patient with apparently dense bones is typical of fluorosis. Fluoride also affects the structure of osteoid and produces a situation similar to osteomalacia, hence the abnormal, indistinct trabecular pattern. However, fluorosis is a generalized poison, and patients do not die of their bone disease, but rather of its other effects on cardiac conduction and the neurotransmitting system.

Vitamin D and Vitamin A Intoxication

Overdosing with various vitamins usually fails to produce any noticeable effect on the skeleton. However, idiopathic hypercalcemia has been reported with hypervitaminosis D and A, although they are quite different in other regards. Both are associated with metastatic soft-tissue calcification, and the former is associated with dense bones, often with dense metaphyseal bands at the ends of long bones (Fig. 84).

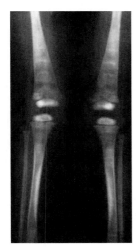

Figure 84 Vitamin D intoxication. Legs in a child whose mother gave him far too much fish liver oil. In the legs, there are many horizontal, sclerotic, metaphyseal bands. Note that the patient also has Erlenmeyer flask deformities.

On the other hand, hypervitaminosis A is now quite commonly seen as a result of the treatment of acne with Retin A (Fig. 85).

The characteristic finding is of an enthesopathy with ossification of paraspinal ligaments and ossification of the origin and insertion of ligaments into the skeleton. This cannot be distinguished from DISH except by the age of the patient. DISH occurs in patients older than 50, when most people have outgrown their acne. In infants, vitamin A intoxification also produces a widespread periosteal thickening resembling Engelmann's disease.

OTHER CAUSES OF DENSE BONES

Probably the commonest cause of dense bones is secondary hyperparathyroidism in renal failure, and this is discussed earlier in this chapter. Hypothyroidism is also associated with dense bones and hyperphosphatasia (or juvenile Paget's disease) is another rare cause of dense bones. Both of these are also discussed elsewhere in this chapter. In all three of these situations, the increased density is usually more often generalized.

A patchy increase in bone density may be seen in metastatic disease, particularly in male patients with prostate cancer and in female patients with breast cancer. However, almost any malignancy can send off blastic metastases, and apparently, (Fig. 86) whether a metastasis is lytic or blastic depends on the release of specific prostaglandins. Some patients with mucus-secreting carcinomas, particularly of the upper gastrointestinal tract, may develop a generalized increase in bone density, although this is rare (Fig. 87).

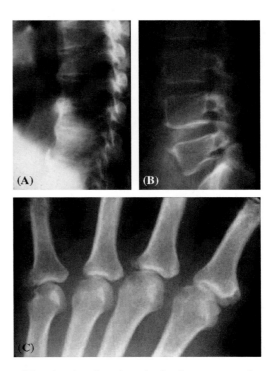

Figure 85 (A) Vitamin A intoxication in a young male patient with acne who was treated with Retin A. The patient has ossification of the anterior long ligament typical of an enthesopathy. (B) Lateral lumbar spine in the same patient showing typical syndesmophytes. (C) Hand in the same patient showing bony overgrowth on both sides of the metacarpo-phalangeal joints.

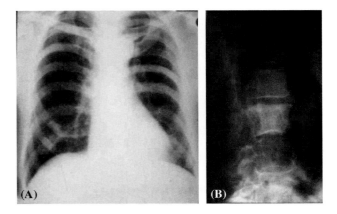

Figure 86 Prostate metastases in two different male patients. (A) Chest X-ray showing patchy sclerotic lesions in a number of ribs. (B) Lateral lumbar spine showing patchy sclerosis in the body of L4.

Finally, there is a rare, sclerotic form of multiple myeloma occurring almost exclusively in middle-aged, black males, and associated with what is called the "Poems syndrome" (Fig. 88).

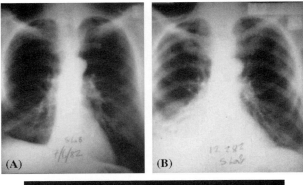

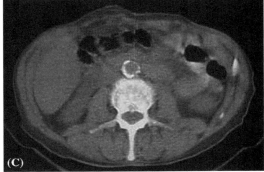

Figure 87 Metastases from a mucus-secreting carcinoma of the esophagus. (**A**) Initial film that shows postsurgical changes of the right base but is otherwise normal (7/82). (**B**) Film taken one month later confirms the increased density of the rib cage that was confirmed by this CT scan of the abdomen, *see* part (**C**). (**C**) CT scan of abdomen confirming the above findings.

POEMS stands for

Polyneuropathy
Organomegaly
Endocrinopathy
Myeloma
Sclerotic bones and skin changes

The subject of metastases and myeloma will be further discussed in chapter 6.

OSTEOGENESIS IMPERFECTA

Osteogenesis imperfecta is almost unique in that the primary abnormality is in the collagen matrix of the bone. Osteogenesis imperfecta is a congenital generalized bone disorder that leads to multiple fractures and deformities of long bones. The exact etiology is unknown but appears to be related to the metabolism of one of the trace metals, possibly zinc, either due to dietary deficiency or because of some enzymatic abnormality. This causes a delay in the maturation of the cross-linkages of collagen in both mineralized and nonmineralized tissue.

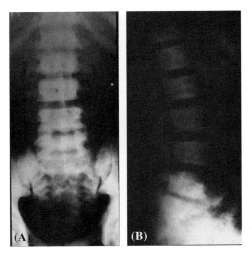

Figure 88 POEMS syndrome. (**A**) AP and (**B**) Lateral lumbar spine in a young male black patient with multiple myeloma and sclerotic lesions throughout the skeleton. *Abbreviation*: AP, anteroposterior.

There are various ways to classify osteogenesis imperfecta, but there appear to be three major forms of the disorder: a congenital variety, a juvenile type, and a delayed form.

Osteogenesis Imperfecta Congenita

The infant is either stillborn or very sickly with grossly deformed limbs due to multiple fractures. Blue sclerae are also obvious (due to the basic defect in the collagen). Radiographically, there are numerous fractures of long bones, a poorly ossified skull with multiple wormian bones, and flattened vertebrae.

Juvenile Osteogenesis Imperfecta

This is the most common form of osteogenesis imperfecta. There is an increasing incidence of fractures with a peak just before adolescence. These children also have blue sclerae and are sometimes deaf. Radiographically, there is marked osteopenia with thin cortices that are noted to be striated due to widened haversian canals. The skull may show typical changes of osteogenesis imperfecta congenita. There will be many fractures, old and new, some associated with excess callus formation.

Osteogenesis Imperfecta Tarda

This is a rare form of matrix disease in which the patient has no fractures as a child and seems to become prone to fractures following very minor trauma in his or her 30s and 40s.

5

Congenital and Developmental Abnormalities

INTRODUCTION

For many of the congenital and developmental diseases of the whole skeleton, there is a classification for different forms of dysplasia, which divides it geographically rather than by age or appearance. This can sometimes be rather confusing. However, this is the way most books on the subject have been published, and this is the traditional way one would look at the X rays. Thus, you need to make a decision about whether the dysplasia involves primarily the epiphysis, the metaphysis, or the diaphysis. Fortunately, the diaphyseal dysplasias are quite easy to separate from the others, since they mainly cause increased density in the bone. Often the epiphyseal and metaphyseal dysplasias appear to overlap. This is because changes in the metaphysis will secondarily cause changes in the epiphysis. However, as a general rule, the epiphyseal dysplasias are somewhat more common than the metaphyseal dysplasias.

EPIPHYSEAL DYSPLASIAS

Chondrodysplasia Punctata or Stippled Epiphyses (Conradi-Hünerman Disease)

This presents at birth. The children have a flat face with a depressed nasal bridge and asymmetrical shortening of their extremities. It is also associated with a scoliosis. There is some evidence that giving coumadin to pregnant mothers will induce Conradi's syndrome in children at birth (1).

Radiographically, the child presents with stippled epiphyses, most typically seen in the hands and feet, but they may occur throughout the body (Fig. 1).

Frequently they will have dysplastic hips with multiple ossification centers, and this may be seen with or without subluxation (Fig. 2A, B).

There appear to be two main types of this condition:

- The rhizomelic form is seen is infants who die of multiple congenital anomalies within a year (Fig. 3).
- The nonrhizomelic forms continue onto adulthood with normal life span. The patients often have vertebral and paravertebral stippling and vertebral anomalies (Fig. 4).

Multiple Epiphyseal Dysplasia (Fairbanks' Disease)

This is an important condition and one of the more common dysplasias that one sees. It usually presents in the second year of life with a waddling gait, and as the children grow, they will complain of painful joints, which have restricted mobility.

Radiographically, the epiphyses are irregular and malformed. The hips are frequently involved (Fig. 5), and the patients have coxa magna, which leads to premature degenerative arthritis (Fig. 6).

The knees and shoulders (2) may also be involved, and the distal femoral epiphyses overgrow, causing mechanical problems in the knee and also leading to premature degenerative arthritis.

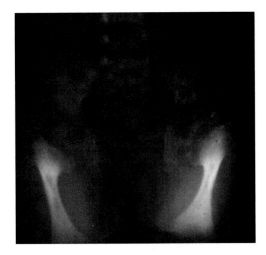

Figure 1 Conradi's syndrome. Note the multiple growth centers in the femoral heads.

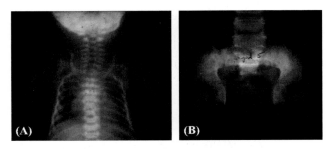

Figure 2 Conradi's syndrome. Note the stippled epiphyses in (**A**) the humeral heads and (**B**) the femoral heads and the dysplastic hip.

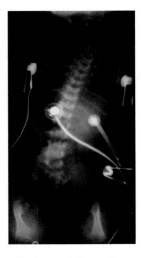

Figure 3 Rhizomelic form of Conradi's syndrome.

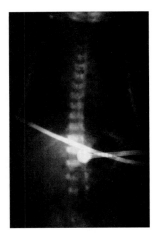

Figure 4 Nonrhizomelic form. Note the multiple growth centers in the spine.

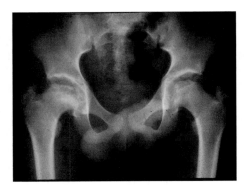

Figure 5 Multiple epiphyseal dysplasia. Note the bilateral coxa magna and deformed epiphyses.

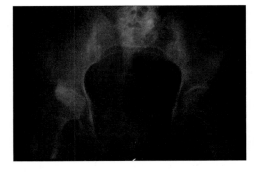

Figure 6 Male patient age 35 with multiple epiphyseal dysplasia who has coxa magna and premature degenerative arthritis.

Spondyloepiphyseal Dysplasia

This is also an important dysplasia because it is basically the main cause of "congenital" scoliosis, which accounts for approximately 5% of patients with scoliosis in the United States. Spondyloepiphyseal dysplasia (SED)

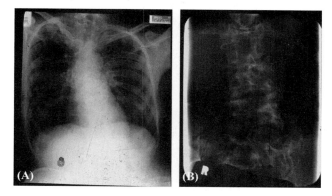

Figure 7 Spondyloepiphyseal dysplasia. The patient has (**A**) a barrel chest, and a severe scoliosis with multiple congenital anomalies in the rib cage and (**B**) a severe scoliosis with multiple congenital anomalies in the lumbar spine.

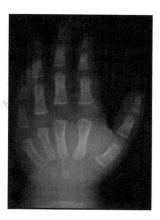

Figure 8 Hypothyroidism. The chronological age is five. The bone age is two.

usually presents at birth. On examination, the children usually are somewhat shorter than expected, and they have a curved spine and a barrel chest (Fig. 7A, B). The knees are involved and they get genu valgum, and deformities can also be seen in the shoulders and other joints. However, the spinal changes are often the most significant.

The hips may be involved and have dysplastic acetabulae, as well as coxa magna, which are caused by malformed femoral ossification centers.

Thus, SED must be also considered when one comes across a young adult who has either bilateral coxa magna, as well as premature osteoarthritis of the hip, or has premature osteoarthritis of the knee and whose femoral condyles appear malformed.

Hypothyroidism

Hypothyroidism is obviously an endocrine disorder and is not a true dysplasia. However, children with this condition are frequently seen by geneticists because their clinicians do not recognize the condition. Hypothyroidism presents clinically with sluggishness, constipation, small stature, and a characteristic "pig-like" facies.

Radiologically, there is retardation of bone maturation that can be severe (Fig. 8).

The patients have small epiphyses, frequently containing multiple ossification centers. The bones, overall, appear to be rather dense (Fig. 9A, B).

Dysplasia Epiphysialis Hemimelica (Trevor's Disease)

Trevor's disease consists of irregular fragmented epiphyses usually involving one joint, particularly the ankle with multiple ossification centers (3) (Figs. 10A, B and 11).

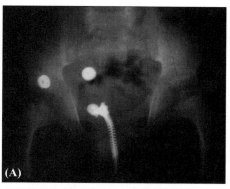

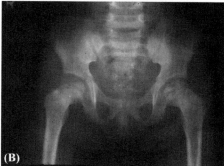

Figure 9 Hypothyroidism. (**A**) This child has a chronological age of six and a bone age of four. Note the multiple ossification centers in the femoral heads. (**B**) Following treatment with thyroxine, the bone age of the femoral heads returns to normal.

It presents in early childhood. It is thought to be a developmental disorder characterized by abnormal growth. It has been seen in other joints, such as the hand and shoulder.

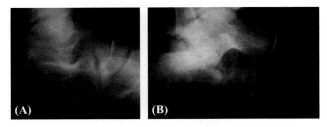

Figure 10 (**A**) Lateral and (**B**) Oblique views of dysplasia epiphysialis hemimelica. Note the multiple growth centers around the talus and calcaneus. Note the tarsal coalition between the talus and calcaneus. The remainder of the skeleton was normal.

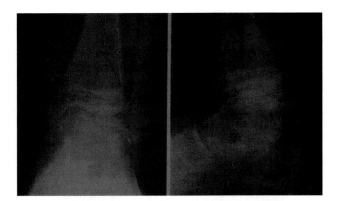

Figure 11 Dysplasia epiphysialis hemimelica—a similar but different patient.

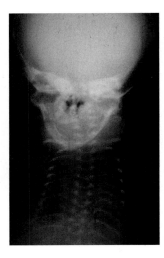

Figure 12 Thanatophoric dwarfism. Note the narrow thorax with flattening of the vertebral bodies.

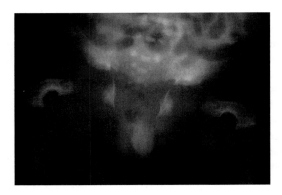

Figure 13 Thanatophoric dwarfism. The femurs are short and bowed and have a "telephone receiver" appearance. Similar findings are present in the tibia.

METAPHYSEAL DYSPLASIAS

This is a very large group of conditions, and well over 300 different syndromes have now been described (4). However, most of these consist of a family or a small group of patients. There are three specific dysplasias that I will describe in some detail. I will also include a brief description of Pyle's disease which is not a true metaphyseal dysplasia.

Thanatophoric Dwarfism

Although this is a very rare condition, Boards' examiners like to show it! It presents at birth with dwarfism, and the children have short extremities and a relatively large head (Fig. 12).

Radiographically, there is a narrow thorax with flattening of the vertebral bodies (Fig. 12), but the major finding is in the long bones, where there are metaphyseal flaring (telephone receiver) bones (Fig. 13).

One interesting differential diagnosis is of an infant at birth showing evidence of a strange dysplasia, whereupon the differential diagnosis between the infantile form of osteogenesis imperfecta and thanatophoric dwarfism becomes important. In the infantile form of osteogenesis imperfecta, the child has short extremities and a large head; the shafts of the bones are wide, but osteopenic, and have multiple fractures. The vertebral bodies are normal.

On the other hand, in thanatophoric dwarfism, there are short extremities and ribs with a large head; the long bones show metaphyseal flaring (telephone receiver), and the bones are dense and without fractures. The vertebral bodies are flattened and notched.

Achondroplasia

This is an important condition, not only for the people involved, but for us to recognize it early. It presents at

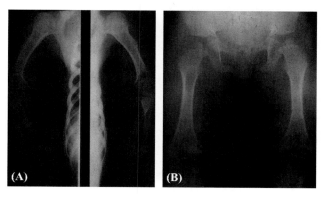

Figure 14 Achondroplasia. (**A**) The arms are short and have enlarged metaphyses. Note the relative sparing of the elbows due to their overall lack of growth when compared to the proximal humerus and distal radius and ulna. (**B**) The legs are short and have enlarged metaphyses and distorted epiphyses.

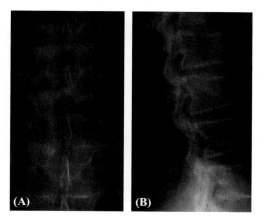

Figure 16 (**A, B**) Achondroplasia. Similar changes can be seen in this lumbar spine in a 27-year-old patient who has severe spinal stenosis in the lower lumbar region with scalloping of the posterior aspect of the lumbar vertebral bodies.

birth with a child who has a disproportionately large head, normal body, and short limbs (Fig. 14A, B).

Radiographically, the spine shows narrowing of the interpedunculate distance in the lumbar and sacral regions (Fig. 15A, B). In the early twenties, this will lead to spinal stenosis, often requiring a wide laminectomy if paralysis is to be avoided (Fig. 16A, B). Patients with achondroplasia have sacral dysgenesis and flaring of the metaphyseal regions of the long bones, and their femoral necks are characteristically shortened. The acetabulae are also usually dysplastic (Fig. 17).

This condition is instantly recognizable, and many achondroplastics out of desperation appear in shows in

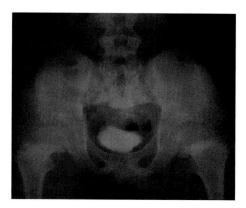

Figure 17 Achondroplasia. There is sacral dysgenesis and flaring of the metaphyseal regions of the long bones, and their femoral necks are characteristically shortened.

which their stature is the attraction. It is doubly regrettable that they are driven to this livelihood because there is absolutely no association between achondroplasia and mental deficiency. Dachshund dogs also have achondroplasia that often leads to premature weakness and even paralysis in their hind legs (Fig. 18).

Hypochondroplasia

This is a forme fruste of achondroplasia, and usually presents somewhat older, often at age five or six. The children are of smaller stature than normal and have short limbs. They will also develop spinal stenosis, and their upper femurs and acetabulae are usually distorted. This is a relatively common condition (Fig. 19A, B).

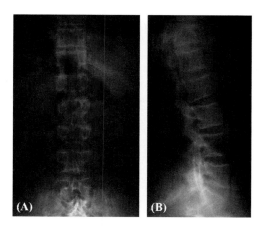

Figure 15 Achondroplasia. (**A**) The vertebral bodies are short and squat with progressive narrowing of the interpedunculate distance from L2 downward so that the spinal canal is extremely narrow at L4 and L5. (**B**) The vertebral bodies are short and squat with progressive narrowing of the interpedunculate distance from L2 downward so that the spinal canal is extremely narrow at L4 and L5.

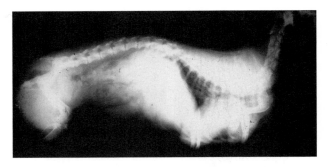

Figure 18 Dachshund dog with the typical in-bred changes of achondroplasia.

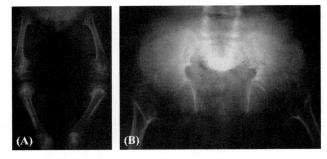

Figure 20 (A) Metaphyseal chondrodysplasia or metaphyseal dystosis of the Jansen type—12-year-old patient. This patient has short limbs with markedly distorted metaphyses and epiphyses. (B) Metaphyseal chondrodysplasia or metaphyseal dystosis.

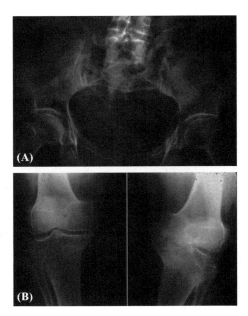

Figure 19 Hypochondroplasia. (A) Note the hip deformity and premature arthritis in the 35-year-old male with hypochondroplasia. The patient also has coxa magna. (B) There are deformities of the metaphyses and epiphyses of both femurs and proximal tibias.

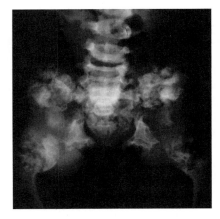

Figure 21 Metaphyseal chondrodysplasia or metaphyseal dystosis of McKusick. This patient also had malabsorption syndrome and renal anomalies.

Metaphyseal Chondrodysplasia or Metaphyseal Dysostosis

There are many different types of metaphyseal chondrodysplasia. Well over 300 different syndromes have now been described, and they are very difficult to differentiate (4). Some of these, like the Jansen type, are possibly associated with hyperparathyroidism, osteopenia, and erosions. There is the McKusick type, which is associated with immunological and intestinal disturbances. Radiographically, they all look remarkably similar, with metaphyseal irregularities, widening, and distortion producing rather short bones (Fig. 20). There are short femoral necks with wide trochanteric regions (Fig. 21).

Often the metaphyseal chondrodysplasias will involve the acetabular roofs, as well as the base of the skull and calvarium. Since this is a very rare group of conditions, I suggest that if you have more interest, read Koslowski's book (4).

Metaphyseal Dysplasia or Pyle's Disease

Usually people with metaphyseal dysplasia have normal height with a normal life expectancy, but they do have knock-knees (genu valgum). Metaphyseal dysplasia is actually a failure of tubulation, that is, a failure of periosteal resorption. Radiographically, there is metaphyseal flaring, and in the distal femurs, there is an Erlenmeyer flask deformity (Fig. 22). They also have widened ribs. This condition is of no clinical importance other than to include it in the differential diagnosis of Erlenmeyer flask deformity.

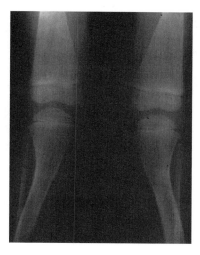

Figure 22 Pyle's disease. Note the typical Erlenmeyer flask deformities with metaphyseal flaring of the distal femur and proximal tibia.

DIAPHYSEAL DYSPLASIAS

Unfortunately, this group of conditions is as divergent as the rest, and the term sclerosing dysplasias, or dense bone dysplasias, could do just as well. There are two generalized conditions in this group, and perhaps ten patchy, sclerotic dysplasias, of which three are somewhat important.

Osteopetrosis

This is also known as marble bone disease or Albers-Schönberg disease, and was first described in 1907. In its purest form, it represents the failure of osteoclastic function, which produces an overall defect in bone modeling. There are two main forms; an autosomal recessive form, which leads to death from anemia in the teens, and an autosomal dominant form, which is more benign (5). In the severe form, there is a failure of both periosteal and endosteal osteoclasis, leading to a lack of remodeling, which is particularly obvious in the metaphyseal regions of long bones (another cause of Erlenmeyer flask deformities of the distal femur), and a lack of bone marrow cavity, and hence, a very sclerotic skeleton (Figs. 23, 24A–C).

In the mild form, because of the osteoclasts malfunction, which is secondary to some exogenous influence that comes and goes, these patients do not die of anemia because their bone marrow cavity exists, and hence, they do not develop anemia (Fig. 25A, B). It was a preconceived notion that the osteoclast abnormality was a lack of actual osteoclasts, either complete or partial, but it is now known that the defect is the lack of an osteoclast-stimulating enzyme (5) (Fig. 23). Attempts have been

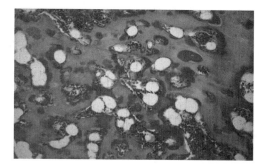

Figure 23 Osteopetrosis. A histological specimen. There is dense bone without any viable osteoclasts.

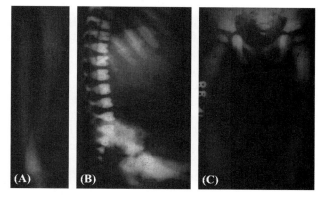

Figure 24 Osteopetrosis. Infantile form. (**A**) The bones are dense with metaphyseal flaring and celery stalking (*the thin black lines running vertically at the metaphyseal ends of the radius and ulna*). Insufficiency fractures are also present. (**B**) The vertebral bodies are dense with no bone marrow. (**C**) Note the metaphyseal flaring and lack of bone marrow as well as celery stalking. The distal femurs are widened, i.e., Erlenmeyer flask deformity.

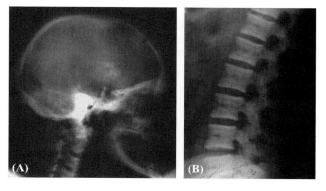

Figure 25 (**A**) Mild form of osteopetrosis with dense bones but with bone marrow cavities in the jaw and calvaria. (**B**) Osteopetrosis. There is bone marrow centrally in the vertebral bodies and in the posterior elements.

made to overcome this problem with the use of bone marrow transplantation, but this is only successful in 50% of the patients, so, obviously, something else is also responsible for the total failure of osteoclastic activity.

In the classical infantile form, the child presents with severe anemia and dense brittle bones with many fractures. In the long bones, there is failure of tubulation or modeling, with flared, widened metaphyses, absolutely white bones with pseudo-fractures, stress fractures, incremental fractures, and true fractures all of which may be present. In infancy, attempts at remodeling occur adjacent to the growth plates, and an appearance of "celery stalking" is apparent (Fig. 24 A, C).

Erlenmeyer flask deformities are seen in the distal femur (Fig. 24C). In the skull, there is total loss of the diploic space and the calvarium is very sclerotic. In the spine, the vertebral bodies are densely white, although the central vascular canal appears as a relative lucency, producing a sandwich-like effect (Fig. 24B). The posterior elements are also densely white. Because of a lack of bone marrow cavity, the liver and spleen enlarge to take over hematopoietic function of the body, and eventually, extramedullary hematopoiesis occurs and presents as large masses of bone marrow growing adjacent to the spine in both the chest and the abdomen. Without successful therapy, the patients die of recurrent infection and from severe anemia in their mid-teens.

The more benign form has several guises from a very mild "bone-within-a-bone" appearance in the spine, and is elsewhere found serendipitously in middle-aged people, to a more advanced sclerotic form where, although the bone marrow is partially present, the calvarium of the skull is thickened and sclerotic. The vertebral bodies are quite dense, although the posterior elements appear normal, and the cortices of the long bones are thickened. The pelvis shows a mixture of dense sclerotic areas with more lucent areas in the iliac wings causing a ghostlike appearance (Figs. 26A, B and 27).

To some extent, this appearance needs to be separated from Engelmann's disease, since neither disease is fatal, this separation is somewhat superfluous. Classically, the adult form of osteopetrosis involves the whole skeleton, whereas classically, Engelmann's disease involves the long bones only.

Engelmann's Disease

Engelmann's disease was first described in 1910 as Engelmann-Camurati disease, and it is due to a failure of periosteal osteoclasis. The patients have normal bone marrow cavities and are not anemic so that they have a normal life span and do not die young. It is also a rare condition and appears to be familial. There appear to be

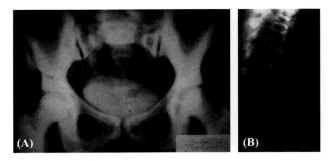

Figure 26 (**A**) Adult form of osteopetrosis with dense bones, involvement of the whole skeleton and the pelvis but with bone marrow cavities in the iliac crest and pubic rami. (**B**) Adult form of osteopetrosis in the same patient. There is adequate bone marrow present in the vertebral bodies and the overall appearance is that of a "bone-within-a–bone."

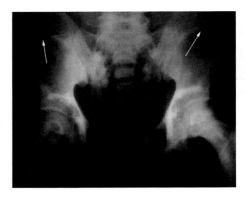

Figure 27 Adult form of osteopetrosis. Note the "ghosting" appearance of the iliac crests suggesting that the metabolic defect comes and goes.

three grades of Engelmann's disease: (*i*) the adult, asymptomatic type, which the commonest, (*ii*) an adolescent and young adult type, in which the patients experience severe bone pain, as well as stress fractures, and (*iii*) an infantile form where the children have bone pain, difficulty in walking, and an abnormal gait (6). Engelmann's disease is a disease of intramembranous ossification, and so, the bones develop thick cortices, as well as thickening of the skull vaults. A few patients have some involvement of the metaphysis, but the majority only have cortical involvement of long bones and no involvement of the axial skeleton (Fig. 28A–D).

Hence, the differentiation from osteopetrosis which has obvious involvement of the spine, ribs, and pelvis, as well as long bones. Incidentally, the old name for Engelmann's disease was "diaphyseal dysplasia." The defect in periosteal resorption leads to a failure of remodeling or tubulation, and thus, these patients also have Erlenmeyer flask

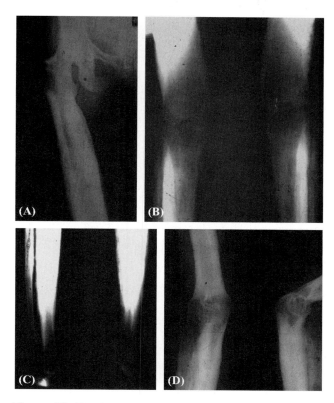

Figure 28 Engelmann's disease. (**A**) The patient has cortical thickening of all the mineralized long bones with sparing of the metaphyses and epiphyses as well as the pelvis. (**B**) Note the surgical excision of the proximal fibula heads bilaterally. (**C**) Note the sparing of the ankle bones. (**D**) Note the resection of the proximal radius bilaterally because of overgrowth.

deformities (7). The two complications of Engelmann's disease that one occasionally sees are incremental fractures (particularly on the outer cortex of the upper femur) and relative overgrowth of the radius when compared with the ulna, and the fibula when compared with the tibia, which may necessitate removal of the radial head at the elbow and the proximal fibula at the knee.

Osteopoikilosis

Most of us have one or more bone islands (enostoses) in our skeleton. However, patients with osteopoikilosis have multiple bone islands, usually mainly grouped around the shoulder and hip girdle (Fig. 29A–D).

It is an entirely benign condition except when a middle-aged male patient is found to have carcinoma of the prostate, and these bone islands are thought to represent metastases. The appearance is usually different; bone islands are smaller and often have distinct margins and frequently a "tail" of bone like a comet speeding into the surrounding trabecular bone. They also do not light up on the bone scan, whereas patients with prostatic metastases have a positive bone scan. The patient with osteopoikilosis also has a normal acid phosphatase. Osteopoikilosis is somewhat common, so you need to be aware of it.

Osteopathia Striata

There are two forms of osteopathia striata, the commoner and benign type affects tall, adolescent children, usually

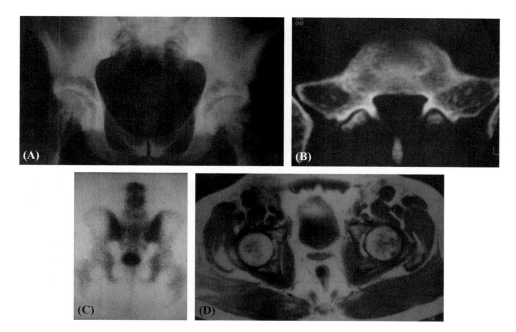

Figure 29 Osteopoikilosis. (**A**) Plain film. Note the multiple bone islands. (**B**) CT scan. (**C**) The bone scan is normal. (**D**) MRI.

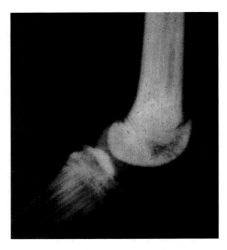

Figure 30 Osteopathia striata. Note the stippled metaphysis in this otherwise normal child.

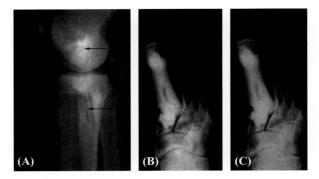

Figure 31 Melorheostosis. (**A**) A 24-year-old asymptomatic female. Note the new bone on the inner aspect of the distal femur (*arrow*) and proximal tibia (*arrow*). (**B, C**) There is dense new bone in the medial cuneiform, first metatarsal, and first proximal phalanx of the great toe.

Table 1 Sclerosing Bone Dysplasias: A Spectrum of Disease

A. Dysplasias of enchondral ossification

    a. Osteopetrosis

    b. Pyknodysostosis

B. Dysplasias of secondary spongiosa (mature bone)

    a. Bone island (enostosis)

    b. Osteopoikilosis

    c. Osteopathia striata

C. Dysplasias of intramembranous ossification

    a. Ribbing's disease

    b. Van Buchem's disease

    c. Worth's disease

    d. Sclerosteosis

D. Mixed sclerosing dysplasias

    1. Affecting enchondral ossification

        a. Dysosteosclerosis

        b. Metaphyseal dysplasia (Pyle's disease)

        c. Craniometaphyseal dysplasia

    2. Affecting intramembranous ossification

        a. Melorheostosis

        b. Craniodiaphyseal dysplasia

    3. Overlap syndromes, i.e., osteopoikilosis, osteopathia/strata, and melorheostosis

Source: From Ref. 9.

male, where their bone resorption does not keep up with their bone formation. The metaphyseal regions of the growing long bones have marked sclerotic striations. This is best seen about the knee (Fig. 30).

Once the growth plates fuse, the striations disappear, and the skeleton reverts to normal. The second and very rare form of osteopathia striata is a syndrome known as Voorhoeve's disease (8). These children have mental retardation, cataracts, deafness, and cranial deformities, as well as striated bones. The striations can once again be seen at the ends of long bones, as well as a fanlike appearance in the pelvis. The ribs, tarsal bones, and base of the skull are also very dense.

Melorheostosis

Melorheotosis is also not uncommon. It is a mesodermal abnormality with linear or segmental new bone formation running in sclerotomes. It often only involves one limb, usually lower, and looks as though someone has poured new bone down the outer margins of the involved bones; say, the distal femur, distal tibia, the outer aspect of the ankle, and the middle cuneiform and third metatarsal (Fig. 31A–C).

Melorheostosis is benign and has no significance. The name derives from the Greek term for flowing honey, and the appearance certainly resembles the patches of honey when spilt that run down a series of kitchen drawers, for example.

If the above syndromes that cause dense bones are not enough for you, there are at least five more rare conditions associated with dense bones, which at least need to be included in this book if only for completeness (Table 1).

Pyknodysostosis is a patchy form of osteopetrosis and is associated with mental deficiency and short-limbed dwarfism. Ribbing's disease, which was thought to be a minor form of Engelmann's disease, is now considered to be a type of chronic recurrent multifocal osteomyelitis (see page 115).

Sclerosteosis occurs only in Africans who have cortical thickening involving long bones, but particularly the skull, face, and mandibles. It is familial, and only about 30 cases have been described. Van Buchem's disease again occurs mainly in people of white South African extraction, with large, endosteal hyperostoses on their skulls, mandibles, ribs, and clavicles, as well as their long bones. This is also extremely rare and is autosomal recessive. Worth's disease is a less severe form of Van Buchem's disease.

Uehlinger's disease is a form of Engelmann's disease associated with skin thickening and is probably because of a generalized mesodermal growth defect. The patients have progressive facial nerve deficits and elevated alkaline phosphatase.

THE MUCOPOLYSACCHARIDOSES

Hurler's Disease

Hurler's disease is classified as Mucopolysaccharidosis I. It presents in the first month of life with the baby having a flat bridge of the nose, flared nostrils, widely spaced eyes, thick lips, large tongue, mental retardation, dwarfism, and hepatosplenomegaly. Radiographically, these children have macrocephaly and cranio-ostosis, with a J-shaped sella (Fig. 32A–D).

They have wide ribs with a low, hook-shaped vertebral body. Hypoplasia of the acetabulae associated with coxa valga is also seen. The long bones are short and wide, the phalanges are short, wide, and bullet-shaped (Fig. 33D). The hands are said to have a characteristic appearance of thickened shafts with tapered ends, and proximal tapering of the metacarpals. However, if one looks at children with

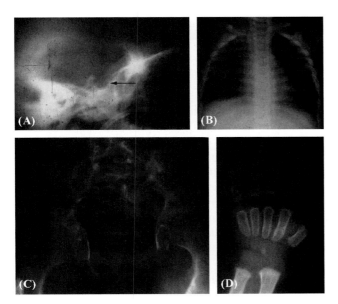

Figure 32 Hurler's disease. (**A**) Note the large skull and J-shaped sella. (**B**) Chest X ray. Note the wide ribs. (**C**) The patient has bilateral coxa valga with dysplastic acetabuli. (**D**) The phalanges are short and bullet-shaped.

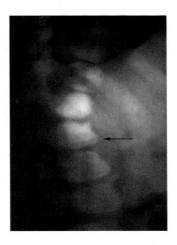

Figure 33 Hurler's disease. Note the "beaking" of L2 with the hook on its lower aspect (*arrow*).

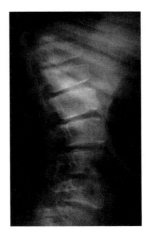

Figure 34 Hurler's disease. Another patient with wedging of many vertebral bodies.

the other mucopolysaccharides, I believe that all the hand X rays are relatively similar.

It is the vertebral bodies that help confirm this diagnosis. They can be fairly normal in size, or somewhat ovoid, except for those at the thoracolumbar junction. L2 is usually hypoplastic and displaced and has a large anteroinferior beak associated with a kyphosis (Figs. 33 and 34).

This helps differentiate Hurler's disease from Morquio's disease, which has a central beak (M for Morquio and middle).

Hunter's Disease

Hunter's disease, mucopolysaccharidosis II, is a forme fruste of Hurler's disease. It presents later and has lesser general features. Often the children will have a large skull with a J-shaped sella (Fig. 35A).

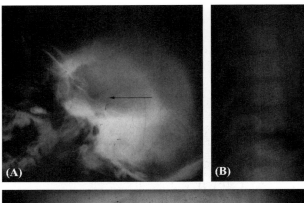

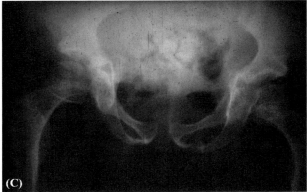

Figure 35 Hurler's disease. (**A**) There is a large head and the patient has a J-shaped sella. (**B**) The vertebral bodies are relatively normal. (**C**) The patient has dysplastic acetabuli with a mild degree of coxa valga.

The vertebral bodies are more inclined to be normal in Hunter's disease, although the hypoplastic acetabulae and coxa valga can still be seen (Fig. 35B, C).

Sanfilippo's Disease

Sanfilippo's disease is a mucopolysaccharide disorder (type III) that is a deficiency of an essential enzyme that breaks down heparin sulfate. Heparin sulfate builds up in the brain causing many symptoms such as hyperactivity, sleep disorders, loss of speech, dementia, and typically death before adulthood.

Morquio's Disease

Morquio's disease is classified as mucopolysaccharidosis IV. This presents rather later than Hurler's disease and is usually not picked up until the second to fourth year of life. It is a form of dwarfism associated with a short spine, prominent joints, and accentuation of the lower part of the

face. The skull is basically normal, unlike in Hurler's disease (Fig. 36A–F). However, odontoid hypoplasia is commonly seen in Morquio's disease (Fig. 36B). The vertebral bodies are often quite flat (universal vertebra plana) and have a classical anterocentral vertebral body beak (Fig. 36C).

It usually occurs at the thoracolumbar junction, and either L1 or L2 is hypoplastic and displaced. Remember, M is for Morquio and middle, whereas Hurler's disease has the anterior vertebral beaks adjacent to the lower end of the vertebral body. The children also have wide ribs.

In the pelvis, the acetabulae are flat, deep, and irregular, and the femoral epiphyses are often irregular. These children also have a short, thick, femoral neck, and coxa valga (Fig. 36D). The long bones show widening of the ends and, once again the hands are said to be characteristic with conical second and fifth metacarpals (Fig. 36E, F). It is often difficult to separate any of the mucopolysaccharides from each other, but the beaking of the anterior end plates of the spine will help. Once again, remember that the central or middle beak is in Morquio's disease, whereas the lower beak is in Hurler's disease.

Maroteaux-Lamy's Disease

Maroteaux-Lamy disease is considered a lysosomal storage disorder, which is part of the mucopolysaccharide disorders (type V). In children affected by this disorder, there is growth retardation by the age of three years. Children affected by this syndrome have coarsening of facial features and abnormalities in the bones of the hands and spine. The intellect is usually normal.

TARSAL COALITION

Although first described in the 18th century, it was not until the advent of X rays that tarsal coalition could be properly characterized. A number of clinical situations alert the orthopedist to the presence of tarsal coalition, and these include peroneal spastic flatfoot and painful rigid flatfoot. Many of the patients with this condition walk with a characteristic in-toeing gait. It is now thought that tarsal coalition is an inherited, autosomal dominant disorder. The overall incidence of tarsal coalition is 1% of the population, and in 60% of these patients, it is bilateral. The two commonest coalitions are talocalcaneal, classically involving the middle facet (48%) and calcaneonavicular (44%). The remainder is rare.

The radiological diagnosis of tarsal coalition initially is based on plain-film findings. The traditional anteroposterior (AP) and lateral views are often useless, although

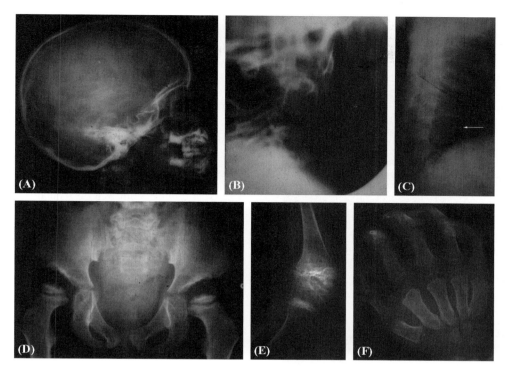

Figure 36 Morquio's disease. (**A**) The skull is normal. (**B**) There is complete absence of the odontoid with a wide atlanto-axial joint. (**C**) There is universal vertebra plana with a "beak" is the middle of each vertebral body. (**D**) There is bilateral coxa valga with hip dysplasia. (**E**) The knee gives the appearance of a metaphyseal dysplasia. (**F**) The metacarpals are somewhat conical, which is said to be characteristic of Morquio's disease.

a recently described sign is highly suggestive of talocalcaneal coalition on the lateral view. This is the so-called "C-sign," which is a C-shaped line formed by the superior articular surface of the talus continued onto the undersurface of the sustentaculum tali. Sometimes, an actual bony bridge can be seen between the talus and calcaneus on the lateral view (Fig. 37A–C).

Talar beaking, which is a traction spur seen on the superior surface of the talonavicular junction, is a common secondary sign of talcalcaneal coalition. A 45° oblique view is very useful for detecting calcaneonavicular coalition, and, in fact, will often tell us if the coalition is fibrous, cartilaginous, or osseous. An axial view (akin to the Harris view of the calcaneus used for fractures) will often show the subtalar joints whether they are fused.

If there is still some doubt, then either CT or MRI can be useful. There has been a controversy in the radiological literature about which one is better. I believe that CT scans are the most useful. The coronal cuts demonstrate talarcalcaneal coalitions and whether they involve the medial or the lateral facets. Reconstructed sagittal and oblique CT scans are useful to confirm calcaneonavicular and other coalitions.

On MRI, the T1 sequences are most sensitive and are still useful if one needs confirmation of the coalition, and if a decision needs to be made about whether the coalition is osseous, cartilaginous, or fibrous.

THE PEDIATRIC HIP

Although a large number of diseases and disorders can affect the hip in children, there are four primary developmental or inherited disorders. These disorders were called congenital hip dislocation, which were later termed as congenital hip dysplasia, and now more correctly called developmental hip dysplasia (DHD); Legg-Calvé-Perthes disease (LCPD); slipped capital femoral epiphysis (SCFE); and coxa vara, coxa valga, and coxa magna (Table 2).

Developmental Hip Dysplasia

This used to be known as congenital hip dislocation or congenital dysplastic hip. Most babies, just after their birth, have an Ortolani test, which is performed to check

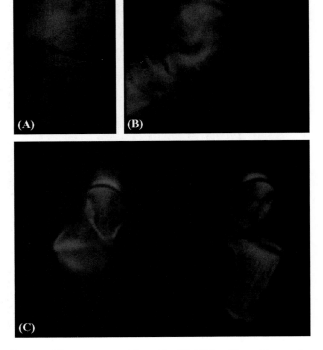

Figure 37 Tarsal coalition. (**A, B**) Plain films. These show fusion between the talus and sustentaculum tali of the calcaneus. This is the commonest tarsal coalition. (**C**) CT scan. This clearly shows fusion between the talus and sustentaculum tali.

Table 2 Differentiation of Pediatric Hip Disease

	DHD	LCPD	SCFE	Coxa vara, coxa valga
Acetabulum	Abnormal	Normal	Normal	Normal
Femoral head	Malformed	Flattened	Slipped	Normal
Upper femoral metaphysis	Wide	Wide	Normal	Normal
Neck/shaft angle	Normal	Normal	Normal	Abnormal

Abbreviations: DHD, developmental hip dysplasia; LCPD, Legg-Calvé-Perthes disease; SCFE, slipped capital femoral epiphysis.

infants for hip dislocation. In a normal neonate, no sound is elicited by this procedure; however, in children with developmental hip dysplasia (DHD), there is often a click. If it is necessary to confirm this, ultrasound is probably the best way to do so (10). However, X rays can be very useful, particularly in the later stages of the condition, once the femoral head is ossified.

The incidence of true developmental dysplasia in the whole population is from 1% to 2%. It is associated with

the white population, breech presentations, six times as common in females, and in first-born infants. It is often bilateral. Three types of DHD have been mentioned below:

- True DHD (teratological)
- The dislocatable hip
- The subluxable hip

In order to assess the radiographs adequately, a number of lines should be drawn and measurements be made. The classical lines are:

1. Hilgenreiner's line is a horizontal line drawn through both triradiate cartilages (Fig. 38A).
2. The acetabular index or the acetabular angle is a line drawn from where the horizontal line and the triradiate cartilage meet, and measures the angle of the acetabulum (Fig. 38A, left hip). Sharp classified this first and noted that in children under the age of 3 years, the angle is often as high as 45°, but by

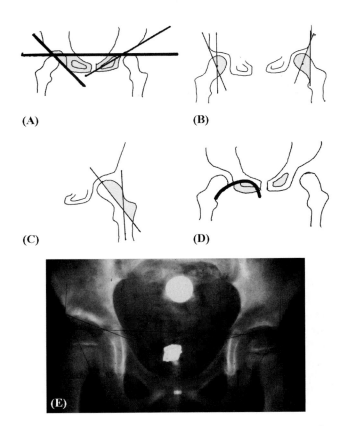

Figure 38 (**A**) Hilgenreiners line and acetabular angle. (**B**) Centre edge angle (two methods). (**C**) Neck shaft angle. (**D**) Shentons line. (**E**) Lines and measurements for developmental hip dysplasia.

14 years of age, the angle drops to 41°, and, in most adults, it is 35°.

3. Center edge angle is an angle drawn between a vertical line, which is dropped through the epicenter of the femoral head, and a second line drawn from this epicenter to the margin of the acetabulum (Fig. 38B). The vertical line is vertical to Hilgenreiner's horizontal line. This measurement was first described by Wiberg. In very young children, it is difficult to measure, but by age five, it measures about 19°. It continues to increase until, in adults, it measures 25° to 30°. Interestingly, the orthopedic community does the opposite and drops a vertical line from the outer margin of the acetabulum, and then an angled line to the center of the femoral head. Obviously these readings are identical (Fig. 38B).

4. Femoral neck/shaft angle: At birth, the upper femur is relatively vertical, and the neck/shaft angle measures 150°. However, as the child bears weight, this angle decreases and in most adults, it is about 130°. This line is reproduced by drawing a vertical line through the femoral shaft, and then a line through the center of the femoral neck (Fig. 38C).

5. Shenton's line is used by most of the medical students as it is easy to remember. Draw a line along the undersurface of the femoral neck and continue it onto the undersurface of the pubic ramus (i.e., the top of the obturator foramen in normal people). This line is said to resemble a Roman arch. This line is broken in someone with DHD (Fig. 38D).

6. Width of space between the vertical component of the ischium and the proximal femur: This measurement really works only if you have a normal side for comparison. If the child has bilateral congenital hip dysplasia, then it is difficult to measure. However, in children with DHD, this space is markedly widened (Fig. 38E).

Radiographically, in very young children, the easiest way to look for DHD is to assess the angle of the acetabulum, which can be done by the naked eye. The second radiographic line to draw is up the shaft of the femur. If a straight line is drawn up the femur and the baby is in a frog-leg position, that is, with the knees abducted, a line drawn straight through the femur should cross that of the acetabulum. If it does not do so, then there is almost certainly displacement present. Once the femoral head has started appearing, a line taken through the femoral neck and femoral head should transect the acetabulum. In most cases of DHD, it lies outside the region of the triradiate cartilage. This line can be drawn with the child at neutral or in abduction. However, the ideal way to diagnose early DHD is by the use of ultrasound (Fig. 39).

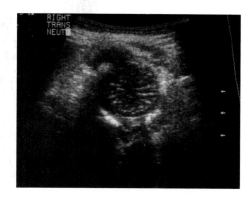

Figure 39 Neonatal hip ultrasound. Normal appearance. Note that the femoral head lies nestled in between the iliac crest and ischial ramus.

Other modalities that can be used to confirm DHD include:

1. Ultrasound was first used to diagnose DHD some 20 years ago. Basically, one can assess the shape of the femoral head and the acetabulum, the position of the labrum, as well as some secondary changes. Recently, 1000 newborn babies had their Ortolani sign, the X rays, and ultrasound compared with each other (Figs. 39, 40, 41). The ultrasound was found to be extremely sensitive, and the authors found that it could detect minor degrees of DHD in children who did not have an audible click. Femoral head coverage can also be shown with ultrasound, and about 55% of the femoral head should be covered by a normal acetabulum. Ultrasonographers use the phrase alpha angle to describe the angle between the straight part of the iliac bone and the acetabulum. All the unstable hips had less coverage. These authors' final conclusion was that ultrasound is extremely sensitive and useful in assessing the neonatal acetabulum (11). Usually the hip is scanned in a transverse-neutral situation. This is easy to do. In a normal hip, the femoral head can be clearly seen, as can the iliac bone and the pubic bone, which make a nice triangle, into which the femoral head fits (Fig. 39). On the other hand, a subluxed femoral head lies somewhat outside this triangle, and the triangle becomes flatter with apparently widening (Fig. 40B). A dislocated femoral head is easy to diagnose because the femoral head can often not be seen within the acetabulum. The two acetabular components are also almost flat, as opposed to being triangular (Fig. 41B).

2. In arthrography, the cartilage anlage can be clearly shown and it can be ascertained whether it lies within the acetabulum (Fig. 42A, B).

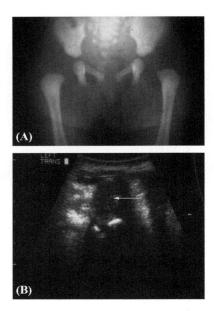

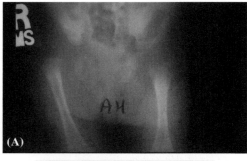

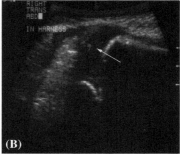

Figure 40 Developmental hip dysplasia. Subluxed femoral head. (**A**) Radiograph shows that the right side is normally aligned but the left upper femur is displaced outward. (**B**) Although the femoral head can be clearly seen (*arrow*), its relationship to the iliac crest and ischial ramus shows it to lie above both of them.

Figure 41 Developmental hip dysplasia. Dislocated hip. (**A**) Radiograph showing a normal left side and a dislocated right side with the upper femur displaced upward and outward. (**B**) The iliac crest and ischial ramus are clearly seen but the femoral head is not (*arrow*).

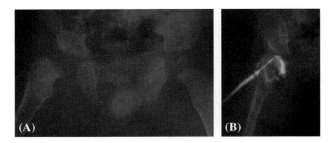

Figure 42 (**A**) Plain film and arthrogram in a child suspected of having developmental hip dysplasia. The left side is normal. The right femoral head is missing and the proximal femur is displaced outward. (**B**) The arthrogram reveals a normal sized femoral head anlage although it is subluxed out of the acetabulum.

3. Nowadays some people recommend MRI, with or without arthrography, which makes this an invasive procedure, and it costs a lot more than ultrasound.

Legg-Calvé-Perthes Disease

Legg-Calvé-Perthes disease (or Legg-Perthes as it is usually known) is basically avascular necrosis of the femoral head in childhood. It is an interesting condition in that it affects males in 80% of cases, it involves the white population, and the children are short in stature and of greater intelligence than normal. The age range in America is between approximately three and seven. The age range in Europe is actually older than this, usually between about 7 and 12. There is no satisfactory explanation for this divergence. Fifteen to 20% of patients with Legg-Calvé-Perthes disease develop it on the other side so that it becomes bilateral, although it may not be synchronous. Similarly, 20% of patients later go on to develop secondary adult avascular necrosis. Although the etiology of Legg-Calvé-Perthes disease is unknown, many of these children develop a tender, swollen hip some three months beforehand, and it is now thought that transient synovitis leads to an effusion that, in turn, leads to compression of the blood supply to the femoral head. In children, the femoral head gets its principle blood supply from the transverse ligament, which runs in the ligament teres into the fovea, and 20% of the femoral head blood supply comes in via the capsular vessels. However, Legg-Calvé-Perthes disease has also been described following trauma in which a child has had an effusion or recurrent effusions, such as can be seen in hemophilia. Thus, an effusion, or transient synovitis, will obviously compress both these sources of blood supply, and this in turn, can lead to avascular necrosis in the femoral head in a young child.

Radiologically, the affected femoral head initially appears to be somewhat smaller and there is increased

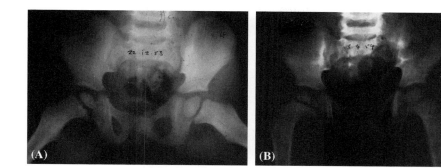
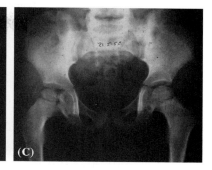

Figure 43 Legg-Calvé-Perthes disease. (**A**) Series of pelvis films taken over two years. In the initial film the left side is normal. The right femoral head is smaller than the left, and the growth plate is widened and the proximal femoral metaphysis thickened. (**B**) 6 months later, there has been continued fragmentation and collapse of the right femoral head. (**C**) 18 months later, the right femoral head is regrowing although the proximal femoral metaphysis remains widened. However, the left femoral head is now showing early signs of Legg-Calvé-Perthes disease.

medial joint space because of the presence of an effusion, and the femoral head itself appears to have some irregular ossification and subchondral fissures.

At two to three months, there is epiphyseal sclerosis with some fragmentation, and the physeal plate itself becomes irregular, with cysts and what I term "erosions" (Fig. 43A). At six to nine months, these metaphyseal cysts enlarge and start to ossify, as a result of which the growth plate widens. The proximal femoral metaphysis also widens to accommodate the new growth plate (Fig. 43B). At this stage, the capital femoral epiphysis is flattened and fragmented. At 12 months, the epiphysis becomes very fragmented and is considerably smaller, but the metaphysis begins to heal.

At 15 to 18 months, the epiphysis itself starts healing with reossification. However, without adequate therapy, which means no weight bearing and long periods of rest, the femoral head remains flattened and distorted. At three-year follow-up, the residual findings can be of a flat femoral head, which has continuing reossification associated with a wide upper femoral metaphysis (Figs. 43C and 44A, B).

Although this diagnosis is easy to make on plain films, some authors did MRI, and Bos et al. (12) have followed them by performing sequential MRIs on 16 children. Their final conclusion was that MRI was helpful and correlated well with the radiographic findings. They also pointed out that MRI is probably a better way to diagnose early Legg-Calvé-Perthes disease than plain films. This is similar to the finding in adult avascular necrosis. Similarly, Egund and Wingstrand (13) performed MRI on 35 children with Legg-Calvé-Perthes disease. They performed arthrography and MRI on all the children. They felt that MRI gave them more information about the femoral head and what was actually happening in it. Ten of the children with sequential MRI showed remodeling of the femoral head.

Slipped Capital Femoral Epiphyses

It is normally known as SCFE (pronounced "skiffy"). Slipped capital femoral epiphyses occur in overweight adolescents, frequently in the black population. It is also

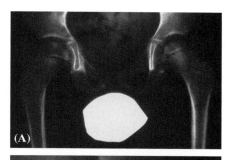
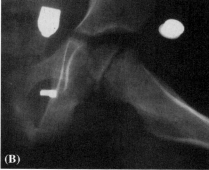

Figure 44 (**A**) Legg-Calvé-Perthes disease. Early signs in an AP pelvis film, which shows a normal right side but the left femoral head is smaller than expected. (**B**) A frog-leg view in the same patient reveals early Legg-Calvé-Perthes disease with fragmentation of the femoral head, widening of the proximal femoral metaphysis, and irregularity of the growth plate.

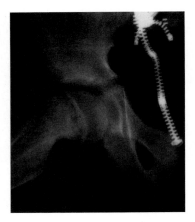

Figure 45 Slipped capital femoral epiphyses—idiopathic. This frog-leg view of the right hip shows that the femoral head has slipped and rotated medially and posteriorly.

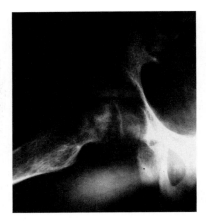

Figure 46 Slipped capital femoral epiphyses in renal failure. This child has severe secondary hyperparathyroidism with an abnormal trabecular pattern, secondary rickets, and with a slipped capital femoral epiphyses on the right.

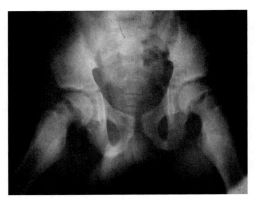

Figure 47 Slipped capital femoral epiphyses in rickets. This child with severe nutritional rickets has all the classical findings of rickets (chap. 4) and with a slipped capital femoral epiphyses on the right.

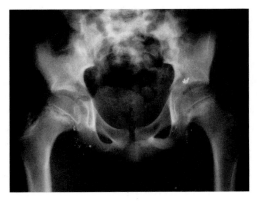

Figure 48 Slipped capital femoral epiphyses following radiation. This child has bilateral coxa magna (see later) with discrete slipped capital femoral epiphyses. Note the retained contrast from a previous lymphogram.

three times more common in boys than in girls. Interestingly, it occurs in an older age group in boys (aged 12–15) than in girls (aged 10–13), where it is associated with the menarche. It is associated with delayed bone age, and 95% of the patients are obese. Similar to Legg-Calvé-Perthes disease, SCFE is bilateral in 25% of patients. It is thought that the etiology is due to trauma, no doubt related to the patients' obesity.

Radiologically, the femoral head classically slips posteromedially (Fig. 45).

A number of lines have also been described in this situation: a line through the middle of the neck does not bisect the femoral head, and a line on top of the neck misses the head altogether. There is frequent widening of the epiphyseal plate. Often the first clue to SCFE is on the frog-leg view or the lateral projection, since the frontal view appears to show a normal position. Apart from the "idiopathic" form of SCFE, there are a number of other causes, and these include renal failure (14) (Fig. 46), rickets (Fig. 47), and radiation therapy (15) (Fig. 48).

Although one considers this a disease of children, obviously it has side effects later on, and, in a recent study, 61 patients were reviewed over 40 years later and it was found that 20% had contralateral SCFE at maturity and 23% later. Of these patients, only two were asymptomatic. On review of the X-ray films, early degenerative arthritis was found in 19% of patients whose slip had been treated and had no obvious deformity on follow-up. The incidence of degenerative arthritis increased to 31% in those patients who were untreated.

If there is any doubt about the presence of SCFE on plain films, either an arthrogram or an MRI can be used to confirm the diagnosis (Figs. 49A, B and 50).

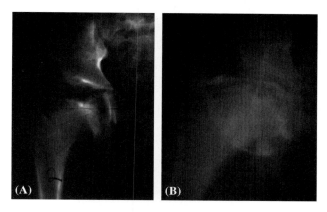

Figure 49 Slipped capital femoral epiphyses. (**A**) Plain film showing a characteristic and severe SCFE. (**B**) The arthrogram confirms the severe slip.

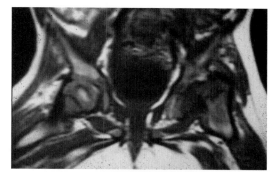

Figure 50 Slipped capital femoral epiphyses in a different child. MRI. coronal PD sequence. The right hip is normal with the normal "bull's-eye" pattern of the femoral head anlage. The left side shows a severe slipped capital femoral epiphyses with the femoral head in the acetabular, and the femoral neck subluxed outward and upward. The femoral head itself is difficult to see.

Coxa Vara

The term coxa vara is used when the shaft of the proximal femur is in marked varus angulation compared with the femoral neck. Radiologically, it almost appears to be at right angle. There is a congenital idiopathic coxa vara, although this is quite rare. Most of the other causes of coxa vara are specific diseases.

Most often, coxa vara is seen in association with osteogenesis imperfecta, fibrous dysplasia, in association with primary and secondary hypoparathyroidism, or with rickets. It is also seen commonly in a number of dysplasias, particularly the epiphyseal dysplasias and chondrodysplasia (Fig. 51).

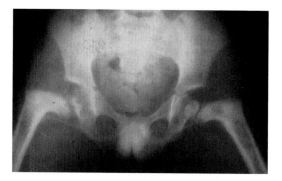

Figure 51 Coxa vara. This young child with renal failure and secondary hyperparathyroidism developed severe bilateral coxa vara shortly after starting to walk.

Coxa Valga

Coxa valga, on the other hand, is a condition associated with children who do not bear weight. Their femoral neck never forms fully, and there is a straight line between the femoral neck and the femoral shaft. The classical example of this is in patients who have cerebral palsy or meningomyeloceles. However, any form of neuromuscular disorder can be associated with coxa valga (Fig. 52).

Coxa Magna

Coxa magna means that the femoral head is large and does not fit properly into the acetabulum. The term usually used to describe it is "covered," implying that the femoral head is larger than the acetabulum. Once again, this is seen primarily in the various dysplasias, particularly the

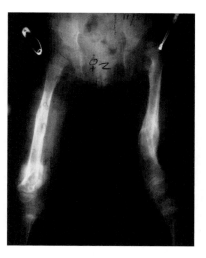

Figure 52 Coxa valga. This two-year-old child with severe cerebral palsy never walked and has bilateral coxa valga with a developmental hip dysplasia on the left.

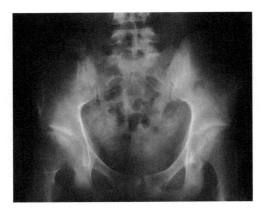

Figure 53 Coxa magna. A 30-year-old man with premature degenerative arthritis has bilateral coxa magna as a result of spondyloepiphyseal dysplasia.

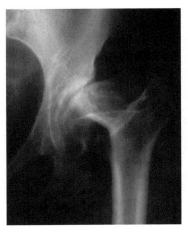

Figure 54 Coxa magna. The classical cause of severe coxa magna is slipped capital femoral epiphyses and this is a case with marked distortion of the left hip, a shallow acetabulum and coxa magna.

epiphyseal dysplasias and spondyloepiphyseal dysplasias (Figs. 53 and 54). However, it can also be seen secondary to both Legg-Calvé-Perthes disease and SCFE.

Proximal Femoral Focal Deficiency

This is an unusual condition that is poorly described in many books except for some specialized orthopedic books. It refers to a congenital anomaly where the femoral head and proximal femoral neck either do not form at all or may form abnormally, and so the child is born with a congenitally short femur.

It has a very characteristic radiographic appearance with apparently a relatively normal acetabulum, but no femoral head, neck, or intertrochanteric region (Fig. 55A–C). There are a number of different classifications, but they are of no concern here.

PEDIATRIC FEET

Many textbooks have been written about pediatric feet. Once again, I intend to simplify the abnormalities into three types. Before we begin, it is necessary to review the anatomy of the foot and to remind you that there are three parts of the foot: the hindfoot, which consists of the talus and calcaneus; the midfoot, which consists of the cuboid, navicular and cuneiforms; and the forefoot, which consists of the metatarsals and phalanges. Each of these bears a normal relationship to the next. This relationship may be abnormal or normal. If it is abnormal, the findings may be a "varus" deformity or a "valgus" deformity. Some other words used in foot congenital abnormalities are "equinus" and "cavus." "Equinus" refers to superior elevation of the hindfoot, and obviously from its derivation, it is meant to

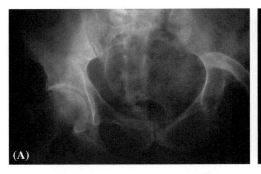

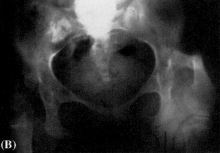

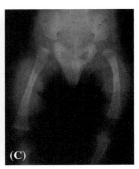

Figure 55 (**A**) Proximal femoral focal deficiency shows a normal right side and a dysplastic proximal femur on the left with a small spike of femoral shaft, which is posteriorly dislocated. (**B**) Bilateral hip deformities with a very short deformed femur on the left with proximal focal femoral deficiency and a basically absent femur on the right. (**C**) Shows a normal right side but a short femur on the left with absent trochanters in another patient.

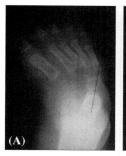
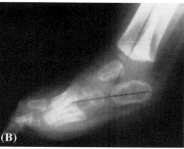

Figure 56 (**A**) Clubfoot. AP view. Note that metatarsals have a distinct varus deformity. (**B**) On the lateral view, the posterior aspect of the calcaneus is elevated, and the child has a high arch (equinocavus).

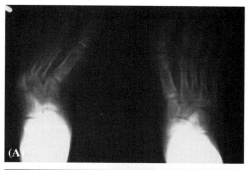

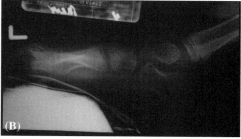

Figure 57 (**A**) Metatarsus varus. The right foot is normal. On the left side, the mid and forefoot are in markedly varus although the lateral view is essentially normal. (**B**) Lateral view appears essentially normal.

look like the heel of a horse. However, this is usually a clinical finding and not a radiological one. Someone who has an increased plantar arch or a high arch is known to have "cavus" foot. There are three other terms that need to be defined. "Talipes" means a severe equinovarus foot, which resembles a horse's hoof and basically describes the underlying findings in clubfoot (Fig. 56A, B).

"Pes planus" means a flatfoot, and this can be seen in many conditions and will not be discussed here further. Finally, the term "vertical talus" means just what it says that although the other bones in the foot are fairly normal, the talus is vertical. This may be an isolated finding or it can be seen in association with a number of dysplasias.

Radiographically, if the alignment of the foot in the AP view is taken into account, a line drawn through the center of the talus should either run through the line of the first metatarsal, or the interspace between the bases of the first and second metatarsal.

Similarly, a line drawn through the length of the calcaneus should transect the space between the fourth and fifth metatarsals. Thus, by definition, a varus deformity occurs when the calcaneal line on the AP view falls outside the 5th metatarsal (Figs. 56A and 57A).

In a valgus foot, a line drawn through the talus is markedly inside any of the metatarsal shafts, although the calcaneal line may be normal.

In the lateral view of a normal foot, the calcaneus subtends an angle of approximately 30° to the ground. The talus subtends an angle of 30° to the calcaneus, and if a line through the talus is drawn down through the foot, it should transect the metatarsals, particularly the first metatarsal.

In a varus deformity, the calcaneus is either horizontal to the ground or even possibly has reversed angulation (equinus). The talar line is parallel to the calcaneal line. In a valgus deformity, the talus is vertical.

Clubfoot

In a clubfoot, the posterior aspect of the calcaneus is elevated. Thus, the calcaneus either is horizontal or actually has a reversed angle (Fig. 56). In clubfoot, the talus is in its normal position, but the metatarsals have a marked varus angulation with respect to the hindfoot, that is, metatarsus varus.

Metatarsus Varus

In this abnormality, the lateral view is essentially normal, with normal talar and calcaneal angles. However, on the AP view the line of the metatarsals swings in markedly so that the calcaneal line, instead of transecting the fifth metatarsal, usually misses the foot altogether.

Vertical Talus

In vertical talus, on the lateral view, the calcaneus is usually horizontal rather than at a 30° angulation, and the talus is vertical (Fig. 58A, B). In order for the foot to accommodate this situation, the forefoot goes into valgus angulation. The patient also has a flatfoot in association with this abnormality (Fig. 59A, B).

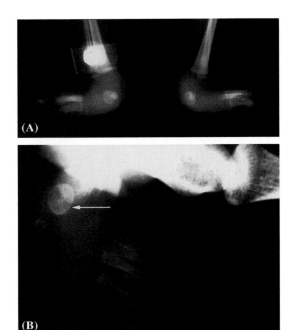

Figure 58 (**A**) Bilateral vertical talus in a very young child. On the lateral view, the talus (*arrow*) is vertical, the calcaneus is horizontal. (**B**) In this oblique view, the vertical talus is more obvious (*arrow*), and the forefoot is in marked valgus angulation with respect to the hindfoot.

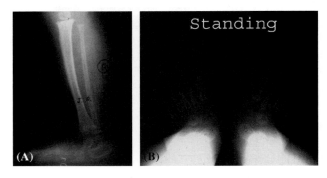

Figure 59 (**A**) Vertical talus is an older child. On the lateral view, the pes planus is easy to see and the talus is almost vertical. (**B**) On the AP standing view, there is marked metatarsus valgus.

SCOLIOSIS

Various types of scoliosis have been reported. Basically, there are idiopathic and structural types of scoliosis. In the United States, idiopathic scoliosis accounts for approximately 80% of the cases. Usually, the primary curve is in the thoracic region and to the right. For those of you who are opera buffs, Rigoletto has his hump, traditionally over his right shoulder. Frequently, there is a secondary curve in the lumbar region, and this is convex to the left. However, not all cases of idiopathic scoliosis have this appearance, and sometimes the primary curve can be convex to the left in the thoracic spine, or the primary curve may actually be in the lumbar region.

A reasonable way to look at the types of scoliosis is to consider them as structural, nonstructural, and transitory. The nonstructural types are those that are corrected on bending sideways, and these are often postural or compensatory, for instance, one leg being shorter than the other. The important group is the structural scoliosis. Idiopathic (or genetic) scoliosis accounts for 80% of these cases and can be divided into infantile, juvenile, and adolescent (Table 3; Fig. 60A, B). In Europe, the infantile type is quite common, whereas in America, the adolescent is by far the most common. The second subgroup is that of congenital conditions such as block vertebrae or hemivertebrae. This represents 5% of cases of scoliosis. Often this is associated with a spondyloepiphyseal dysplasia. The third group comprises neuromuscular disorders, and these may be neuropathic, which include poliomyelitis, cerebral palsy, and meningomyeloceles or myopathic, which includes muscular dystrophies, amyotonia, and Friedreich's ataxia. The fourth group is caused by neurofibromatosis. The fifth group is of certain mesenchymal disorders, including congenital conditions such as dwarfism, Morquio's disease, and Marfan's syndrome. There are also acquired mesenchymal disorders, including juvenile chronic arthritis and adult rheumatoid arthritis. Also, some people would consider Scheuermann's disease and osteogenesis imperfecta in this group. The sixth group includes trauma, with scoliosis following fractures, dislocations, radiation, surgery, or burns (Figs. 61A, B and 62).

The final subgroup is transitory scoliosis, and this is usually associated with sciatic nerve problems, hysterical patients, or inflammatory scoliosis. Inflammatory scoliosis can be seen associated with a spinal abscess or a spinal tumor, such as osteoid osteoma (Fig. 63A, B).

Probably the most interesting cause of scoliosis is radiation therapy. This occurred in the early days in the management of Wilm's tumors, where the radiation was confined to one side of the abdomen including one-half of the spine, thus damaging the growth plates on the side of the vertebral bodies and causing a scoliosis.

Nowadays, the radiation field includes both sides of the spine, and so the child will still be of short stature and have markedly deformed vertebral bodies with compression, increased density, and markedly irregular growth plates, but there would be no evidence of a scoliosis.

Table 3 Types of Scoliosis

A. Nonstructural scoliosis, i.e., corrects on bending sideways
   1. Postural
   2. Compensatory, i.e., due to a short leg, for example
B. Structural scoliosis
   1. Idiopathic (genetic) 80%
      a. Infantile
      b. Juvenile
      c. Adolescent
   2. Congenital (5%)
   3. Neuromuscular
      a. Neuropathic
         i. Polio
         ii. Cerebral palsy
         iii. Meningomyelocele
      b. Myopathic
         i. Muscular dystrophy
         ii. Amyotonia
         iii. Friedreich's ataxia
   4. Neurofibromatosis
   5. Mesenchymal disorders
      a. Congenital
         i. Dwarfism
         ii. Marquio's disease
         iii. Marfan's syndrome
      b. Acquired
         i. Juvenile chronic arthritis
         ii. Rheumatoid arthritis
      c. Others
         i. Scheuermann's disease
         ii. Osteogenesis imperfecta
   6. Trauma
      a. Fracture
      b. Irradiation
      c. Surgery
      d. Burns
C. Transitory scoliosis
   1. Sciatic
   2. Hysterical
   3. Inflammatory
      a. Associated with abscess
      b. Associated with tumor, i.e., osteoid osteoma

Source: From Ref. 16.

Osteochondroses

Over 50 different osteochondroses have been described, and many of them have eponyms. More recently, it has

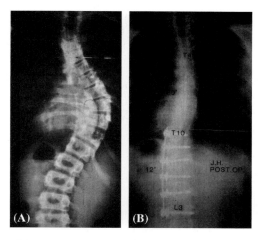

Figure 60 (**A**) Idiopathic scoliosis. There is a primary curve convex to the right in the lower thoracic region, and a secondary curve convex to the left in the lumbar region. No congenital anomalies of the spine are apparent. (**B**) Postoperatively, the primary curve has been reduced from 60° to 20°. Note the Allen fixation device on the left of the lower spine (note both films are "reversed" and viewed as from the patient's back).

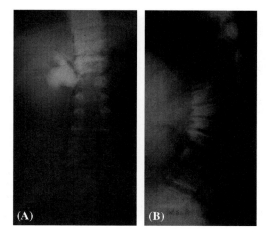

Figure 61 (**A**) Radiation scoliosis. In the frontal view, there is a discrete scoliosis convex to the left. Note the large hypertrophied solitary right kidney in this patient who received radiation therapy for a Wilms' tumor on the left, which was subsequently removed. (**B**) Lateral view shows the extensive abnormalities of the vertebral bodies caused by radiation.

become obvious that many of these conditions are not really related. In fact, they could be subdivided into those osteochondroses that really represent true avascular necrosis, those conditions that are actually avulsion phenomena from various ligamentous insertions, and finally, osteochondritis dissecans.

Group I consists of the osteochondroses, which are due to true avascular necrosis. The most common of these is probably Legg-Calvé-Perthes disease of the femoral head

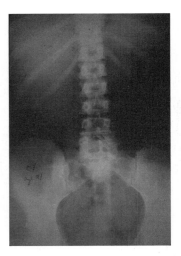

Figure 62 AP lumbar spine in another patient who received radiation for a left sided Wilms' tumor. Although the spine is spared, note the decreased size of the left hemi pelvis secondary to radiation.

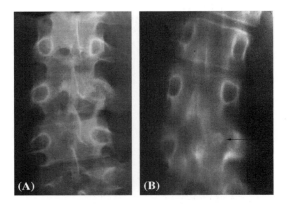

Figure 63 (A) Scoliosis caused by an osteoid osteoma. The curve is away from the tumor. The plain film is unremarkable. (B) The sclerotic nidus of the tumor can be clearly seen on this tomogram (*arrow*).

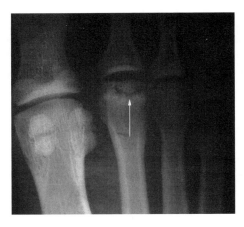

Figure 64 Freiberg's disease. Note the fracture through the second metatarsal head with flattening.

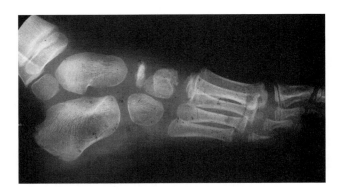

Figure 65 Kohler's disease. This is controversial with many people thinking it a normal variant. In this lateral foot X ray, the tarsal navicular is noted to be flattened and sclerotic. In my clinical experience, 80% of these reverse and return to normal, although 20% continue to have a flat navicular often developing secondary degenerative changes in later life.

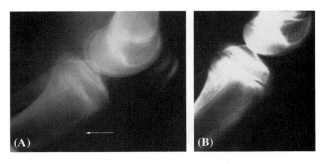

Figure 66 (A) Normal. In the normal knee the growth centers that make up the tibial tubercle grow downward (*arrow*). (B) Osgood-Schlatter's disease. However, as a result of repeated avulsion injuries in an athletic child, the growth center will grow upward in the line of the patella tendon (*arrow*).

(which has just been discussed) and Panner's disease of the capitellum lunate (see later in this chapter for a fuller description). Some people would include Freiberg's disease of the second or third metatarsal head, but most people now consider this as posttraumatic (Fig. 64).

Two other examples of true avascular necrosis in this group are Kienböck's disease of the lunate (Fig. 73 for a full description), and Kohler's disease of the tarsal navicular. All of these represent true avascular necrosis. Both Panner's disease and Kienböck's disease will be discussed in more detail at the end of this chapter (Fig. 65).

The second group of osteochondroses are avulsion injuries. The classical example is Osgood-Schlatter's disease of the tibial tubercle, which is an avulsion of the insertion of the patellar tendon (Fig. 66A, B).

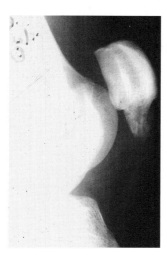

Figure 67 Sinding-Larsen disease. This is the opposite of Osgood-Schlatter's disease and the avulsion injury causes extra ossification off the lower pole of the patella.

Similarly, at the other end of the tendon, Sinding, Larsen, and Johannson described a chronic avulsion of the lower pole of the patella, giving a beak-like appearance to the bone (Fig. 67).

Sever's disease of the posterior calcaneal apophysis has also been ascribed to an avulsion phenomena. However, most of us doubt that this condition even exists (Fig. 68). The third group of osteochondroses is a condition called osteochondritis dissecans. Although this is most commonly seen in the knee, it can be seen in virtually every other joint in the body, although it is

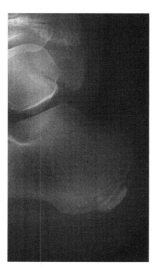

Figure 68 Sever's disease describes a very dense appearing calcaneal apophysis, but I believe that this is simply a case of delayed maturation of that growth center.

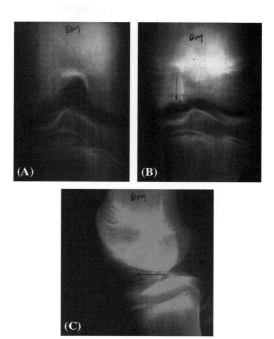

Figure 69 (**A**) Osteochondritis dissecans. Intercondylar notch view. (**B**) AP view. (**C**) Lateral view of the left knee. This is a young patient with classical osteochondritis dissecans affecting the lateral aspect of the medial epicondyle (LAME). Note the irregularity and fragmentation of this region in all three views (*arrows*).

next most common in the talus and, after that, in the shoulder. Osteochondritis dissecans is probably a form of avascular necrosis. It has also been ascribed to the failure of fusion of multiple growth centers, although I think it might, in fact, be a combination of the two. In the knee, the classical place is seen in the lateral aspect of the medial epicondyle (this spells LAME), and it is usually anterior (Fig. 69A–C). It is difficult to diagnose in young adolescents because the epiphyses will have many scattered growth centers, which may appear as osteochondritis dissecans. In such a case, an MRI of the knee will exclude the condition (see later).

Osteochondritis dissecans can be seen anywhere in the knee; the second commonest site is apparently on the undersurface of the patella, but it can also be seen on the tibial plateaus, and on the lateral femoral epicondyle.

The second commonest site of osteochondritis dissecans is in the ankle, where it involves the lateral dome of the talus (Fig. 70).

Classically, it involves the lateral aspect of the talus. A similar condition can be seen on the medial aspect, but this is almost certainly secondary to trauma and inversion injuries (Fig. 71A–D). The third commonest site is on the humeral head.

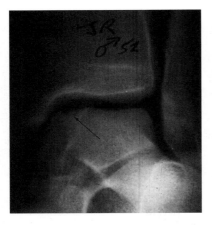

Figure 70 Osteochondritis dissecans of the talus. There is a discrete defect on the medial dome of the talus in this 52-year-old male (*arrow*).

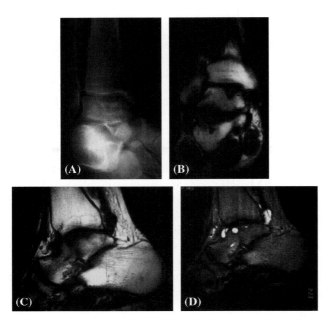

Figure 71 (**A**) Right ankle (mortise view). Classical but severe osteochondritis dissecans of the medial dome of the talus in this 28-year-old male. (**B**) Right ankle (coronal MRI). (**C**) Sagittal PD. (**D**) Sagittal fat saturation. The defect can be clearly seen in all these views. On this sagittal fat saturation slice, the collapse of the subchondral surface with cyst formation can also be seen.

MRI IN THE OSTEOCHONDROSES

There are a number of situations where MRI can be useful in assessing the viability of the bone and cartilage in patients with osteochondritis. We have already mentioned

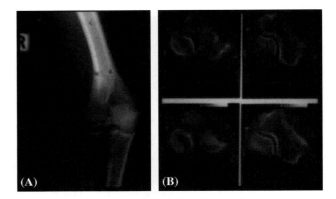

Figure 72 Panner's disease. There is fragmentation of the capitellum that is better seen on the CT scan (**B**) than on the plain film (**A**).

Legg-Calvé-Perthes disease, but the workup of patients with both Panner's disease and Kienböck's disease can be aided by an MRI. In general, dead bone has very low intensity (black) on all sequences on MRI, and living bone follows the bone marrow signal, which is high on T1, intermediate on delayed T2, and of low intensity on fat saturation sequences. In Panner's disease, which is osteochondritis of the capitellum, MRI can show the viability of the bone and the contours of the articular surfaces. There are two types of Panner's disease—a childhood type that is probably a growth defect and usually resolves, and the more characteristic adolescent type that usually persists. On plain films, there is irregularity of the articular surface (often posteriorly) as well as patchy lucencies within the capitellum. This can be confirmed by a CT scan (Fig. 72A, B).

In the early sequences on MRI, the capitellum appears hypointense, but on later T2 sequences, there is a mix of low intensity (dead bone) and high intensity because of a fracture line forming between the dead bone and the underlying living bone (Fig. 73A–C).

However, if there is some attempt at healing due to surgical intervention, the central intensity returns to normal (Fig. 74A, B).

A recent article discusses the natural progression of osteochondritis dissecans of the capitellum by studying 16 patients with early Panner's disease for four years. Seven patients in group 1 had subchondral flattening without fragmentation and four of these resolved completely. Group 2 (9 patients) had flattening with fragmentation, and only one of these healed completely suggesting that once the capitellum has fragmented, healing is unlikely.

Kienböck's disease is avascular necrosis of the lunate and occurs as a result of repetitive trauma and is often seen in gymnasts. It is also said to be associated with a short ulnar. Plain films in the early stages of Kienböck's

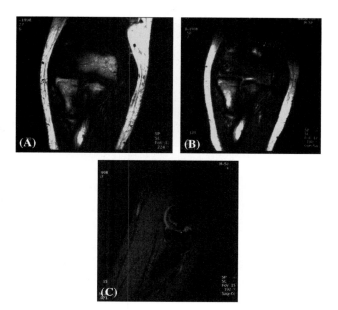

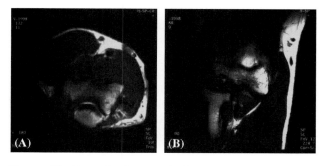

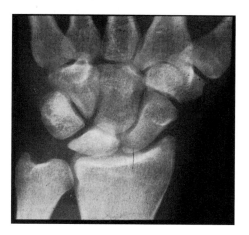

Figure 75 Kienböck's disease. Plain film. This shows the typical radiographic appearance with increased density and partial collapse of the lunate diagnostic of Kienböck's disease.

Figure 73 Panner's disease. (A–C) These three MR images show a mixed intensity area on the anterior surface of the capitellum with fragmentation and loose body formation.

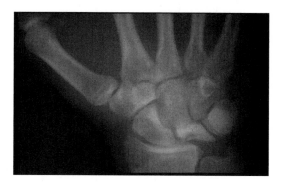

Figure 76 Kienböck's disease. Plain film in another patient showing more advanced collapse.

Figure 74 Panner's disease. (A, B) MRI in another patient shows a more chronic appearance with the main bony fragment apparently having normal bone marrow signal suggesting that it is surviving.

disease show that the lunate has increased density in comparison to the other carpal bones (Fig. 75). As the disease progresses, the lunate collapses and fragments.

MRI will show marked loss of marrow signal in the lunate, which appears black on all sequences (Fig. 76). The patient illustrated also had an old fracture of the scaphoid with avascular necrosis of the proximal pole, which also shows up as being hypointense on MRI (Figs. 77 and 78A, B).

This second case also has avascular necrosis of the proximal pole of the scaphoid and the lunate is abnormal. In an interesting surgical paper, 39 patients who underwent surgical shortening of the radius for Kienböck's disease were followed-up for four years. As a result of the operation, the pain had decreased in 90% and grip strength improved in 50% of the patients.

Of more interest is the use of MRI in the evaluation of osteochondritis dissecans. This has already been discussed to some extent above. However, MRI is able to differentiate between living and dead bone, and to some extent determine whether the bony fragments are viable and whether they are in the process of healing. Classically, osteochondritis dissecans in the knee affects the LAME, and although plain films show the lesion, MRI can better evaluate the various changes in marrow signal as well as evaluate the extent of the lesion because on many occasions, the plain films only show a subchondral defect (Fig. 79A, B).

More importantly, MRI can look for any evidence of healing after surgical intervention. This has been

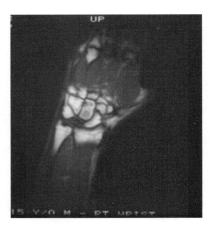

Figure 77 Kienböck's disease. MRI showing complete lack of signal in the lunate suggesting total avascular necrosis and bone death.

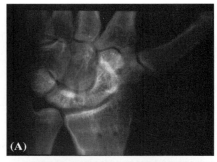

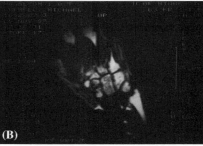

Figure 78 Kienböck's disease. Plain film and MRI in a different patient who has both Kienböck's disease and avascular necrosis of the scaphoid. (**A**) The plain film shows increased density in both bones. (**B**) The MRI shows a signal void in both bones typical of avascular necrosis.

somewhat controversial. A number of early papers suggested that many of these lesions had healed on the basis of MRI criteria. However, in a number of recent papers, a group of 15 patients were followed, 14 of whom had a high signal intensity line between the bony fragment and the underlying bone. All of these proved unstable at the time of surgery. In fact, the high signal line represents a

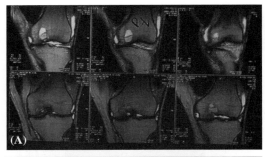

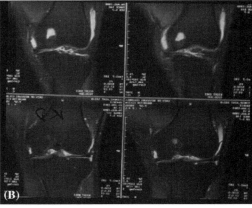

Figure 79 (**A**, **B**) Osteochondritis dissecans of the knee. The MRI shows significant subchondral cystic changes in the lateral aspect of the medial epicondyle with irregularity of the subchondral bone as well a small chondral defect.

fracture line with separation of the viable bone from the osteochondral fragment. This is similar to the MRI appearance seen in avascular necrosis in the femoral head. On the other hand, healing can also be demonstrated on MRI by bony bridging between the fragment and the underlying bone. In a recent paper on the long-term follow-up of osteochondritis dissecans of the knee, 22 knees were followed for an average of 34 years: 45% had poor results and 55% considered their results excellent following surgical intervention.

HOLT-ORAM SYNDROME

This is an autosomal dominant syndrome first described in 1960 and has an incidence of 1 in 100,000 births. However, most cases are due to spontaneous mutation in the gene that codes for transcription factor TBX5, located on the long arm of chromosome 12. This results in abnormalities of the upper extremity and in cardiac abnormalities. Upper extremity involvement is always present and results in aplasia or hypoplasia of the radial, carpal, or thenar bones. In approximately three-quarters of the patients, associated cardiac deformities are also present, most commonly an atrial or ventricular septal defect.

POLAND SYNDROME

Incidence estimates of Poland syndrome range from 1 in 100,000 to 1 in 10,000 live births and include underdevelopment or absence of the pectoralis major as well as the overlying breast tissue. The right side is affected twice as often as the left. Patchy absence of hair on the underside of the ipsilateral arm has also been reported. Webbing of the fingers of the ipsilateral hand, rib anomalies, and a small elevated scapula (Sprengel's deformity) are associated deformities.

NAIL-PATELLA SYNDROME

Nail-Patella syndrome is also called Fong's disease, hereditary onychoosteodysplasia (HOOD syndrome), and Iliac-Horn disease. This syndrome affects ectodermal and mesodermal tissues and has an incidence of approximately 1 in 50,000 live births. The syndrome includes underdevelopment which is the result of a mutation in the gene for transcription factor LMX1B, located on the long arm of chromosome 9q34. The classic tetrad includes fingernail dysplasia, absent or hypoplastic patellae, the presence of posterior conical iliac horns, and hypoplasia of the radial heads. Kidney disease and glaucoma are now part of the syndrome, and most of the morbidity is due to the nephropathy.

MARFAN'S SYNDROME

This is an autosomal dominant connective tissue disorder and has a prevalence in the range of 1 in 10,000 to 1 in 5000. Abnormalities in fibrillin-1 gene (chromosome 15) are the most common known mutations. TGFβ signaling pathway may represent a final common pathway and has also been implicated. The Ghent criteria have superceded the Berlin criteria and the diagnosis is now based on family history, genetic analysis, and the evaluation of six organ systems (skeletal, ocular, cardiovascular, pulmonary, skin, and dural). Skeletal manifestations include tall, thin stature with long limbs (arm span to height ratio > 1.05), pectus excavatum that requires surgery or pectus carinatum, arachnodactyly, scoliosis greater than 20°, reduced extension of the elbows (<170°), protrusio acetabula, and dural ectasia as well as prominent abnormalities in other organ systems.

A number of other congenital or hereditary conditions are considered elsewhere in this book. Hemophilia, thalassemia, and sickle cell anemia, for example, are discussed earlier in Chapter 3. This chapter will close with the discussion of an unusual yet not uncommon condition: fibrous dysplasia.

FIBROUS DYSPLASIA

This is another condition that is presumably congenital in origin and is related to abnormal bones. It may be monostotic, with only small areas of abnormality or the whole bone involved; or polyostotic, in which case a whole limb or side of the body may be involved. If associated with sexual precocity, fibrous dysplasia is known as Albright's syndrome.

The radiographic appearances are characteristic, with loss of the normal trabecular pattern, widening of the bone with scalloping of the inner surface of the cortex, and an overall smooth "ground glass" texture to the bone. If fibrous dysplasia occurs in a long bone there may be bowing; in a rib, fibrous dysplasia produces a "soap bubble" appearance; and if it occurs in the femoral neck, fibrous dysplasia leads to a characteristic "shepherd's crook" deformity. The complications of fibrous dysplasia include pathologic and incremental fractures, curious irregular speckled new bone formation resembling popcorn within a normal bone, and an increased incidence of sarcomatous change particularly following previous radiotherapy, which was a mode of treatment 30 years ago. The more localized forms of fibrous dysplasia fill in spontaneously without any sequelae.

REFERENCES

1. Hall JF, Pauli RM, Wilson KM. Maternal and fetal sequelae of anticoagulation during pregnancy. Am J Med 1980; 68:122–140.
2. Ingram RR. The shoulder in multiple epiphyseal dysplasia. J Bone Joint Surg Br 1991; 73(2):277–279.
3. Luisiri A, Silberstein MJ, Sundaram M, et al. Dysplasia epiphysialis hemimelica. Orthopedics 1985; 8(9):1170–1175.
4. Koslowski K, Beighton P. Gamut Index of Skeletal Dysplasia, Second Edition, 1995, Springer, Berlin and New York.
5. Milgram JW, Jasty M, Osteopetrosis. A morphological study of twenty-one cases. J Bone Joint Surg Am 1982; 64(6):912–929.
6. Grey AC, Wallace R, Crone M. Engelmann's disease: a 45-year follow-up. J Bone Joint Surg Br 1996; 78(3):488–491.
7. Kaftori JK, Kleinhaus U, Naveh Y. Progressive diaphyseal dysplasia (Camurati-Engelmann): radiographic follow-up and CT findings. Radiology 1987; 164(3):777–782.
8. Voorhoeve N. L'image radiologique nan encore decrite d'une anomalie du squelette. Acta Radiol 1924; 3:407–427.
9. Greenspan A. Sclerosing bone dysplasias—a target-site approach. Skeletal Radiol 1991; 20(8):561–583.
10. Terjesen T, Anda S. Ultrasound measurement of femoral anteversion. J Bone Joint Surg Br 1989; 71(2):237–239.
11. Harcke HT. Imaging methods used for children with hip dysplasia. Clin Orthop Relat Res 2005; 434:71–77.
12. Bos CF, Bloem JL, Obermann WR, et al. Magnetic resonance imaging in congenital dislocation of the hip. J Bone Joint Surg Br 1988; 70(2):174–178.

13. Egund N, Wingstrand H. Legg-Calvé-Perthes disease: imaging with MR. Radiology 1991; 179(1):89–92.

14. Madeira IR, Machado M, Maya MC, et al. Primary hyperparathyroidism associated to slipped capital femoral epiphysis in a teenager. Arg Bras Endocrinol Metabol 2005; 49(2):314–318.

15. Liu SC, Tsai CC, Huang CH. Atypical slipped capital femoral epiphysis after radiotherapy and chemotherapy. Clin Orthop Relat Res 2004; (426):212–218.

16. Kiem. Adapted with permission from Clinical Symposia 1978; 30(1):1–30. Copyright c 1978, CIBA-Geigy Corporation.

6

Bone and Soft Tissue Tumors

INTRODUCTION

Rather than memorize a list of tumors both common and uncommon, an organized approach to their clinical and radiological features is useful. However, it has been estimated that the average radiologist will only see one osteogenic sarcoma or osteosarcoma (OGS) in his or her whole lifetime. The most important parameters in the diagnosis of a bone tumor are the age of the patient, the site of the tumor, and its appearance. The sex of the patient is of little help since more tumors occur in male patients then in female patients with the usual ratio being 2:1.

The age of the patient is important since most tumors have a fairly limited age range. So, for instance, eosinophylic granuloma, Ewing's sarcoma, and metastatic neuroblastomas occur largely in young children, chondroblastoma and osteoid osteoma in adolescents, and giant cell tumor and OGS in young adults. At the other end of the spectrum, multiple myeloma and metastases occur mainly in older patients. With respect to malignant tumors, Ewing's sarcoma is mainly seen below the age of 20 years, OGS seen from ages 15 to 25 years, parosteal OGS 25 to 40 years, chondrosarcoma 30 to 45 years, and undifferentiated pleomorphic sarcoma (UPS) after the age of 50 years.

The site of the tumor is also important, although the majority of primary bone tumors occur in the metaphysis of long bones. An epiphyseal lesion in a child is usually caused by one of three things: eosinophylic granuloma, Brodie's abscess, and chondroblastoma. In someone older than 40 years, an epiphyseal lesion is either due to multiple myeloma or a metastasis. Diaphyseal lesions are usually bone marrow tumors, so depending on the age of the patient—Ewing's sarcoma, lymphoma, multiple myeloma, and metastatic disease in chronological order. The only tumor that characteristically goes from the metaphysis into the epiphysis is a giant cell tumor. Some tumors that extend from the metaphysis into the diaphysis include fibrous dysplasia, unicameral bone cysts (UBCs), and a sessile osteochondroma. The remainder of primary tumors in long bones occur in the metaphysis itself. With respect to flat bones, all bets are off, although chondroid tumors occur more commonly in the pelvis and shoulder girdle than osteoblastic or fibroblastic lesions.

Finally, the appearance of the tumor is important—does it contain trabeculae (in which case it is probably osteoblastic) or cartilaginous calcifications (then use the word "chondro" in the name of the tumor)? Does it have a "ground-glass" appearance? This is classically seen in fibrous dysplasia but can also be seen in other fibrous tissue tumors as well as in brown tumors of hyperparathyroidism. If it appears lucent then it may contain fluid (UBC), blood [aneurysmal bone cyst (ABC) or arteriovenous malformation], or solid myxomatous tissue. The margins are important—thick sclerotic margins imply long-standing and benign tumors: no margins imply aggressive behavior, although not necessarily malignant. Always remember infection that can appear aggressive. The term "expansile" is loosely used since bone cannot expand, but what does happen is that the inner endosteal cortex gets eroded while the periostium is laying down bone on the outside. Thus, expansibility implies a non-aggressive and benign condition, although OGS can also be expansile.

Putting all these things together—age, site, and appearance should at least suggest either a benign or a malignant process. Some people more correctly use the terms non-aggressive and aggressive. If the tumor appears benign, there are some lesions we term "leave-me-alone" lesions and these include fibrocortical defects, fibrous dysplasia, intraosseous lipomas, bone islands, and osteomas. These need no further management once the radiological diagnosis has been made, hence "leave-me-alone." Some other lesions require follow-up without surgical intervention, for instance, benign enchondromatous calcifications in the proximal or distal metaphysis of a humerus or femur in older patients: three months, six months, and yearly follow-up, unless the patient starts developing pain. Once again, remember the old medical aphorism—at least do no harm. So, sort out the benign from the malignant bone tumors and you will be helping the patient as well as the clinician.

TUMORS OF OSTEOBLASTIC ORIGIN

Osteoma Bone Islands and Enostoses

Bone islands and osteomas can be found in people of almost any age, although they are rare below the age of 10 years. They are equally common in both sexes, and most of us have at least one bone island somewhere in us. Bone islands can occur in any flat or long bone but seem to be more common in the metaphyseal ends of the long bones and in flat bones such as the pelvis. Osteomas occur in and around the skull. The classical osteoma occurs in one of the sinuses and is frequently seen in a frontal sinus (Fig. 1).

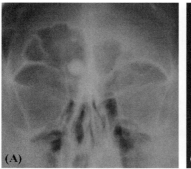
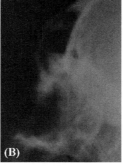

Figure 1 Classical osteoma in a frontal sinus. (**A**) AP view. This is still attached to the underlying bone. (**B**) Lateral view. This is still attached to the underlying bone. *Abbreviation*: AP, anteroposterior.

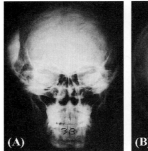
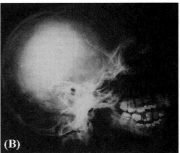

Figure 2 Osteoma in the parietal bone of the skull. (**A**) AP view. (**B**) Lateral view. *Abbreviation*: AP, anteroposterior.

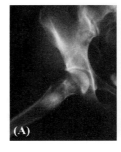
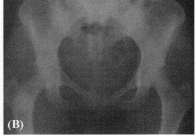

Figure 3 Osteoma or giant bone island in the upper right femur. (**A**) Frog-leg view. (**B**) AP view. *Abbreviation*: AP, anteroposterior.

If it loosens from its anchor, it can drop off and obstruct the sinus causing sinusitis and ultimately osteomyelitis. In the flat bones of the vault of the skull, osteomas usually appear as a dense, sclerotic area often described as "ivory." Both osteomas and bone islands are entirely benign, and the only reason for operating is for cosmetic reasons or if they obstruct the outlet of one of the sinuses. Bone islands can grow to quite an extraordinary size when they are known as giant bone islands. While these are growing they are usually positive on a bone scan. The differential diagnosis between a small bone island and a metastasis, however, is usually based on the fact that on a bone scan a metastasis will have high intensity but a bone island will not light up (Figs. 2–4).

The classical appearance of a large bone island is as follows: at least three of the sides are smooth but the other side has a meteor-like effect with normal trabeculae running into the bone island itself (Fig. 5).

Osteoid Osteoma

These are also probably not real tumors since they are inclined to disappear after four or five years. The classical age range is from 20 to 30 years. They occur twice as commonly in male patients as in female. The vast majority

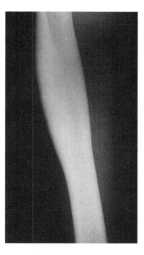

Figure 4 Osteoma of the midshaft in the right femur; note the cortical thickening. This could just as easily be a healed stress fracture, an undetected osteoid osteoma, or sclerosing osteomyelitis of Garre.

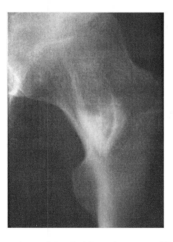

Figure 5 Giant bone island. Note that two sides are smooth, but the proximal margin blends into the underlying trabecular pattern like a meteor.

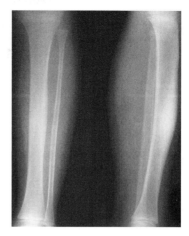

Figure 6 Classical osteoid osteoma in the mid-tibia shaft with a 1-cm central lucency and marked sclerotic reaction surrounding it.

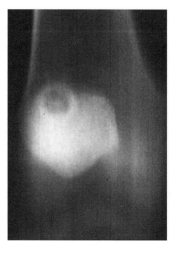

Figure 7 Osteoid osteoma in the patella. This is a tomogram and shows that the nidus contains some mineralization.

of osteoid osteomas are in the metaphyses of long bones such as the tibia and femur, although they may occur in the midshaft of one of these bones (Fig. 6).

They also occur in bones such as the patella, talus, and posterior elements of the spine (Figs. 7 and 8).

Osteoid osteomas have been found in the talus but they are rarely described in the skull or clavicle.

Two types of osteoid osteoma are described: the cancellous and the cortical type. The cancellous type is typically seen in the upper femur (Fig. 9), where it can occur in the femoral calcar. The central lucency is actually

the nidus of the tumor. The cortical appearance is what one sees in the long bones with a large sclerotic reaction, although the nidus may not be seen on plain films. A CT scan or an MRI may help. The treatment is to leave them alone and treat the pain, which classically occurs at night, with salicylates. The tumor will disappear in four to six years. However, surgeons like removing these lesions when they can. In a nice review article from the Mayo Clinic, they discussed 67 patients of whom 48 were male. The age range was 8–53 years, although the mean was 20 years, and the patients usually presented with pain which worsened at night. Of the tumors, two-thirds were cortical and one-third medullary, although a few were intra-articular. Intra-articular osteoid osteomas appear to arise within the actual lining of the joint. The overall

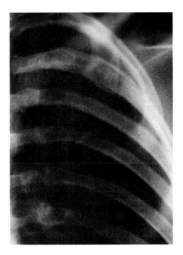

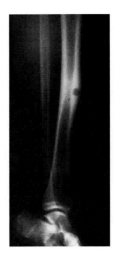

Figure 8 Osteoid osteoma in the rib. Note the mineralization within the nidus but little sclerotic reaction surrounding it similar to Figure 7. Both of these are examples of the cancellous type of osteoid osteoma.

Figure 10 Classical osteoid osteoma in the midtibia.

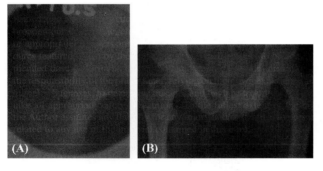

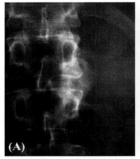
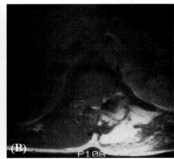

Figure 9 Osteoid osteoma in the femoral calcar. (**A**) Tomogram of right hip. The nidus is seen to lie with the femoral calcar. (**B**) AP of pelvis. The nidus is seen to lie with the femoral calcar. This patient had had two earlier biopsies of his femoral neck until they saw the nidus in the calcar! *Abbreviation*: AP, anteroposterior.

Figure 11 Osteoblastoma in the left posterior aspect of L1. (**A**) Plain film. The plain film shows expansion of the lateral mass containing ossification. (**B**) MRI. The MRI shows a large expansile tumor invading the pedicle, transverse process, and lamina of L1 extending into the soft tissues. *Abbreviation*: MRI, magnetic resonance imaging.

concept is that osteoid osteomas are a benign inflammatory reaction rather than a true tumor (Fig. 10).

they are expansile and lytic and expand out to one side or the other. As I mentioned, they do occur in flat bones and long bones, although this is even rarer (Figs. 11–13).

Osteoblastomas

Osteoblastomas are rare. The majority occur in the second and third decades, and they are mainly seen in the spine (over 60%). However, they have also been rarely seen in long bones and even in flat bones.

In the spine they characteristically appear to have their epicenter within the pedicle and extend forward into the body and backward into the lamina. They may become so extensive that the vertebral body collapses, but usually

Osteosarcoma

OGS can be conveniently subdivided into five types:
Conventional type
  Pathological subtypes

- Telangiectatic
- Small cell
- Large cell
- Central low grade.

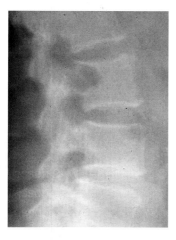

Figure 12 Osteoblastoma in the L2 vertebral body. This discrete lytic lesion extends from the pedicle forward into the vertebral body, which is characteristic of a small osteoblastoma.

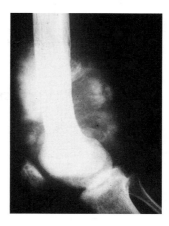

Figure 14 Conventional osteogenic sarcoma. There is a large soft tissue mass containing "sunray" spiculation and producing dense sclerosis in the underlying bone.

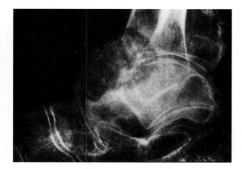

Figure 13 Osteoblastoma in the talus. There is a large expansile, basically lytic lesion destroying the upper surface of the talus and containing ossification.

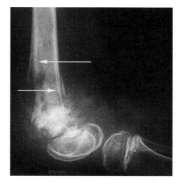

Figure 15 Conventional osteosarcoma. This tumor is more destructive and lytic and has produced classical Codman's triangle (*arrows*). Note the involvement of the growth plate.

Parosteal type
Periosteal or juxtacortical type
High-grade surface OGS
Secondary OGS

- Paget's disease
- Fibrous dysplasia
- Bone Infarcts
- Radiation
- Orthopedic instrumentation

The conventional type of OGS classically occurs between the age of 10 and 25 years and is twice as common in males as in females. It represents 20% of all malignant bone tumors. It occurs in the metaphysis of long bones and approximately 70% occur at the knee of which 60% occur in the distal femur. On plain films it rarely appears to cross the growth plate. Its radiological appearance will vary from being very lytic and destructive to being completely sclerotic. Approximately 60% of the patients have periosteal

elevation that is known as a Codman's triangle and about 15% show what is known as sunray spiculation (Figs. 14 and 15). In flat bones, OGS can be entirely sclerotic (Fig. 16).

The treatment nowadays is to give chemotherapy and irradiation, and the five-year survival rate is now in the region of approximately 40%.

The central low-grade OGS occurs in a somewhat older age group and usually consists of some discrete lytic and blastic areas in the metaphysis of a long bone. The five-year survival rate following adequate treatment and excision is approximately 80% (Fig. 17).

Epiphyseal involvement was said to never occur in OGS; however, with the advent of MRI, epiphyseal involvement is found to occur in approximately two-thirds of the patients (Fig. 18).

There is a rare condition called osteosarcomatosis in which a patient develops multiple OGS. The tumors may be synchronous or metachronous with the tumors all starting together or starting separately over several

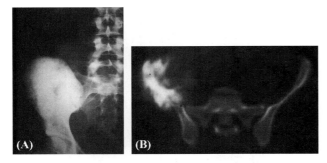

Figure 16 Osteosarcoma in the pelvis. (**A**) Plain film. There is an extensive sclerotic lesion involving almost the entire right iliac wing. The differential diagnosis in a younger patient would include Ewing's sarcoma (see below). (**B**) CT scan. There is an extensive sclerotic lesion involving almost the entire right iliac wing. *Abbreviation*: CT, computed tomography.

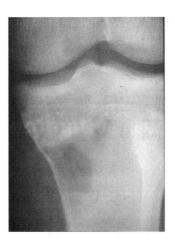

Figure 17 Central low-grade osteosarcoma. There is a discrete patchy destructive lesion involving the medial metaphysis of the proximal tibia and extending into the soft tissues in this 22-year-old male. Note the patchy mineralization both in the bone and in the soft tissue components.

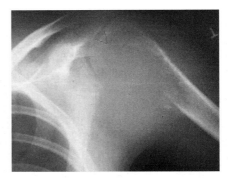

Figure 18 Lytic osteosarcoma involving both the metaphysis and the epiphysis in this 23-year-old Jehovah's witness who refused all therapy. This was probably a telangiectatic type of osteosarcoma.

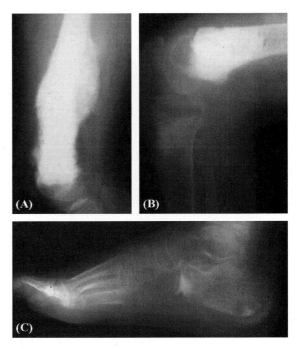

Figure 19 Osteosarcomatosis. This 12-year-old girl developed a series of osteosarcomas over a few months so this is the metachronous variety. (**A**) Left femur—first tumor. (**B**) Right femur—next tumor. (**C**) Left calcaneus with probably two separate osteosarcomas, which appeared six months later.

months. There appear to be two subtypes of this already rare tumor. The first subtype is in children younger than 18 years, in which case the tumor is extremely malignant and the five-year survival rate is 0%. The second subtype, which is not quite as common, usually has bilateral symmetric lesions and the five-year survival rate is not so serious (Fig. 19).

The telangiectatic OGS is a pathological term and not a radiological finding. Radiologically, telangiectatic OGS are usually more lytic than blastic. They have the same prognosis as conventional OGS. The other subtypes are entirely pathological diagnoses (Figs. 18 and 20).

OGS can and frequently do metastasize to other bones. They also may metastasize to the lungs where they can cavitate or ossify (Fig. 21), and rarely they will cause hypertrophic osteoarthropathy (Fig. 22).

Parosteal Osteosarcoma

Parosteal OGS have a very characteristic appearance, although they are relatively rare; they represent only

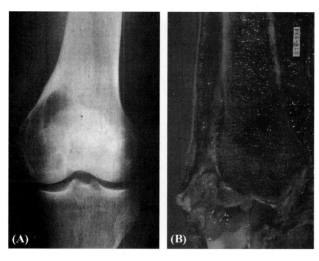

Figure 20 Telangiectatic type of osteosarcoma. (**A**) Plain film. On the film the differential diagnosis would suggest a giant cell tumor (see below) but this was, in fact, a telangiectatic type of osteosarcoma. (**B**) Pathological specimen shows the large central hemorrhage, which extends into the anterior soft tissue and is typical of a telangiectatic type of osteosarcoma.

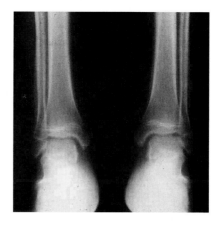

Figure 22 Hypertrophic osteoarthropathy in the lower legs in a child caused by metastatic osteosarcoma. Note the parallel periosteal reaction running along both the distal tibias and fibulas.

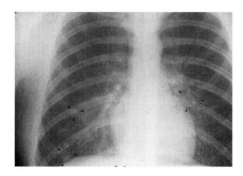

Figure 21 Multiple pulmonary metastases from osteosarcoma. Some have cavitated (*arrowheads*) and some have ossified.

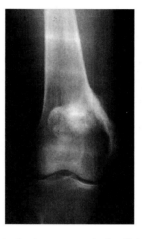

Figure 23 Parosteal osteosarcoma in the distal femur. There is sclerotic new bone adjacent to the medial cortex of the femur in this 29-year-old male. This was resected and he has had no recurrence for over 20 years.

1% of all malignant tumors. Their age range is somewhat older than that found in case of conventional OGS, i.e., between 25 and 40 years. They are metaphyseal and 75% of them occur in the lower femur. The radiological appearance looks as though someone has poured some bone on the outer aspect of the distal cortex of the femur (Fig. 23).

If one can find the periosteal line (which is lucent because it is a fibrous tissue), this will be shifted away from its normal anatomical position. The importance of this finding is that in myositis ossificans, the periostium remains in its normal position (Fig. 24).

The usual management is local excision or amputation and the five-year survival rate is 90%.

Periosteal or Juxtacortical Osteosarcoma

The periosteal OGS is even rarer than the parosteal osteosarcoma. It occurs in patients generally older than 50 years and is usually more destructive and is metadiaphyseal. The five-year survival rate is approximately 60%, which is in-between the conventional and parosteal survival rates (Figs. 25 and 26).

High-Grade Surface Osteosarcoma

Finally, the high-grade surface OGS is extraordinarily rare. Most of them occur on the anterior surface of the tibia

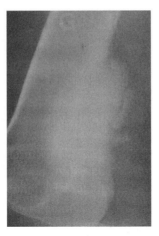

Figure 24 Parosteal osteosarcoma. This is much more extensive and has invaded the intramedullary canal of the femur, thus increasing the risk of metastases.

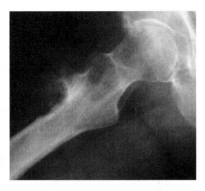

Figure 25 Periosteal osteosarcoma. This 56-year-old male presented with increasing pain in his right hip. There is an extrophic lesion scalloping the outer cortex of the underlying femur, typical of periosteal osteosarcoma.

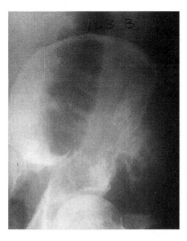

Figure 26 Periosteal osteosarcoma in the pelvis of a 70-year-old male. This lesion almost has the appearance of an osteochondroma except that it contains ossifications rather than calcifications.

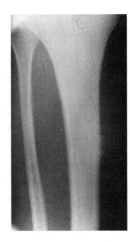

Figure 27 High-grade surface osteosarcoma. This 40-year-old physician presented with sudden pain and swelling in his midtibia. There is a discrete perpendicular periosteal reaction and soft tissue swelling seen on the medial aspect of the tibia. He died of multiple metastatic disease within a year.

where they produce a perpendicular, fluffy periosteal new bone appearance with a soft tissue mass. Differential diagnosis lies between a surface OGS and the very benign finding of a periosteal hematoma. However, the five-year survival rate is almost 0% (Fig. 27).

Secondary Sarcomas

Secondary sarcomas are described in a number of different situations, although probably the most commonly seen secondary sarcomas are following irradiation or in association with Paget's disease. The radiation threshold for a secondary sarcoma to occur is over 60 Gy. A radiation sarcoma occurs in patients older than 40 years in an area that had been irradiated many years previously. They could also be seen following the use of thorium and other radioactive substances. Treatment is relatively useless and the two-year survival rate is basically 0%. Radiation sarcomas are usually destructive rather than blastic and the majority occur following radiation for breast cancer and so are seen around the shoulder (Figs. 28 and 29).

Occasionally, radiation-induced soft tissue OGS can also be seen (Fig. 30).

The sarcomas seen in association with Paget's disease are discussed in section "Paget's Disease" of chapter 4.

CHONDROID TUMORS—TUMORS OF CARTILAGINOUS ORIGIN

Chondroblastoma (Codman's Tumor)

These represent approximately 1% of all benign tumors and occur entirely in children from the age of 5 to 15 years.

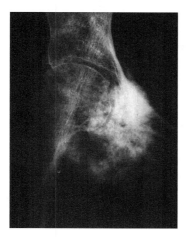

Figure 28 Radiation-induced osteosarcoma. This young female received over 90 Gy to her pelvis for a cervical cancer nine years previously. There is a destructive, expansile, sclerotic lesion involving her right anterior acetebular column as well as pubic and ischial rami. On biopsy this was found to be an osteosarcoma.

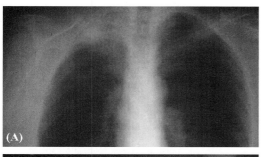

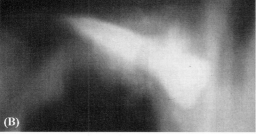

Figure 29 Radiation-induced osteosarcoma. This elderly lady received a high dose of radiation to her right axilla for breast cancer. Nine years later she developed this radiation-induced osteosarcoma of her clavicle. (A) Chest X-ray. (B) Tomogram of her clavicle showing marked sclerosis of the bone with a large soft tissue mass.

They are twice as common in boys as in girls. They occur within the epiphysis and typically are seen in the proximal humerus, proximal femur, and the distal femoral and upper tibial epiphyses. The radiological findings are of a lucency with clear-cut sclerotic margins, often containing

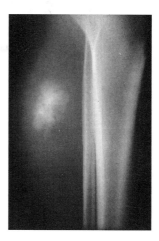

Figure 30 Soft tissue osteosarcoma secondary to radiation in a 45-year-old male who was complaining of pain and swelling in his calf. He had received over 80 Gy for an Ewing's sarcoma, which had been cured over 30 years previously.

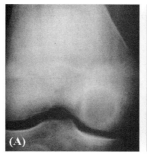 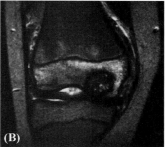

Figure 31 Chondroblastoma. (A) Plain film. There is a well-circumscribed lesion in the medial femoral condyle in this 16-year-old boy. (B) MR. This shows the characteristic mixed pattern of low and high intensity seen on all sequences. *Abbreviation*: MR, magnetic resonance.

patchy calcifications. The MR appearance is well marginated, usually round tumor in the epiphysis with mixed signal on all sequences (Fig. 31).

Characteristically, they contain patchy areas of high signal on the delayed T2 and fat-suppressed sequences (Fig. 32).

Chondroblastomas also have one unique characteristic as they may cause a periosteal reaction distal to the tumor (Fig. 33).

They can also cross the growth plate if they recur or if they get very large (Fig. 34).

The treatment is curettage but if left alone, they seem to disappear. They are entirely benign.

Two points should be made: The differential diagnosis of a solitary epiphyseal lucency in children is between three entities—chondroblastoma, Brodie's abscess, and eosinophylic granuloma. The second point is that some

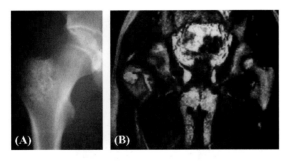

Figure 32 Chondroblastoma. (**A**) Plain film. There is a mixed blastic/lytic lesion seen in the greater trochanter of the right femur. This is an apophysis and is equivalent to an epiphysis. (**B**) MRI. This again shows a mixed low and high signal intensity lesion in the greater trochanter of the right femur. *Abbreviation*: MRI, magnetic resonance imaging.

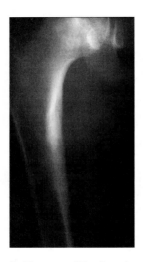

Figure 33 Chondroblastoma. Distal periosteal reaction. The chondroblastoma is in the humeral head and not seen well on this film. The periosteal reaction is on the medial side of the upper humerus and distal to the tumor.

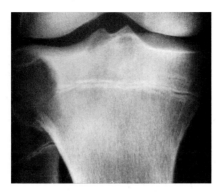

Figure 34 Chondroblastoma. This large chondroblastoma crosses the growth plate in this 15-year-old female.

people consider the clear cell chondrosarcoma, which occurs in the epiphysis of young adults to be the malignant version of the chondroblastoma.

Osteochondroma (exostosis)

These are common, representing 25% of all benign bone tumors. It is thought that most of us have at least one exostosis in our skeleton. They can be seen at any age but are usually seen below the age of 30. They are metaphyseal and grow away from the growth plate. Solitary osteochondromas occur almost entirely in the long bones and at least 60% are seen near the knee or shoulder (Figs. 35 and 36).

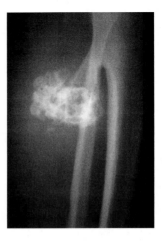

Figure 35 Osteochondroma proximal tibial metaphysis. The large bony stalk can be seen as well as the prolific cartilaginous cap. Note that this is pointing away from the growth plate.

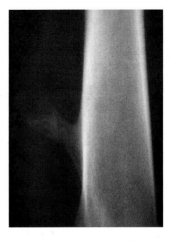

Figure 36 Osteochondroma in the distal femur. This one appears only to have a bony component although on CT or MRI a cartilaginous cap may be seen. This could be considered as an exostosis. *Abbreviations*: CT, computed tomography; MRI, magnetic resonance imaging.

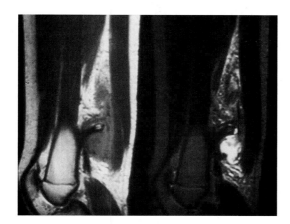

Figure 37 Ostechondroma seen in two sagittal sequences on an MRI showing a large soft tissue reaction in the soft tissue overlying the tumor. This turned out to be a bursa. *Abbreviation*: MRI, magnetic resonance imaging.

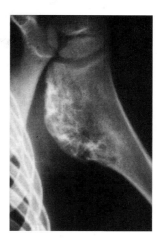

Figure 38 Sessile osteochondroma. This is a typical sessile osteochondroma involving the medial metaphysis of the proximal humerus in a young boy. Note the mixed cartilaginous and bony elements.

Radiologically, they have two components: a bony component where the bone marrow of the long bone is contiguous with the bone marrow of the osteochondroma. They may have a cartilaginous cap, which may or may not calcify. It is thought that they occur as a result of a physeal plate fracture where the fragment rotates away from the joint.

Solitary osteochondromas may turn malignant although the actual incidence of malignancy is controversial. In my opinion, malignancy occurs in less than 1 in a 1000 solitary osteochondromas. In fact, a more common complication is bursitis occurring over the tip of the osteochondroma (Fig. 37).

If an osteochondroma appears to start growing or if there is any suggestion of malignant change, an MRI is the imaging technique of choice. The conventional wisdom is that if the cartilaginous cap seen on MRI or CT is greater than 2 cm, malignancy needs to be excluded by biopsy.

Two points also need to be made with respect to osteochondromas. Solitary osteochondromas can be seen elsewhere such as in flat bones and will occasionally occur in the spine. The second point concerns the rather curious appearance of what is known as a sessile osteochondroma, which appears to be caused by a slowly developing flat osteochondroma originating at a growth plate. The vast majority of these are seen in the proximal humerus and femur, although they have been described elsewhere (Fig. 38).

The complications of a sessile osteochondroma include bowing of the long bone particularly the arm and distortion of the adjacent joint. The second complication is an increase in risk of malignancy: This is said to be as high as 10%.

Hereditary Multiple Osteochondromatosis

This is largely a familial condition, although approximately 10% of people have no family history. The child is shorter than expected, so this condition is usually diagnosed early, often in children younger than 10 years. Forty percent of patients have deformities of their forearms, 10% have leg length discrepancies, 8% have angular deformities of various joints, and 25% have a poor functional rating in at least one joint (Fig. 39).

Many of these patients have sessile osteochondromas in the proximal femurs. However, the main problem with multiple osteochondromatosis is the increased incidence of malignancy. The overall risk is said to be 1% per long bone lesion and 5% per flat bone lesion turning into a chondrosarcoma per patient (Fig. 40).

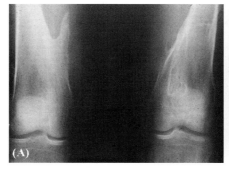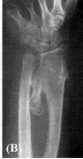

Figure 39 Multiple osteochondromatosis. (**A**) Knee. Note that all the lesions are growing away from the growth plate and are causing Erlenmeyer flask deformities of the femurs. (**B**) Wrist in the same patient. Note that all the lesions are growing away from the growth plate.

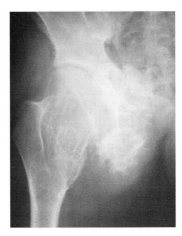

Figure 40 Chondrosarcoma arising in a sessile osteochondroma in a different patient with multiple osteochondromatosis.

Enchondroma

These are relatively common lesions accounting for 10% of benign bone tumors. Usually found between the ages of 10 and 40 years, they are twice as common in male patients. They classically occur in the small bones of the hands (over 70%) (Fig. 41), but they can be seen in almost any long bone where they seem to originate in the metaphysis and spread down into the diaphysis (Fig. 42A).

However, in the phalanges they can also extend into the epiphysis. Radiologically, they are lucent usually with some expansion and thinning of the cortex. Many of them contain calcifications, particularly those that are seen in the long bones, although those seen in the fingers rarely have visible calcifications (Fig. 41). The calcifications are described as having a typical "arcs and whorls" appearance (Fig. 42B). The treatment varies as to where the tumor is. If it is a solitary enchondroma occurring in a phalanx, it is usually either left alone or treated with curettage. If it occurs in the upper humerus or femur and associated with bone pain, then curettage is necessary to

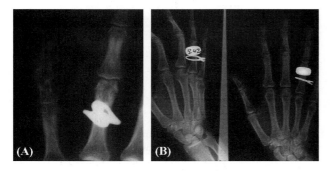

Figure 41 Enchondroma. (**A, B**) Plain films in two different patients showing a well-circumscribed somewhat expansile lytic lesion in the phalanges, typical of an enchondroma.

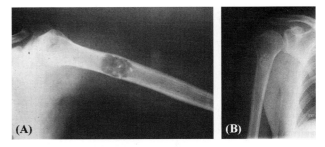

Figure 42 Benign enchondroma in an upper humerus in two different patients (**A**) 32 year old man with renal failure (note the widening of the a-c joint) with an incidental finding of a benign enchondroma containing multiple calcifications. (**B**) 56 year old man showing the typical "arcs and whorls" appearance of calcified chondroid tissue.

exclude malignant change. Conventional wisdom teaches that enchondromas in the hand are benign but at the end of long bones they should probably be considered to be premalignant. If they are not painful and occur as an incidental finding, then a follow-up X-ray should be taken at six months and then yearly.

Enchondromatosis (Ollier's Disease)

This is considered to be a developmental disorder or a dyschondroplasia. These patients have multiple enchondromas, and it is a familial condition. There is a high risk of malignant change with Ollier's disease. Radiologically, the enchondromas appear to be mixed with osteochondromas (Fig. 43).

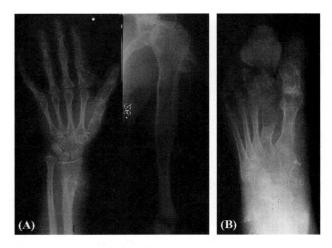

Figure 43 Multiple enchondromatosis (Ollier's disease). (**A**) Arm. Note the marked distortion of the skeleton caused by both multiple enchondromas and multiple osteochondromas. (**B**) Foot in the same patient. Note the marked distortion of the skeleton caused by both multiple enchondromas and multiple osteochondromas.

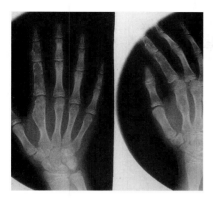

Figure 44 Multiple enchondromatosis in a single ray. Note the enchondromas in the second metacarpal and all three phalanges of the index finger.

Multiple Enchondromatosis in a Single Ray

The most common form of enchondromatosis is a group of enchondromas running down a ray in the hand (Fig. 44).

This situation also has an increased risk of malignant change and the ray needs to be excised.

Maffucci's Syndrome

This is a combination of multiple enchondromas with multiple hemiangiomas (Fig. 45). It is extremely rare and patients die of malignant change in the hemiangiomas.

Periosteal or Juxtacortical Chondroma

This is a relatively rare tumor, although it seems to be relatively common in the small bones of the hands. As

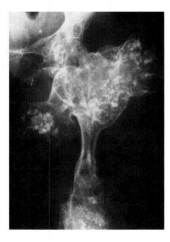

Figure 45 Maffucci's syndrome. Note the multiple enchondromas, multiple osteochondromas, and phleboliths, which are typically seen with hemangiomas.

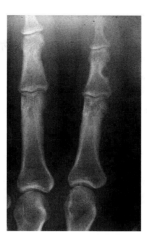

Figure 46 Periosteal chondroma. This is a typical example seen in a phalanx.

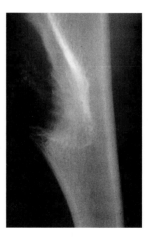

Figure 47 Periosteal chondroma. This is a much larger lesion seen in the proximal humerus of a 14-year-old boy. Note the invagination into the bone and the central calcifications.

opposed to occurring within the intramedullary canal (enchondroma) or on the exterior of the bone (osteochondroma), the periosteal chondroma occurs in the periostium where it appears as an expansile lesion with scalloping of the outer cortex of the bone but producing an outer bony margin. The majority of them have a cartilaginous matrix containing calcifications. Periosteal chondromas are mainly seen in the phalanges but they can occur in metaphyseal sites elsewhere such as the proximal humerus or femur (Figs. 46 and 47).

Histologically, they are very similar in appearance to both the cartilaginous cap of osteochondromas and the cartilaginous matrix seen in enchondromas. The differential diagnosis can be difficult because in long bones, they appear to be much more aggressive than they really are.

Chondrosarcoma

The majority of chondrosarcomas are soft tissue tumors. They usually present as a large soft tissue mass frequently adjacent to a joint, but they can occur in the soft tissues of the arms and legs and in the retroperitoneum. There are a number of subtypes of chondrosarcoma, including a central chondrosarcoma, a dedifferentiated chondrosarcoma, and a clear cell chondrosarcoma.

Chondrosarcomas represent 20% of all malignant tumors and occur in an older age group than OGS', being seen most frequently between the ages of 35 and 50 years. They are also twice as common in males as in females. They may occur as a primary lesion or secondary to a preexisting benign lesion such as an enchondroma or osteochondroma. In flat bones, such as the pelvis and shoulder girdle, they are frequently "central" in location (Fig. 48).

In long bones, they are usually metaphyseal and are frequently seen in the upper femur and the upper humerus as well as in the pelvis and shoulder girdle (Fig. 49).

The radiological appearance of a chondrosarcoma is that of a large soft tissue mass often with a dense bony reaction in the underlying bones, although obviously the tumor can also infiltrate and destroy the bone (Fig. 50).

They are slow growing and frequently contain calcifications, which may be in the matrix or be dysplastic. The treatment is usually chemotherapy and radiation therapy followed by surgery, if possible. The prognosis is poor in spite of their being slow growing. The five-year survival rate is less than 40%.

One of the subtypes of chondrosarcoma is known as a central chondrosarcoma, which occurs usually in the

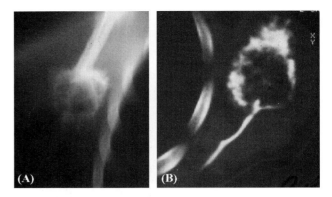

Figure 49 Chondrosarcoma in the left scapula of a 28-year-old professional athlete. (**A**) Tomogram. There is a moderately large mass expanding and destroying the tip of the scapula blade. Note the central calcifications. On biopsy, this was a grade I chondrosarcoma. (**B**) CT scan. *Abbreviation*: CT, computed tomography.

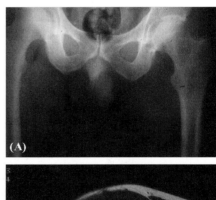

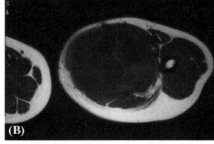

Figure 50 Typical soft tissue chondrosarcoma occurring in the proximal thigh of a 64-year-old male. (**A**) Plain film shows no abnormality apart from the soft tissue mass. (**B**) MR shows a huge mass destroying and displacing the adductor muscles. *Abbreviation*: MR, magnetic resonance.

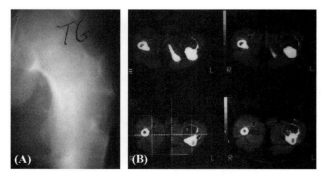

Figure 48 Chondrosarcomas. (**A**) Plain film. There is a large densely calcified mass surrounding the left femoral neck in this 40-year-old man. It has been growing slowly enough to have produced marked bony buttressing. (**B**) Four slices from a CT scan. *Abbreviation*: CT, computed tomography.

proximal end of the humerus or femur and occurs as a result of secondary malignant change in a long-standing enchondroma (Fig. 51).

The patient starts complaining of increasing pain and an X-ray will show enlarging lucent areas around the

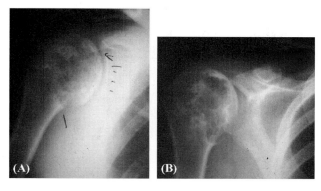

Figure 51 Central chondrosarcoma involving the proximal humerus. (**A**) On the external rotation view, there is marked destruction of the humeral head with an associated mass. (**B**) On the next film note the central calcifications suggesting that this began as an enchondroma.

calcifications. An MRI is the ideal method of evaluating whether a benign enchondroma has turned into a chondrosarcoma.

Another interesting problem with chondrosarcomas is they can "dedifferentiate" where a grade I relatively slow-growing chondrosarcoma will undergo rapid and aggressive malignant change and will become an undifferentiated pleomorphic sarcoma in which the prognosis is very poor (Fig. 52).

Clear cell chondrosarcomas are rare. They usually occur in patients younger than 40 years. They are consid-

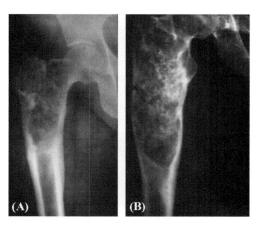

Figure 52 Chondrosarcoma, which has dedifferentiated. (**A**) Initial film. The patient was a 53-year-old female who was complaining of pain in her right hip and this lesion was seen. On biopsy, it was found to be a grade I chondrosarcoma. The patient was lost to follow-up. (**B**) Film taken two years later shows that the lesion has become much more aggressive and that a pathological fracture has occurred. On biopsy, the chondrosarcoma had dedifferentiated into an undifferentiated pleomorphic sarcoma and the patient died within three months.

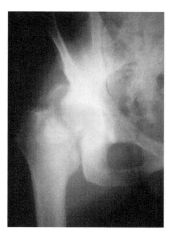

Figure 53 Clear cell chondrosarcoma. The right femoral head of this 27-year-old man has basically been destroyed. A large soft tissue mass can also be seen.

ered to be the malignant version of the chondroblastoma. There are fewer than 50 cases in the world literature. They occur almost exclusively at the epiphyseal ends of a long bone, particularly the proximal femur and humerus, although they have been rarely described in flat bones (Fig. 53).

The radiological appearance is that of an expansile, destructive lesion involving the epiphysis and often containing calcifications. They appear to have relatively sclerotic margins before they become very destructive. Histologically, they are a grade I chondrosarcoma. Once again I would stress that these are very rare.

FIBROUS TISSUE TUMORS

Fibrocortical Defect and Nonossifying Fibromas

This heading also includes nonossifying and ossifying fibromas, all of which are similar histologically, although fibrocortical defects are generally less than 2 cm in length. Fibrocortical defects are the typical "leave-me-alone" lesion and represent 25% of benign bone tumors. They can be multiple and even familial. There is some overlap with other fibrous tissue conditions, including brown tumors of hyperparathyroidism. They are usually found between the age of 10 and 20 and disappear by the age of 30. They have an equal sex incidence and are generally metaphyseal, occurring characteristically at the lower end of the femur, both ends of the tibia, and in the distal end of the fibula (Fig. 54).

Radiologically, they have a "soap-bubble" appearance and occur on the edge of the bone where they appear to split the cortex. They tend to fill in with age by sclerosis

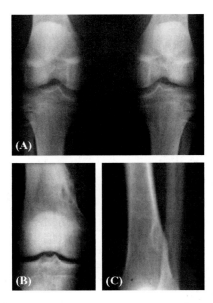

Figure 54 Fibrocortical defect. (**A, B**) Plain films of the knee in two different patients showing typical fibrocortical defects on the medial distal femoral metaphysis. (**C**) Ankle in a different patient showing a healing fibrocortical defect in the distal tibial metaphysis.

and ossification. Fibrocortical defects usually have clear-cut margins and are somewhat expansile. Small fibrocortical defects are usually higher than they are wide. Nonossifying fibromas are often 5 to 10 cm in size and extend further into the intramedullary cavity from their original subcortical position (Figs. 55 and 56).

Some of the nonossifying fibromas actually ossify and hence become ossifying fibromas.

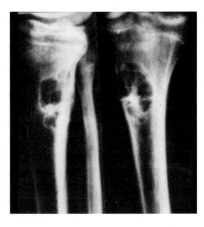

Figure 55 Nonossifying fibroma. A much larger well-defined lytic lesion containing central ossification so this could be an ossifying fibroma.

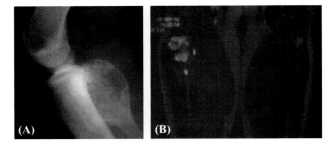

Figure 56 Nonossifying fibroma. (**A**) Plain film. Note a very large expansile lesion in the proximal fibula containing both ossification and lytic areas. (**B**) Coronal MRI. The MRI shows a mixed intensity expansile lesion. *Abbreviation*: MRI, magnetic resonance imaging.

Chondromyxoid Fibroma

This is a variant of nonossifying fibroma, which cannot be distinguished radiologically, but histologically are found to contain chondroid tissue and myxoid tissue intermixed. They are not as common as nonossifying fibromas. However, they have a very similar radiographic appearance (Fig. 57).

The vast majority occur in the metadiaphyseal regions of the long bones but occasionally can be seen in the ribs, the hands, and the feet. Radiologically, they have a geographic border with clear-cut margins and a sclerotic rim. Occasionally they can be septated.

Desmoplastic Fibroma

Whereas fibrocortical defects are extremely common, desmoplastic fibromas are extremely rare. They mainly

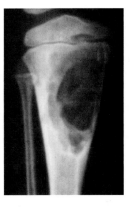

Figure 57 Chondromyxoid fibroma. This 10-year-old male presented with pain in his right knee and this large well-demarcated lytic lesion with the proximal tibia. The differential diagnosis would include a nonossifying fibroma, ossifying fibroma, or a chondromyxoid fibroma. On biopsy, it was found to be the latter.

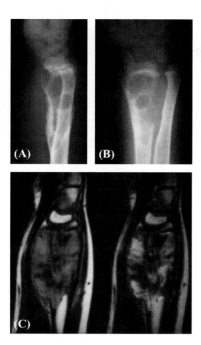

Figure 58 Desmoplastic fibroma in a distal radius. (**A**) Plain film—lateral, shows a large, septated, expansile, destructive lesion. (**B**) Plain film—AP, shows a large, septated, expansile, destructive lesion. (**C**) MRI—proton density sequence shows a rather well organized mixed intensity lesion. *Abbreviations*: AP, anteroposterior; MRI, magnetic resonance imaging.

occur in individuals younger than 30 years and have an equal sex incident. They can occur in any bone in the body but are more typical in the pelvis and long bones. In the long bones they are metadiaphyseal (Fig. 58).

Radiologically, they are lytic, appear to be aggressive, expansile, and frequently have trabeculae running through them.

There is a wide zone of demarcation. Approximately 10% of such cases present with a pathological fracture. Treatment is excision with clear margins and bone grafting, although 25% recur. Desmoplastic fibroma has a complicated differential diagnosis because of its aggressive appearance, and the differential diagnosis ranges from aneurysmal bone cyst, giant cell tumor, and fibrous dysplasia to more aggressive cortical lesions.

Elastofibroma Dorsi

This is a nonmalignant, lentiform, slow-growing pseudo-tumor consisting of fibroelastic and adipose tissue occurring in the shoulder and lying between the scapular and thoracic wall musculature. It is seen largely in older women and is often found serendipitously on CT scans since the majority of the patients are asymptomatic.

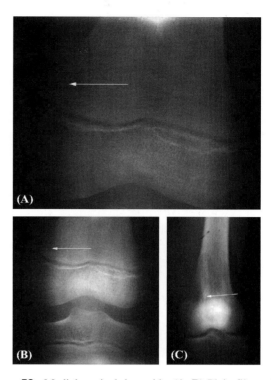

Figure 59 Medial cortical desmoids. (**A**, **B**) Plain films of the distal femur in two different adolescents showing the loss of cortex on the medial metaphysis with a suggestion of a soft tissue mass and periosteal reaction (*arrows*) very reminiscent of an early osteosarcoma.

Medial Cortical Desmoid

This has been included for the sake of completeness. This is a "tug" lesion where the adductor magnus inserts into the posterior medial corner of the distal femur (Fig. 59).

This is a very important lesion for the radiologist to know because it is entirely benign. Histologically, the cells appear to be malignant if the lesion is biopsied, and the pathologist will frequently make the diagnosis of a fibrosarcoma or OGS. Medial cortical desmoids are usually bilateral and symmetrical and occur in tall, thin athletic adolescent children. If there is any doubt about the diagnosis, the child should be taken off all athletic activities and the leg x-rayed again three weeks later.

Malignant Fibrous Histiocytoma (Undifferentiated Pleomorphic Sarcoma)

The old name for this tumor was fibrosarcoma and then approximately 20 years ago it became known as malignant fibrous histiocytoma. Nowadays the better name is considered to be undifferentiated pleomorphic sarcoma (UPS). These tumors represent 25% of malignant tumors

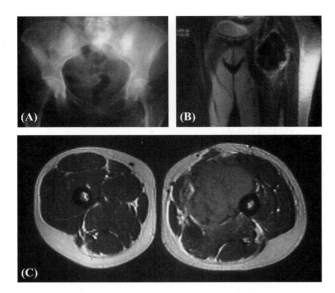

Figure 60 Undifferentiated pleomorphic sarcoma. (**A**) Plain film. The plain film shows some periosteal reaction along the left medial femoral calcar. (**B, C**) MRI scan. The MRI shows a large inhomogenous mass apparently arising from the proximal femoral cortex. *Abbreviation*: MRI, magnetic resonance imaging.

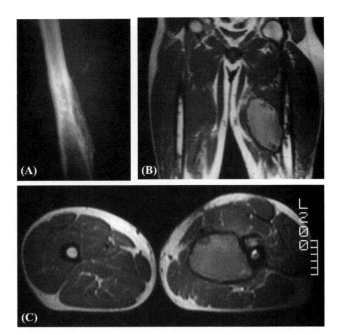

Figure 61 Undifferentiated pleomorphic sarcoma. (**A**) Plain film. The plain film shows a distinct periosteal reaction and large soft tissue mass adjacent to the medial aspect of the distal femur in this 74-year-old male. (**B, C**) MRI scan. The MRI shows a fairly homogenous mass with an apparent capsule. This is actually an MR artifact known as "phase shift" and the tumor was not found to be encapsulated. *Abbreviations*: MRI, magnetic resonance imaging; MR, magnetic resonance.

and occur in older age groups mainly in the soft tissues. The age range is classically 45–60 years, and they have an equal sex incidence. UPS occur primarily in the soft issues adjacent to long bones (Figs. 60 and 61), but if they should occur in a long bone (<5%), they are seen in the metaphysis, classically around the knee, elbow, or shoulder (Fig. 62).

They are slow growing and present as a large soft tissue mass. Occasionally, this mass may have dystrophic calcification within it. The treatment is surgery, and the prognosis is poor with the five-year survival rate being approximately 30%. UPS has an increased incidence following burns, radiation therapy, and even possibly, following orthopedic implants, although this is controversial. The correct workup of these tumors is an MRI and biopsy.

One final comment concerns a very rare entity known as "infantile fibrosarcoma." These classically occur within the first year of life and are seen mainly in the thigh where the baby develops a huge soft tissue mass (Fig. 63).

If left alone these lesions tend to go away by themselves. However, the surgeons have a habit of removing them surgically.

SOLITARY CYSTS AND OTHER LESIONS

Unicameral Bone Cysts

These cysts represent 10% of benign bone tumors. They are usually found in children between the age of 4 and 14, but they can persist up to the age of 50. Most UBCs regress spontaneously and disappear by the age of 20. They are three times as common in boys as in girls and they are metadiaphyseal. Seventy-five percent of UBCs classically occur in the upper humerus and femur. Radiologically, they are central in long bones, start close to the epiphyseal plate in young children but will slowly migrate down into the mid-diaphyseal region (Fig. 64).

In approximately 20% of UBCs, a floating fragment can be found lying within the cyst. If the child's arm is manipulated, this fragment can be seen to move within the cyst because of its being fluid filled (Fig. 65).

The fallen fragment occurs presumably because of a previous fracture through the cyst itself. UBC causes thinning of the cortex with expansion; they often have poor margins in spite of being entirely benign. They occur very rarely in flat bones. The treatment is classically to excise them, but it has been recently discovered that if three steroid injections (hydrocortisone 25 mg each over six weeks) are given into the cyst, the vast majority will regress. UBCs will also heal if the patient sustains a fracture through the cyst. Solitary bone cysts are generally considered to be "leave-it-alone lesions."

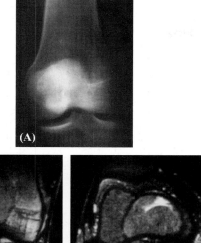

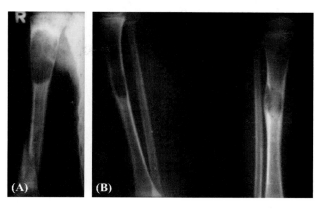

Figure 64 Unicameral bone cyst. (**A**) Humerus. AP film in an eight-year-old with a typical UBC: centrally placed, lytic, expansile, scalloping the inner margins of the cortices in the upper humerus in a young child associated with a long spiral fracture. (**B**) Two views of the right tibia in a young child with a typical unicameral bone cyst. *Abbreviations*: AP, anteroposterior; UBC, unicameral bone cysts.

Figure 62 Undifferentiated pleomorphic sarcoma or fibrosarcoma arising in a long bone. (**A**) Plain film shows no major abnormality. The MR scan (**B**, **C**) shows a large apparently encapsulated tumor of the distal medial femoral condyle. These are T2-weighted sequences showing a more mixed internal signal. *Abbreviation*: MR, magnetic resonance.

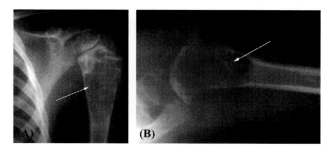

Figure 65 Unicameral bone cyst. (**A**) AP view. The films show a typical UBC with a floating fragment (*arrows*) presumably as a result of a previous fracture. (**B**) Axillary view. The films show a typical UBC with a floating fragment (*arrows*) presumably as a result of a previous fracture. *Abbreviations*: AP, anteroposterior; UBC, unicameral bone cysts.

Aneurysmal Bone Cyst

These are relatively rare and occur in patients aged 6 to 25 years. They are more commonly seen in female patients. The majority of aneurysmal bone cysts occur in the metaphysis of long bones, although they can occur in the posterior elements of vertebral bodies and in flat bones (Fig. 66).

The tumor is "aneurysmal" in both pathological and radiological terms with a "blowout," equivalent to an aneurysm seen in a blood vessel. They have a fairly characteristic, highly expansile radiological appearance (Fig. 67).

The treatment is curettage, but it is important to beware of bleeding, and most of the time the feeding vessels should be thrombosed prior to operation.

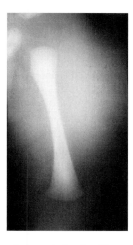

Figure 63 Congenital or infantile fibrosarcoma. There is a huge mass surrounding the femur in this six-month-old baby. On biopsy, it was thought to be a fibrosarcoma, but the parents refused any surgical procedure, and within another six months the child was normal. However, an important differential diagnosis needs to be considered in this situation and that is of Ewing's sarcoma.

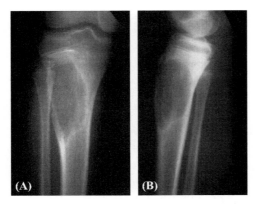

Figure 66 (**A**, **B**) Aneurysmal bone cyst. There is an expansile, eccentric, lytic lesion on the lateral aspect of the proximal tibia with well-defined sclerotic margins. The differential diagnosis would include nonossifying fibroma.

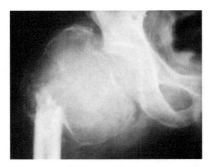

Figure 67 Aneurysmal bone cyst. This large, expansile lesion in a young male adult was found to be an aneurysmal bone cyst secondary to a chondroblastoma.

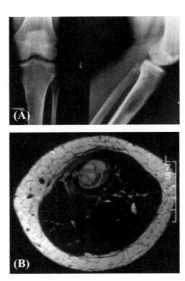

Figure 68 Aneurysmal bone cyst. (**A**) Plain film, AP and lateral views show an expansile, lytic lesion on the medial margin of the metadiaphyseal region of the left upper tibia. (**B**) An axial MRI shows the characteristic fluid-fluid levels, which make the diagnosis easy. *Abbreviations*: AP, anteroposterior; MRI, magnetic resonance imaging.

There is a controversy about whether aneurysmal bone cysts are primary or secondary. The vast majority are probably secondary, often to a giant cell tumor, fibrous dysplasia, chondroblastoma, or nonossifying fibroma. ABCs are basically benign, but if they are irradiated, they can undergo malignant change. One final comment about aneurysmal bone cysts—they frequently contain fluid-fluid levels on CT scans and MRI (Fig. 68).

Conventional wisdom has that fluid-fluid levels occur primarily in aneurysmal bone cysts and telangiectatic OGS, but they have also been seen in simple bone cysts and in soft tissue hemangiomas as well as some other malignant vascular tumors.

Giant Cell Tumor

These represent 15% of benign bone tumors and occur mainly between the ages of 25 and 35 years. They usually occur after the epiphysis closes, although can rarely be

seen before. They are twice as common in men as in women. Giant cell tumors are eccentric and typically involve both the epiphysis and metaphysis and appear to start within the growth plate itself, growing up into the epiphysis and down into the metaphysis. At least 50% of giant cell tumors occur around the knee (Fig. 69), but they can be seen at the end of other long bones particularly the proximal humerus and the distal radius. They have also

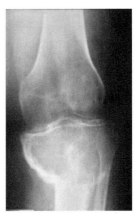

Figure 69 Giant cell tumor. There is a somewhat eccentric, lytic lesion of the proximal tibia in this 24-year-old man, which extends both up into the epiphysis, extending to the subchondral bone, and down into the metaphysis, which is a hallmark of a giant cell tumor. There was also a pathological fracture, which is how it presented.

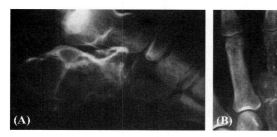

Figure 70 Giant cell tumor in two different patients in different sites. (**A**) The calcaneus is expanded and lytic with a few remaining trabeculae, but the lesion has extended to the subchondral bone at the calcaneal-cuboid joint again, typical of a giant cell tumor. (**B**) Proximal phalanx of the long finger. This lytic, expansile tumor extends from the subchondral bone and has fractured, which is how it presented.

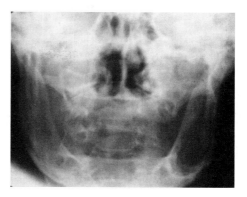

Figure 71 Adamantinoma in a jaw. There is a large, lytic, expansile tumor in the left mandibular ramus. There is a large differential diagnosis for this appearance, but this turned out to be an angioblastoma.

been seen in flat bones as well as some unusual places like the patella (Fig. 70).

In the spine they occur in the posterior elements. Radiologically, they are eccentric and expansile and have a soap-bubbly, lobulated appearance with poor margins and often contain trabeculations. They are lucent and have poor margins with a gradual gradation from the tumor into the normal bone. There is little periosteal reaction. The treatment nowadays is surgery and curettage and washing out the site carefully with phenol, and now less than 5% will recur. Giant cell tumor is another tumor that should not be irradiated because it can become malignant. One final comment about benign giant cell tumors of bone: approximately 2% of them will send out benign pulmonary metastases. The primary site is usually the distal radius and 60% of the original tumors had local recurrence. There is an interval of at least four years between the diagnosis of the primary tumor and the appearance of metastases. The metastases themselves are benign, but the management of these metastases with recurrent lung resections may ultimately kill the patient from pulmonary insufficiency.

Adamantinoma

This is the same as ameloblastoma or malignant angioblastoma of the jaw. The vast majority of these lesions occur in the jaw, but Adamantinomas can also be rarely seen in the tibia (Fig. 71).

They occur at any age from 15 to 70 years and have an equal sex incidence. Although they have mainly been described in the tibia, a few have been seen in the fibula and humerus. They are inevitably diaphyseal (Fig. 72).

Their radiological appearance can vary from a well-defined lucent area with a ground-glass appearance

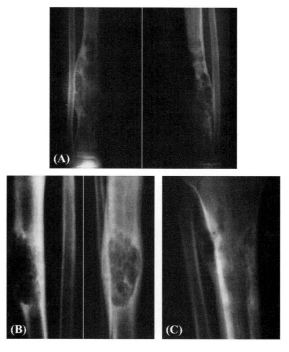

Figure 72 Adamantinoma in the tibia: three examples in three different patients showing the range of radiographic appearances from very aggressive (**A**) to very benign (**C**). (**A**) There is a large, aggressive, destructive lesion in the distal tibial diaphysis associated with a large soft tissue mass. This turned out to be a UPS associated with an adamantinoma. (**B**) A much more benign soap-bubbly lesion in the midtibia in an adolescent. The differential diagnosis would include nonossifying fibroma and aneurysmal bone cyst. (**C**) A very benign-appearing lesion in the upper tibia in a young man, which was thought to have fibrous dysplasia radiologically but on biopsy proved to be an adamantinoma. *Abbreviation*: UPS, undifferentiated pleomorphic sarcoma.

(similar to fibrous dysplasia) to a lobular, lytic, disruptive lesion with course trabeculae and a honeycomb appearance. The treatment ranges from curettage to amputation, depending on the pathology. The more aggressive tumors should be treated similar to UPS. They have a 60% five-year survival rate but may send out metastases. The differential diagnosis of an adamantoma from fibrous dysplasia can be difficult. Fibrous dysplasia is typically seen in a young male patient and there is anterior bowing of the tibia with a ground-glass appearance. An adamantoma will often have a more aggressive moth-eaten appearance and be associated with a periosteal reaction. Unfortunately, there are also a number of other similar conditions, including osteofibrous dysplasia of the tibia, which can make the differential diagnosis even more difficult.

Osteofibrous Dysplasia of the Tibia

This was first described by Campanucci in 1976. It is a rare lesion and occurs in the tibia. Sixty percent of the patients are younger than five years and the majority are boys. It is usually diaphyseal, causing deformity of the bone with bowing and enlargement (Fig. 73).

The radiographic appearance is similar to that of adamantoma except for the age, and it only involves the anterior cortex of the tibia where it appears to be intracortical, causing thinning and expansion. The classical treatment is excision but it may regress by itself, and it appears to stop growing by the age of 15.

VASCULAR TUMORS OF BONE

Hemangioma

Hemangiomas represent 1% of all tumors including soft tissue tumors. However, hemangiomas of bone, apart from those occurring in the spine, are quite rare. They can be found at any age, although the majority are found between the ages of 40 and 60 years.

In the vertebral bodies they cause a characteristic vertical striation and occur in approximately 12% to 20% of the normal population (Fig. 74).

In long bones they are inclined to be expansile, soap-bubbly lesions, and are often multiple with a honeycomb pattern (Fig. 75).

Hemangiomas may contain phleboliths. They are usually asymptomatic and mainly benign.

Histologically, hemiangiomas consist of five types. The cavernous type has large thin-walled vessels. The venous type has large venous channels with thick-walled vessels. The arteriovenous malformation is usually small and subcutaneous and often the vessels are thrombosed. The capillary type is spongy and only contains capillaries. The mixed type is usually a mixture of cavernous and capillary vessels. Most hemangiomas are intramuscular and mainly found in the third and fourth decades.

Haemangiomatosis/Lymphangiomatosis

This is a rare syndrome involving the skeleton and occurring in young people who have multiple lesions occurring at different times. It resembles multifocal

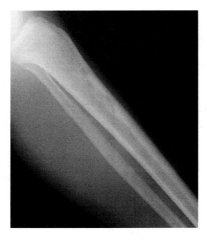

Figure 73 Osteofibrous dysplasia of the tibia in a 15-year-old girl. There is a mixed sclerotic and lytic lesion involving the anterior cortex of the tibia with a very benign appearance and that remained virtually unchanged over the course of several years.

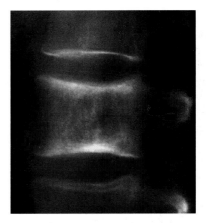

Figure 74 Hemangioma in a vertebral body. Note the vertical trabecular pattern with an overall sclerotic appearance ("corduroy" pattern) and not extending into the posterior elements typical of a benign hemangioma. The differential diagnosis would include Paget's disease in older patients, although this extends posteriorly to involve the pedicles.

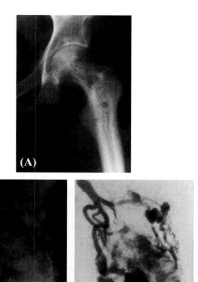

Figure 75 Hemangioma. (**A**) Plain film. The plain film shows a mixed blastic and lytic appearance in the proximal femur without any obvious extension into the soft tissue and no periosteal reaction. (**B, C**) Angiogram. The angiogram shows it to be a cavernous hemangioma.

eosinophylic granuloma, and so a biopsy is usually necessary to separate the two conditions.

Hemangioendothelioma

This is another rare hematological tumor, which often has various secondary endocrine effects, such as causing osteomalacia by destroying vitamin D.

Radiologically, there are loculated, expansile tumors with vascular channels, which have a soap-bubble appearance with sclerotic margins. They occur during the second or third decade, more commonly in men than women, and are located mainly in the metaphysis. Lesions can occur in the calvarium, spine, femur, tibia, and feet and often present with pain and swelling.

Hemangiosarcoma/Angiosarcoma

These are rare and resemble all of the other soft tissue tumors or bony sarcomas without any specific findings to help with the diagnosis. They basically resemble any UPS.

LIPOID TUMORS

Lipomas

These benign lipoid tumors are very common. The vast majority are seen in the subcutaneous tissues of the head, neck, and proximal extremities and are entirely benign. They can occur at any age and in both sexes, but the commonest presentation is in women in their 40s and 50s. They are usually easy to identify on plain films because of their increased, well-circumscribed, and lucent appearance. On CT scans they are easy to identify, because the Hounsfield units are identical to fat. On MRI they may or may not be encapsulated, and they follow the signal of subcutaneous fat (Fig. 76).

If they are not encapsulated, they can be difficult to differentiate from the surrounding fat and only a clinical examination will confirm the diagnosis.

Lipomas have been described all over the body, including the theca, breast, pleura, and brain.

There are two subtypes of lipoma: the intramuscular lipoma has an increased propensity for going malignant, and although most are solitary, a few patients will present with multiple intramuscular lipomas, which have a higher risk of malignancy in the order of 1% to 4%. The majority are benign and have the plain film, CT, and MR findings outlined above (Fig. 77).

Those that do undergo malignant change have an altered MR pattern, which is discussed below.

The intraosseous lipoma is considered to be relatively rare, but we see at least one a month. They are, in fact, relatively common in the calcaneous where they have a characteristic appearance with a fairly well-defined lucent lesion containing a ring of ossification just under the bony margins inside the lipoma itself (Fig. 78).

CT scan and MR imaging will confirm the diagnosis (Fig. 79).

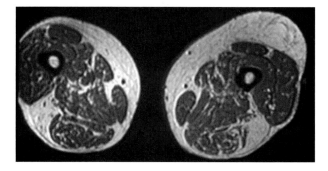

Figure 76 Lipoma MRI. This is the typical appearance of a benign lipoma in the subcutaneous tissue of the anterior left upper thigh. This one appears to be somewhat encapsulated. *Abbreviation*: MRI, magnetic resonance imaging.

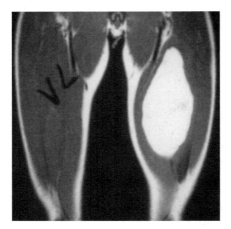

Figure 77 Intramuscular lipoma. MRI. There is a large featureless lipoma within the anterior musculature of the left thigh. It does not contain any fibrous tissue strands or solid masses so it is entirely benign. *Abbreviation*: MRI, magnetic resonance imaging.

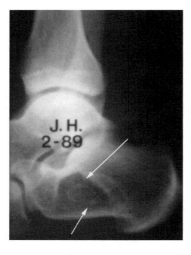

Figure 78 Intraosseous lipoma in a calcaneus. There is a well, demarcated, lytic lesion with a discrete ring of calcification just inside its margins (*arrows*), which is pathognomonic of an intraosseous lipoma.

There are no reports of malignant change of intraosseous lipomas in the literature. They occur classically in the calcaneous but can be seen elsewhere in the skeleton such as the proximal femur and proximal humerus.

Hibernoma is a rare form of benign lipoma that is secondary to proliferation of hibernating fat cells. It is benign and slow growing and often well encapsulated. Most occur near the shoulder girdle and ribs but can be seen in the extremities, and they resemble lipomas except that they are of lower signal intensity on T1 than the

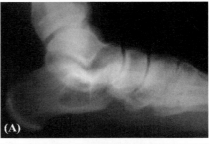

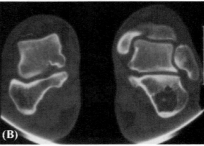

Figure 79 (**A**) Intraosseous lipoma in a different patient. (**B**) Coronal CT scan. The study confirms that the lesion consists of fat. Note the central calcifications. *Abbreviation*: CT, computed tomography.

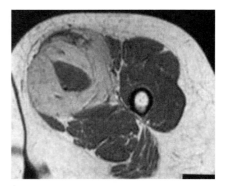

Figure 80 Hibernoma. Although similar in appearance to a lipoma, the fat is noted to be somewhat darker than the surrounding subcutaneous fat.

subcutaneous fat and possibly slightly higher intensity than fat on the fat-suppressed sequences. They are entirely benign (Fig. 80).

Differentiation Between a Benign Lipoma and Early Malignant Change

This can be difficult but as a general rule, lipomas should only contain fat. However, some of the larger ones will contain fibrous tissue bands. On MRI there should be no signal whatsoever within the lesion. Hence, early malignant change can be identified by increasing high signal on the fat-suppressed sequences. Also, another suspicious change would be to see increased thickening of the fibrous tissue bands to greater than 3 mm as well as irregularity of the bands and alteration of the fat density itself.

Liposarcomas

These are the third most common soft tissue sarcomas after UPS and chondrosarcoma. The majority are indistinguishable from other soft tissue tumors, and plain films are rarely helpful in their diagnosis although 10% to 15% contain dystrophic calcification. MRI shows a soft tissue mass. Seventy-five percent occur in the extremities (mainly in the legs) but 20% occur in the retroperitoneum where they are difficult to manage (Fig. 81).

Although there are five histological subtypes, only two have reasonably characteristic MRI findings.

The well-differentiated liposarcoma has up to 75% fat content and contains strands, nodules, and septa within it. They represent 50% of liposarcomas and are of low malignant grade (grade I) with a 60% to 70% five-year survival rate (Fig. 82).

The myxoid liposarcoma has a characteristic MR appearance (20% of liposarcomas) with a homogenous low signal on T1 and a uniformly high signal on the fat suppression sequence (Fig. 83).

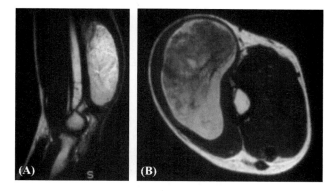

Figure 82 Well-differentiated liposarcoma. (**A**) and (**B**) are MRI images. This large tumor mainly appears to consist of benign fat. However, the upper part of the lesion contains fibrous tissue strands as well as an apparent mass suggesting early malignant change. *Abbreviation*: MRI, magnetic resonance imaging.

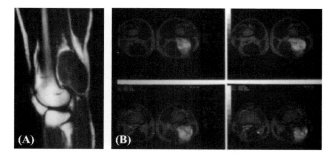

Figure 83 Myxoid liposarcoma. (**A**) MRI—sagittal, proton density image showing a large homogenous mass lying behind the knee with a signal similar to that of muscle. (**B**) MRI—four axial fat saturation slices showing that the mass remains relatively homogenous and now demonstrates very high signal. *Abbreviation*: MRI, magnetic resonance imaging.

TUMORS OF MARROW ORIGIN

Ewing's Sarcoma

This represents approximately 6% of all malignant bone tumors, and although it can be seen at any age, over 70% of Ewing's sarcoma occurs before the age of 20. It is twice as common in males than in females and classically involves the diaphysis of long bones but can also be seen not uncommonly in the pelvis, ribs, and skull. Twenty-five percent of the patients have fever and 90% have an elevated sedimentation rate. The classic radiological appearance is of a permeative lesion in the mid-diaphysis with a substantial periosteal reaction (Fig. 84).

This occurs in layers and is described as "onion skin." The margins may have a Codman's triangle, similar to

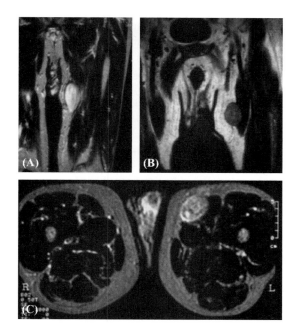

Figure 81 (**A, B, C**) Liposarcoma. These three MRI images show a well-defined mass in the anterior upper thigh, which could be any soft tissue sarcoma. However, on biopsy this proved to be a liposarcoma. *Abbreviation*: MRI, magnetic resonance imaging.

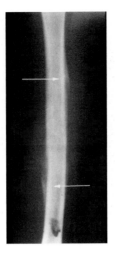

Figure 84 Ewing's sarcoma. There is a long premeative lesion in the middiaphysis of this femur with a periosteal reaction and associated soft tissue swelling. Note the Codman's triangles (*arrows*).

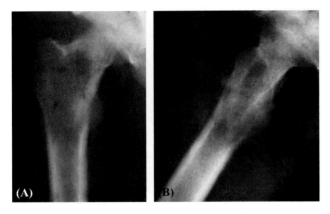

Figure 85 Ewing's sarcoma. (**A**) AP. The femoral neck shows a permeative, lytic, destructive lesion with a periosteal reaction and Codman's triangles. (**B**) Oblique. The femoral neck shows a permeative, lytic, destructive lesion with a periosteal reaction and Codman's triangles. *Abbreviation*: AP, anteroposterior.

those seen in OGS. The tumor is destructive and osteolytic and metaphyseal, as well as diaphyseal involvement can be seen in long bones (Fig. 85).

However, Ewing's sarcoma may elicit a blastic response and, in fact, involvement of the pelvis may be entirely blastic (Fig. 86).

CT and MRI are not particularly useful, although pre-operative MRI will determine the full extent of the tumor. The five-year survival rate is about 60% with active treatment using chemotherapy, radiation therapy, and immuno-therapy. Following excision there is a 20% local recurrence rate and 25% send off pulmonary metastases.

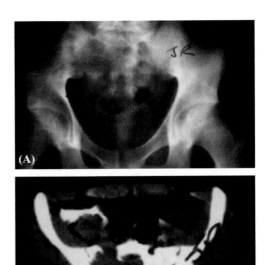

Figure 86 Ewing's sarcoma in the pelvis of this 20-year-old man. (**A**) Plain film. Note the mixed sclerotic, lytic appearance of this pelvis with a large, lucent, destructive area in the right sacrum. (**B**) CT confirms the lytic area as well as the sclerosis in the right iliac bone with a discrete periosteal reaction. *Abbreviation*: CT, computed tomography.

Lymphoma of Bone

This is a complex subject since people are unable to come up with nomenclature that everyone accepts. There is reticulum cell sarcoma, which is probably the same as non-Hodgkins lymphoma (NHL), there is Hodgkins lymphoma and non-Hodgkins lymphoma, and there are sub-types such as giant cell lymphoma of bone.

In general, lymphoma of bone occurs in 10% to 15% of patients with lymphoma where it can be the only finding initially. Those cases are probably all non-Hodgkins lymphoma. The age range is 15–40 years, and it is largely seen in the spine, flat bones, and ribs but can also occur in the proximal humerus and femur (Fig. 87).

It is usually solitary, and in the spine, it can lead to either an ivory vertebra (dense vertebral body) or a ver-tebra plana (flat vertebral body) (Fig. 88).

In flat bones, lymphoma is usually permeative with a mixed sclerotic and lytic pattern. The prognosis depends on the disease elsewhere, although solitary osseous involvement has a 60% five-year survival rate.

Reticulum cell sarcoma and giant cell lymphoma of bone are both subtypes of non-Hodgkins lymphoma. They usually involve long bones such as the femur, upper tibia but also can involve the ribs and clavicles (Fig. 89).

The age range is 20–40 years and it is twice as common in males. The appearance is of a permeative destructive

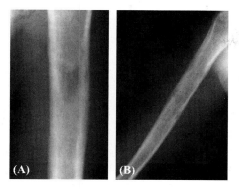

Figure 87 Non-Hodgkins lymphoma in two different patients. (A) Plain film of the proximal shaft of the femur in a 40-year-old man. There is a destructive, lytic, permeative lesion with a discrete periosteal reaction. (B) Plain film of the right humerus in a 29-year-old woman that shows similar changes. Both lesions were found to be due to non-Hodgkins lymphoma.

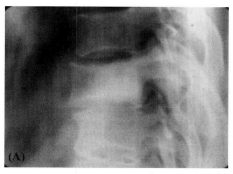

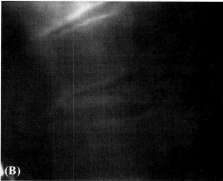

Figure 88 Lymphoma in the spine. (A) "Ivory" vertebra. (B) Vertebra plana.

lesion, involving both cancellous and cortical bone with a discrete periosteal reaction. Pathological fractures occur in 30%. Again the five-year survival rate remains over 60% if the lesion remains solitary.

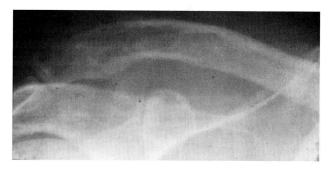

Figure 89 Reticulum cell sarcoma in the distal clavicle of a young medical student. Note the permeative, destructive lesion in the distal clavicle with associated soft tissue swelling.

MULTIPLE MYELOMA AND PLASMA CELL DYSCRASIAS

A.   Major pathological varieties of importance

   1. Solitary plasmacytoma
   2. Multiple myeloma
   3. Primary macroglobulinemia (Waldenstrom)
   4. Amyloidosis

B.   Secondary nonpathological varieties

   5. Chronic inflammatory processes such as hepatitis, chronic Tuberculosis, Subacute Bacterial Endocarditis, and Systemic Lupus Erythematosus
   6. Neoplasia, lymphoma, leukemia, and carcinoma of pancreas and prostate
   7. Drug reactions, penicillin, and new cytotoxic drugs

C.   Idiopathic

Multiple Myeloma

Multiple myeloma is the most commonly occurring bone tumor, accounting for 40% of all malignant tumors compared with 20% for OGS and 20% for chondrosarcoma. It can be seen at almost any age but 75% of the patients are aged between 50 and 70 years. It is twice as common in males, and the signs and symptoms include backache, bone pain (90%), unexplained osteoporosis (10%), weight loss, and weakness. The classical radiological finding is of punched-out lytic areas with clean-cut margins (Fig. 90).

These are most commonly seen in the skull, clavicle, ribs, and shoulder girdle. Generalized osteoporosis of undetermined origin is the presentation in 5% to 10% of patients with multiple myeloma and pathological fractures occur in 50% of patients (Fig. 91).

In the spine, multiple myeloma may present as a vertebral plana (Fig. 92).

Patients with multiple myeloma have abnormal plasma proteins with a wide M band in 90% of patients and Bence Jones proteins in the urine in 60% of patients where the

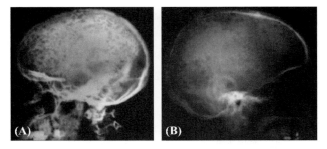

Figure 90 (**A, B**) Multiple myeloma. Two lateral skull films in different patients showing the typical "punched out" lytic areas in the calvarium.

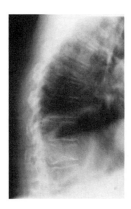

Figure 91 Multiple myeloma. This 48-year-old woman presented with severe, widespread osteoporosis of unknown etiology. On biopsy she turned out to have multiple myeloma.

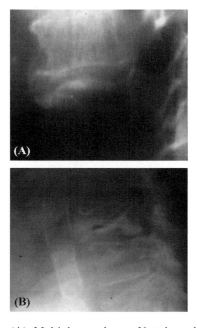

Figure 92 (**A**) Multiple myeloma. Vertebra plana in two different patients with multiple myeloma. (**B**) Shows a vacuum phenomena in the vertebral body itself, which is said to be a characteristic of multiple myeloma.

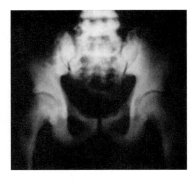

Figure 93 Multiple myeloma. Sclerotic myeloma in a 48-year-old African-American male patient.

proteins precipitate at 50°F but disappear at 80°F. The accepted five-year survival rate is 20% but some patients with multiple myeloma survive for many years. There is a very rare form of sclerotic multiple myeloma with mixed blastic (predominantly) and lytic disease. This almost exclusively occurs in young African-American males aged between 20 and 40 years (Fig. 93).

Solitary Plasmacytoma

Solitary plasmacytoma (SP) is a rare form of solitary multiple myeloma. In the skeleton it appears much more benign and the lesions are expansile and lytic with clear-cut margins, often looking like and occurring at the same sites as a giant cell tumor (Fig. 94).

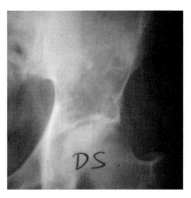

Figure 94 Solitary plasmacytoma in a 39-year-old dentist. There is a somewhat expansile, lytic area in the roof of the acetabulum in this otherwise normal man. The differential diagnosis would include giant cell tumor, aneurysmal bone cyst, and metastases, but on biopsy it turned out to be a solitary plasmacystoma. Eight years later, he developed a similar lesion in his tibia and 10 years after that he developed multiple myeloma.

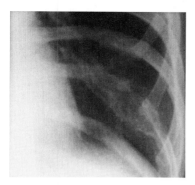

Figure 95 Solitary plasmacytoma. This expansile, destructive lesion in the rib occurred in an otherwise healthy 48-year-old man. The differential diagnosis would include enchondroma, chondromyxoidfibroma, and fibrous dysplasia in a younger patient and metastases or Paget's disease in an older patient.

Sixty percent are metaphyseal in long bones, but they can also be seen in the pelvis and posterior elements in the vertebral bodies (Fig. 95).

Solitary plasmacytoma often occurs in younger patients aged 30 to 50 years but will inevitably progress into multiple myeloma. Incidentally, SP is actually much more common in the soft tissues of the neck, sinuses, and upper respiratory tract. There is also a rare osseous variant of SP with multiple SPs occurring years apart.

Amyloidosis

This is considered to be a plasma cell dyscrasia and occurs in 10% to 15% of cases with multiple myeloma with which it overlaps (Fig. 96).

Primary amyloidosis only rarely involves bones, but secondary amyloid deposits can be seen in the synovium in patients in renal failure who are on long-standing dialysis. Otherwise primary amyloid deposits are seen in the heart, liver, spleen, and kidneys.

Leukemia

Adults with leukemia rarely show skeletal changes although synovial involvement in leukemia is not uncommon. Also, occasionally, discrete lucencies and periosteal reaction can be seen in about 10% of adults. On the other hand, 50% to 70% of children have bone changes that classically are seen in the metaphysis where radiolucent lines may occur or generalized osteopenia can be seen (Fig. 97).

Patchy osteolytic changes have also been described (Fig. 98).

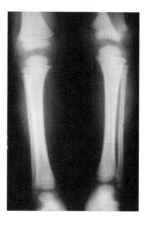

Figure 97 Leukemia. There are discrete lucent areas in the distal ends of both the tibia and fibula associated with a periosteal reaction and "celery stalking" typical of leukemia.

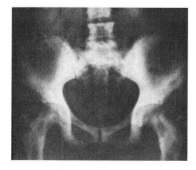

Figure 96 Amyloidosis. There is increased density in all the visualized bones in this patient with primary amyloidosis. Although probably metabolic in origin, both sclerotic lesions and lytic areas have been described in this condition.

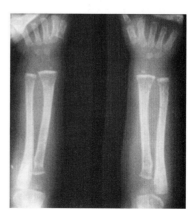

Figure 98 Leukemia. Similar changes are present in the metaphyses of both ends of the radius and the ulna.

SYNOVIAL TUMORS

Like any other tissue, synovium can be associated with any number of benign and malignant tumors. In the benign category, lipomas, hamartomas and hemangiomas all can occur. There are two specific benign tumors of synovium, which will be discussed in detail: pigmented villonodular synovitis (PVNS) and synovial osteochondromatosis. In the malignant category, the classical synovial aggressive tumor used to be known as a synovioma or a synovial chondrosarcoma but is now known as a synovial sarcoma.

Pigmented Villonodular Synovitis

This is a benign proliferation of synovium, which undergoes metaplasia and histologically contains a fibrous stroma, histiocytic infiltrate, hemosiderin, and giant cells. Histologically, it looks the same as a giant cell tumor of the tendon sheath. Approximately 70% of them contain hemosiderin but you can see PVNS totally without pigment or totally pigmented. Grossly, the tumor appears purple because of the pigment, and on MR, hemosiderin is of low intensity on all sequences, so PVNS is usually easy to diagnose. There is a controversy about whether PVNS actually represents a true tumor or possibly some response to a posttraumatic incident. PVNS occurs mainly in younger and middle-aged males and mainly in large joints such as the knee, ankle, hip, and shoulder but can also be seen in small joints, such as the wrist and even the temperomandibular joint (Fig. 99).

In a large joint, the first radiological finding is of soft tissue swelling, and then erosions can occur at the synovial insertions into the bone (Fig. 100).

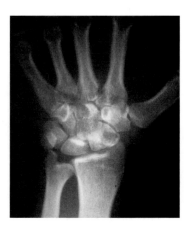

Figure 99 Pigmented villonodular synovitis. This 25-year-old man was complaining of pain and swelling on the radial aspect of his wrist. The plain film shows patchy osteopenia in the distal radius and erosions of the scaphoid, trapezium, and other carpal bones.

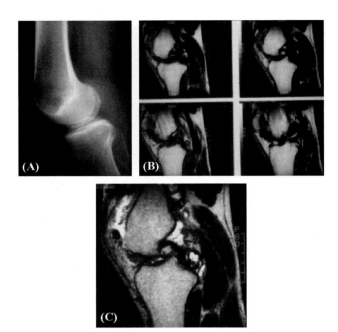

Figure 100 Pigmented villonodular synovitis in a 39-year-old man. (**A**) Plain film. This appears relatively normal apart from soft tissue swelling. (**B**) Set of sagittal proton density images from an MRI. These images show bony erosions with synovial hypertrophy, which is mainly of low intensity due to deposition of hemosiderin. (**C**) Single sagittal slice shows the low intensity synovial hypertrophy in the suprapatellar pouch, in the intercondylar notch, posteriorly, as well as the large effusion. *Abbreviation*: MRI, magnetic resonance imaging.

The synovial proliferation can destroy articular cartilage so that joint space narrowing, erosions, and soft tissue swelling can be seen that can mimic virtually any form of arthritis. Clinically, PVNS presents with pain and swelling frequently with loss of range of motion, particularly if it occurs in the intercondylar notch of the knee where it interferes with flexion and extension by encasing the cruciate ligaments (Fig. 101).

On MRI, the synovial proliferation becomes obvious with synovial thickening and often frond-like masses can be seen throughout the joint. Since the majority are pigmented, the diagnosis is relatively easy to make.

The differential diagnosis is made if the hemosiderin pigment is seen within the synovium, although young male patients with hemophilia also deposit hemosiderin in their synovium. The radiological features and clinical features of hemophilia are different from those of a patient with PVNS. If pigment is not present, then the differential diagnosis is of any synovial tumor. The prognosis is excellent if the whole synovium of the involved joint can be removed, but this is usually difficult, if not impossible, in the knee where intra-articular radioactive strontium can be given to ablate the tumor. However, on the

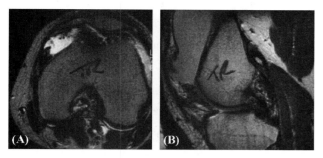

Figure 101 Pigmented villonodular synovitis in a 28-year-old male. (**A**) MRI—axial. (**B**) MRI—sagittal. The images show marked synovial hypertrophy with low-intensity fronds and a huge effusion. The best place to appreciate the low intensity on these images is posterior to the PCL. *Abbreviations*: MRI, magnetic resonance imaging; PCL, posterior cruciate ligament.

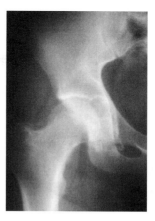

Figure 102 Synovial osteochondromatosis. This single AP view of the hip in a 40-year-old male shows multiple, discrete loose bodies surrounding the femoral neck. *Abbreviation*: AP, anteroposterior.

whole, the recurrence rate following surgical removal is less than 10%. PVNS is entirely benign and will only turn malignant if external radiation is used, after which the tumor turns into an UPS.

Synovial Osteochondromatosis

This is another tumor caused by benign proliferation of synovium, which metaplases into villae that initially calcify and then ossify and fall off into the joint, forming osteochondral loose bodies. It occurs more commonly in men and in patients aged between 20 and 40 and also usually involves large joints such as the knee, hip, and shoulder (Fig. 102), but can occur elsewhere. The clinical presentation is of pain swelling, locking, and loss of range of motion. The radiological features are of multiple loose bodies. Synovial osteochondromatosis is entirely benign. In the knee joint particularly, multiple loose bodies can interfere with motion. They can also migrate into a Baker's cyst if one is present (Fig. 103).

There is a controversy about whether synovial osteochondromatosis is a primary proliferation of the synovium or is secondary to trauma. I believe that it is a benign metaplasia of the synovium. The differential diagnosis would be of osteochondral loose bodies following trauma or in association with osteochondritis dissecans, but there should be a bony defect seen on the plain films in both of these conditions.

Synovial Sarcoma

This is a malignant synovial tumor, and was originally known as a synovioma and then as a synovial chondro-

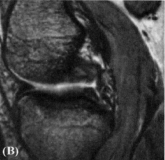

Figure 103 Synovial osteochondromatosis in a 28-year-old male. (**A**) Plain film: Note the soft tissue swelling and joint effusion as well as the multiple small loose bodies lying posteriorly. (**B**) Sagittal MRI through the intercondylar notch confirms the presence of multiple small loose bodies lying posteriorly. *Abbreviation*: MRI, magnetic resonance imaging.

sarcoma. It will no doubt shortly be reclassified as an UPS. The classical age range is given as 20–40 years, and 60% of such cases occur in patients younger than 40 years. But I have seen both younger and older patients who developed synovial sarcomas. Seventy percent are calcified on plain films, and 60% show evidence of bone destruction. At least 90% are soft tissue tumors arising from the synovium surrounding a tendon sheath or ligamentous insertion into a bone rather than occurring in the synovium of the joint (Fig. 104).

There is a basic rule of 60s for synovial sarcomas: 60% occur in females, 60% in the leg (mostly below-the-knee), and 60% below the age 40. It presents and looks like any

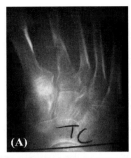
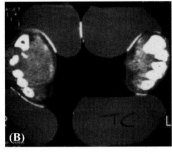
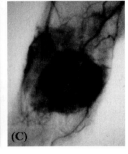

Figure 104 Synovial sarcoma. This 19-year-old girl presented with a painful, bleeding mass on the undersurface of her right foot. (**A**) Plain film. This shows the destruction of the base of the first and second metatarsal as well as a large soft tissue mass. (**B**) CT scan confirms the large mass and shows that it is surrounding the second metatarsal and encroaching on the first and third. Note the soft tissue calcifications. (**C**) Angiogram. This shows the extremely vascular nature of the tumor. *Abbreviation*: CT, computed tomography.

of the other soft tissue tumors, although it has a propensity to invade adjacent bones fairly quickly, particularly in the foot. But most are indistinguishable from any other aggressive soft tissue tumor (Fig. 105).

METASTASES

Although metastases are seen 20 times as commonly as all bone tumors put together, there are relatively few comments to be made about them. Metastases can be blastic, lytic, or mixed in appearance, which depends largely on the type of prostaglandin secreted by the primary tumor. Thus, lung and breast metastases are usually lytic, and metastases from the prostate usually blastic, but if, for example, a prostatic carcinoma invades the bladder, then prostatic metastases can become lytic (Figs. 106–108).

If a breast tumor is adequately treated by either chemotherapy or surgery, then the metastases can become blastic or mixed.

Most metastases occur in places where there is a good blood supply and adequate bone marrow so that they will be seen most often in the metaphyseal ends of long bones as well as in flat bones. In the spine, they frequently involve the pedicles in contradistinction to multiple myeloma, which usually does not. Metastases rarely involve the mandible whereas metastases can.

A few oddities can also be mentioned: lung cancer can send off metastases to curious places such as the anterior cortex of the tibia (known as intracortical metastases), the tufts of the fingers, and the metacarpal heads. Breast cancer can also send off peripheral metastases. A "bullseye" or target metastases can be sent off by thyroid cancer or other endocrinological cancers.

Metastases in children are quite rare, although one exception is that in children younger than five, neuroblastomas can send out multiple small permeative lytic metastases. Although metastases are very common, there is very little else to say about them.

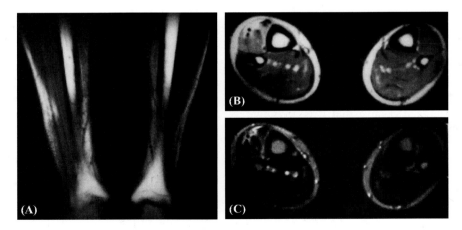

Figure 105 Synovial sarcoma. All of these images show a discrete mass lying in the soft tissues of the anterior lower leg. This is best seen on the axial images. The patient was a 32-year-old female. (**A**) MRI—proton density, coronal. (**B**) MRI—proton density, axial. (**C**) MRI—fat saturation, axial. All of these images show a discrete mass lying in the soft tissues of the anterior lower leg. This is best seen on the axial images. The patient was a 32 years and female. *Abbreviations*: MRI, magnetic resonance imaging.

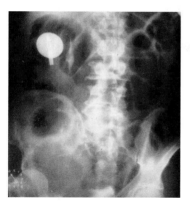

Figure 106 Metastases from bronchogenic carcinoma. There is a large destructive lesion involving much of the lower half of the right iliac bone, typical of a metastasis. The patient had a bronchogenic carcinoma.

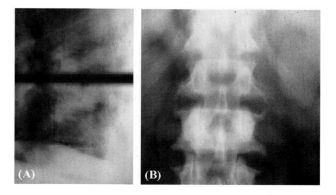

Figure 108 Prostatic metastases in two different patients. Both of these images show patchy areas of increased density, typical of blastic metastases. The patchy nature and focal areas of sclerosis are more typical of metastases than of Paget's disease. (**A**) Lateral thoracic spine. (**B**) AP lumbar spine. *Abbreviation*: AP, anteroposterior.

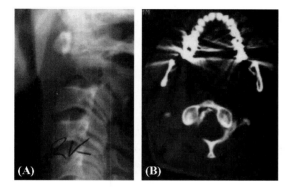

Figure 107 Metastases from unknown primary. This young 34-year-old man presented with neck pain and was found to have destruction of the C2 vertebral body. The primary was later found to be a renal cell carcinoma. (**A**) Plain film. (**B**) CT scan *Abbreviation*: CT, computed tomography.

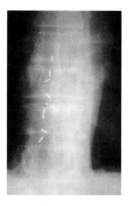

Figure 109 Metastases to pedicle in a patient with bronchogenic carcinoma. Note that the left pedicle of one of the mid-thoracic vertebral bodies is missing, and the paraspinal lines are widened. Multiple myeloma only rarely involves the pedicles and is very rarely associated with soft tissue swelling.

Another point should be made and that is the differential diagnosis between metastatic disease of the spine and osteoporosis. On the whole, metastases involve the pedicles, whereas osteoporosis does not (Fig. 109).

Metastases are usually associated with a soft tissue mass and osteoporosis is not. Also, if there are multiple end-plate fractures, the diagnosis is usually osteoporosis or multiple myeloma rather than metastatic disease.

If metastases are suspected, do a nuclear medicine bone scan and not a bone survey. This is unlike that in suspected multiple myeloma where bone scans are negative at least 80% of the time.

7

Orthopaedic Hardware, Total Joint Replacements, and Their Complications

COMPLICATIONS OF ORTHOPEDIC SURGERY

Surgical complications can be basically subdivided into mechanical and probably unavoidable and genuine errors. Mechanical complications include loosening and fractures of the device as well as infection. Operative surgical errors can be subdivided into malposition of the orthopedic device, the wrong site, the wrong side, and even the wrong patient! In the spine, spinal fusion or performing laminectomies at the wrong level is a relatively common problem—particularly in the mid-thoracic region, although it can occur elsewhere (Fig. 1).

In a recent review (1) of surgery on the wrong site, 126 fully documented cases have been recorded since 1996. Forty-one percent of these cases were orthopedic, 76% wrong body part or site, 13% wrong patient, and 11% wrong surgical procedure. It has been estimated that one in four of all orthopedists who have been in practice for 25 years or more will perform at least one wrong site surgery.

Operative mistakes can happen. Encountering problems during the actual operation does occur (Figs. 2 and 3), although most are not serious. Mechanical failure of various devices, rods, and screws is not uncommon and is obviously not the orthopedists' fault (Figs. 4 and 5).

From a radiologist's point of view, we should try to understand the procedure and what the orthopedist is trying to accomplish. A good example of this is given later in this chapter with the use of a template for assessing the correct position of the prosthetic humeral

head following total shoulder replacement. The radiologist also needs to be aware of the various complications of the procedure and to look for them carefully. However, you cannot blame the surgeons for every bad result (Fig. 6) and some occur serendipitously (Fig. 7).

However, the most important complication is infection. Drez et al. (2) reviewed the incidence of infections following arthroscopy. In 1985, 120,000 arthroscopies were performed with 105 complications and a 1% incidence of infection. Similarly, in 1986, although a lot more arthroscopies were performed, the rate of infection remained between 1% and 2%. However, in obese patients this increased to 18%, in diabetic patients to 10%, in patients on steroids to 16%, and in debilitated patients to 23%. There was also a relationship between the incidence of infection and the length of stay in the hospital: 1% incidence of infections at one day, 2% at seven days, and 3.5% at two weeks. The average cost of managing infections per patient ranges between $10,000 and $100,000. The Centers for Disease Control (CDC) estimates that there are 80,000 plus deaths from hospital-acquired infections per year. In another article, Maurer, et al. (3) reviewed their findings in 24 patients with open tibial fractures. They all underwent external fixation from 7 to 230 days. Seven patients developed one or more infected pin sites. All 24 patients went on to IM nailing and five went on to develop infection around the nail.

Pin track infections have a characteristic appearance. Initially, placing a pin in a bone compresses the surrounding

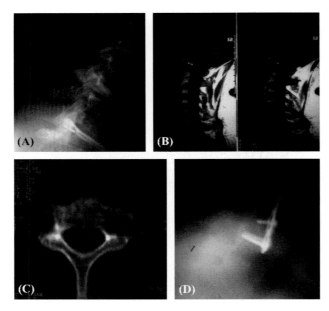

Figure 1 (A) Plain film. This young patient had metastatic osteogenic sarcoma invading the body of C7. It was decided to plate from C6 to T1. This film was taken postoperatively. The plate goes from C5 to C7. (**B**) MRI. (**C**) CT scan. (**D**) Plain film. *Abbreviations*: MRI, magnetic resonance imaging; CT, computed tomography.

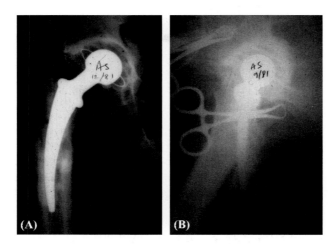

Figure 2 (A) Malposition. AP view of a total hip replacement three weeks after placement. What is wrong with this picture? You should not have cement and cortical bone apparently overlying each other. (**B**) A lateral view shows that the femoral component protrudes through the posterior cortex. *Abbreviation*: AP, anteroposterior.

bone and usually produces a somewhat sclerotic ring seen end on. If this becomes infected, this sclerotic ring (a sequestrum) becomes surrounded by infected and destroyed bone (an involucum). Once established, this has a characteristic appearance (Fig. 8).

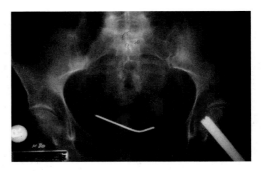

Figure 3 Improper surgical method. This elderly patient presented with "rusty urine." She had a fixed pin placed in her left hip 20 years before. The guide wire was not removed and, on placement of the pin, it had been pushed into the pelvis where it eventually migrated into the bladder.

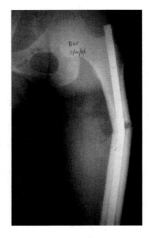

Figure 4 Fractured intramedullary rod.

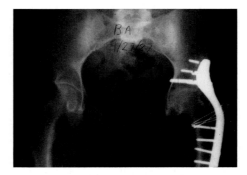

Figure 5 Fractured screws in a hip fusion with a long cobra plate.

Initially, an irregular lucency surrounds the pin. Once the pin is removed the infection becomes more obvious (Fig. 9). Similarly, the progression of the infection can be followed radiologically (Fig. 10). There is a high

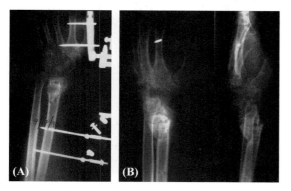

Figure 6 (**A**) Film with external fixator on. Patient problem: This patient undid the screws holding his external fixator in position to show his friends how he could move his wrist. (**B**) Film with external fixator removed.

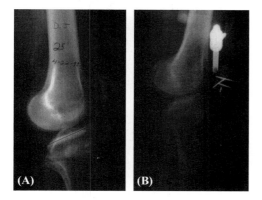

Figure 7 (**A**) Surgical complication during an ACL repair. Normal patella. (**B**) Fractured patella. *Abbreviation*: ACL, anterior cruciate ligament.

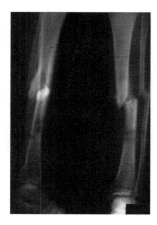

Figure 8 Infected pin track with "ring" sequestrum. AP and lateral views of a left tibia and fibula with an infected pin track. Note the sclerotic ring is caused by inserting the pin (sequestration) and the "ring" of lucency around it, signifying infection. *Abbreviation*: AP, anteroposterior.

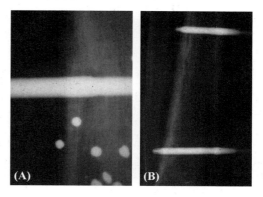

Figure 9 (**A**) Pin track infection. Initial film showing destruction of both cortical and trabecular bone surrounding the pin as well as a discrete periosteal reaction (note the many BBs in the soft tissues). (**B**) Following removal of the middle pin—the infection becomes more obvious.

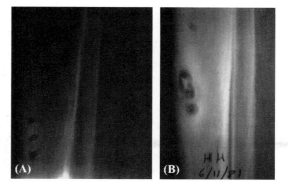

Figure 10 (**A**) Pin tract infection. Initial film is normal. (**B**) Later film shows a typical "ring" sequestration.

correlation between loosening of the pin and development of infection. In the literature, the overall infection rate of inflamed pins is 10% to 14%. Maham et al. (4) reviewed the results of 214 pin tracks in 42 patients. Forty-two percent of these pins were inflamed, 23% were loose, and 75% of pin tips cultured positive for bacteria: *Staphylococcus epidermidis* 90%, *Staphylococcus aureus* 37%, and *Escherichia coli* in 10%. These authors also suggest that all inflamed, infected, or loose pins should be removed. Remember that the overall incidence of infection following any orthopedic procedure is 2%—and look for it (Fig. 11).

COMPLICATIONS OF SPINAL SURGERY

The literature contains numerous articles on the complications of spinal surgery and a recent overview article quoted a 0.1% → 0.3% mortality and overall morbidity of

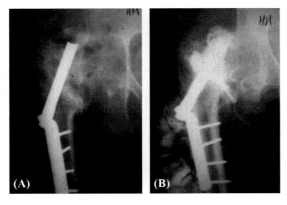

Figure 11 (**A**) Plain film shows marked destruction of both sides of the joint. Infected hip six months following placement of a fixed pin and plate. (**B**) Arthrogram showing large sinus tracts (looking like a barium enema!). The bacteria was *Staphylococcus aureus*.

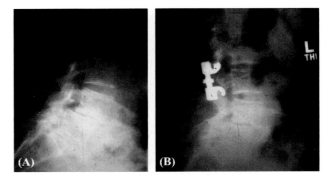

Figure 12 (**A**) Wrong level. Initial film showing that the degenerative disc disease is at L5/S1. (**B**) Postoperative, L4/5 had been fused instead of L5/S1.

3.5%. Deep vein thrombosis and thrombophlebitis occurred in approximately 2% to 3% cases with pulmonary embolism occurring in 1%, nerve root damage in 0.2% to 0.5%, and dural tears in approximately 1%. While in Minnesota, one of my residents and I reviewed (5) the complications of thoracolumbar spine surgery in 1500 patients who were operated on between 1985 and 1995. Their mean age was 42 (6–85 years). Of this group, there were nearly 900 patients who had at least a two-year follow-up and whose charts and radiography were available. There were 434 women and 464 men. The preoperative diagnosis included scoliosis in 10%, pain in 5%, fractures in 5%, failed previous surgery in 17%, and degenerative disc disease in 63%. Nineteen types of instrumentations were used including Texas Scottish Rite in 29%, Steffee Plates in 32%, and Cotrel Dubousset rods in 21%.

The overall complication rate was 49% but this included minor problems such as skin sepsis and residual pain. Of the important complications, infection occurred in 8% (of which 3% had deep infections). Twenty-four percent developed a neuropathy, 1% paralysis, and there were three deaths. Early complications included infection, paralysis, and malpositioning (Fig. 12).

Later complications included loosening, pseudarthrosis, and instrument failure (Figs. 13–15).

Secondary degenerative changes usually occur either below or above the level of the fusion although they can be seen anywhere in association with the instrumentation (Figs 16 and 17).

Radiographic complications included loosening in 16% (Fig. 18), malposition in 5%, instrument failure in 5%, fractures in 3%, pseudarthrosis occurred in 13%, and secondary degenerative changes in 17%. Surgical complications in the immediate perioperative period included

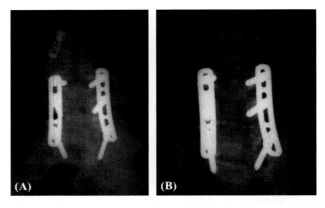

Figure 13 (**A**) Early postoperative film which is normal. (**B**) Film taken one year later shows loosening of all three screws on the left—note the black lines surrounding the screws.

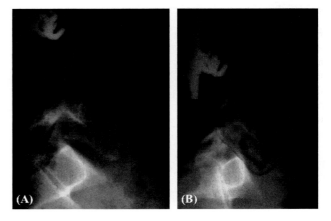

Figure 14 (**A**) Hinging. An early postoperative film in a patient with a long spinal fusion: note the alignment of L4-5. (**B**) A film taken three years later shows that the lamina hooks have slipped, there is hinging of L4-5, and the facet joints have widened.

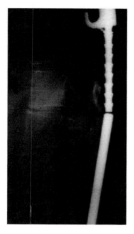

Figure 15 Fractured Harrington rod.

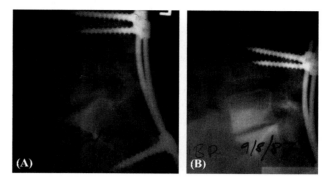

Figure 17 (**A**) Degenerative change. Early film showing degenerative disk disease at L5/S1. (**B**) A film taken one year later shows increase degenerative disc disease at L5-S1.

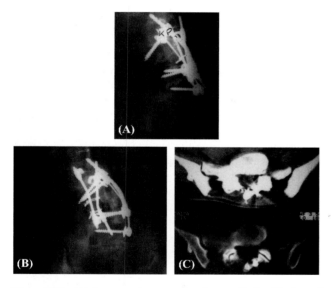

Figure 16 (**A**) Increase degenerative change. Early AP view of a complex spinal fusion in a patient with a severe kyphoscolosis: note that the SI joint appears normal. (**B**) A film taken four years later shows severe degenerative joint disease in the right Sacroiliac joint. (**C**) The finding of (**B**) was confirmed on the CT scan. *Abbreviations*: AP, anteroposterior; SI, sacroiliac; CT, computed tomography.

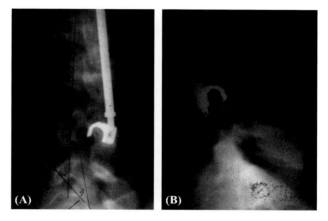

Figure 18 (**A**) Complications with lamina hooks. This one has fallen off the rod. (**B**) In a different patient, this hook has fallen off the lamina.

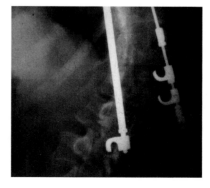

Figure 19 Failure of instrumentation with one rod and several hooks protruding through the skin.

pneumonia, tear of a nerve root, and hardware protruding through the skin (Fig. 19).

In scoliosis surgery, there is a mortality rate of 1% to 2% and this climbs higher with reoperation. Significant nerve injuries occur in 1.5%, paraplegia in 0.5%, pseudarthrosis in 10%, and infection in 1% despite antibiotic prophylaxis. Boachie-Adjei et al. (6) reported on the complication rate in 46 patients who received a Luque segmental instrumentation, with 39 patients having an arthrodesis down as far as the sacrum. The complication rate was 48%, there were three deaths (6%), the rods broke in 10%, the hooks came out in 4%, infection occurred in 9%, and pseudarthrosis in 6%. Following simple laminectomy rather than spinal fusion, there was a 2.4% infection rate. However, if antibiotics are used, this can drop to virtually zero.

Some final conclusions can be drawn both from a radiological and an orthopedic point of view. If spinal fusion is performed, posterior lateral bony fusion significantly decreases the complication rate. On the other hand, the complication rate increases after revision surgery. Low back surgery in general is associated with a high complication rate including postoperative pain, neuropathy, infection, instrument failure, and pseudarthrosis.

RADIOLOGY OF TOTAL JOINT REPLACEMENT

Virtually every joint in the body has been replaced by a prosthesis at one time or another from the temperomandibular joint to the first carpometacarpal joint. But the commonest joint replacements used today are for the major joints—the hips, knees, and shoulders. Less common are elbow and ankle joint replacements. Complications seen following total joint replacements in each of these anatomic sites are similar, so I feel that an initial overview is in order.

There are six major complications that can be seen following total joint replacement, namely, loosening, infection, fractures, dislocations, heterotopic bone formation, and foreign body reactions. Loosening is probably the most common complication occurring in 2% to 5% of hip and knee prostheses and much more commonly in the others. It can be symptomatic or asymptomatic and if the radiologist diagnoses loosening and the patient is asymptomatic, the orthopedist may simply watch the joint over months or years. Infections occur in approximately 2% of total joint replacements. They have a biphasic occurrence with some occurring within the first six months of the implant and the majority occurring four to six years after or even later. The radiological plain film diagnosis of infection in joint replacement can be difficult because of the metal. A computed tomography (CT) scan or magnetic resonance imaging (MRI) can help if there is extensive infection present (i.e., out of the area where the metal artifact is a problem), but the most reliable method of diagnosing an infection in a joint replacement is nuclear medicine. Usually, a combination of a bone scan with an indium 111 white cell scan or a gallium scan will provide the correct diagnosis.

Fractures of the prosthesis used to be common in the old days. However, now that the majority of the prostheses are made of titanium and vanadium and are manufactured under precise conditions, these fractures have become rare. On the other hand, periprosthetic fractures are not uncommon, particularly adjacent to the distal end of the femoral prosthesis in total hip replacements (THRs).

Today, many of the fractures are secondary to true trauma and not to a surgical problem with the prosthesis itself. Dislocations used to be far more common than they are today but they do still occur. Again, there is a biphasic pattern with some occurring in the immediate postoperative period and others occurring –four to six years later. The most commonly seen dislocations today occur at the hip joint and the majority of them are due to the prosthesis being misaligned: for example, the acetabular prosthesis being placed too vertically. Another complication that can be seen particularly in association with replacement of the larger joints is heterotopic bone formation. In the old days, this was commonly seen following THR (and reported in as many as 40% of THRs in some series) but now that the pathophysiology has been better understood, heterotopic bone formation is much less common. It occurs in people who are "bone formers," i.e., in patients with significant osteophytosis, patients with disseminated idiopathic skeletal hyperostosis (DISH) (discussed elsewhere in this book), and patients with ankylosing spondylitis or in acromegaly. If the patient with one of these conditions is identified preoperatively, then there are various methods of managing the situation successfully. These include ibuprofen and other nonsteroidal anti-inflammatory drugs (NSAIDs) as well as the use of low-dose radiation. Finally and probably the most interesting complication is known as "aggressive granulomatous disease," although a better name is probably "granulomatous foreign body reaction," but this has become commonly known as "particle disease" in the recent radiological literature. Although this complication can be seen in any joint, it is more commonly seen around the hip and knee joints as well as in association with silicone prostheses elsewhere in the body. This condition will be dealt with separately at the end of this section.

Total Hip Replacement

The history of hip operations for severe osteoarthritis of the hip started in the 1920s with a girdlestone procedure where the femoral head and synovium (which contains the majority of the nerve endings) were totally resected (Fig. 20).

Hence, the patient had no pain but had a short leg and an unstable hip. Then Smith Peterson introduced a metal cup placed between the patient's femoral head and acetabulum (Fig. 21).

The metal cup ground down any remaining cartilage and the hip joint ended up virtually fused.

The first two-part total hip replacements (THR) were performed in the mid 1930s, principally by Charnley in England and Judet in France. These were mainly metal on metal and failed relatively quickly. Further experiments were made with other materials including ceramics and

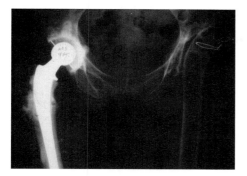

Figure 20 Girdlestone procedure. The left femoral head has been resected and the trochanteric region has migrated upward producing a 3-in shortening of the left leg.

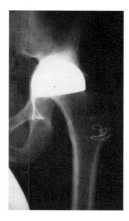

Figure 21 Cup arthroplasty. The cup placed between the patient's native acetabulum and a preshaped femoral head. This example shows virtual total fusion of the hip joint.

plastics, but it was not until the 1960s that the modern THR was introduced and had at least an acceptable five-year survival rate if not a reasonable one. Since then the mechanical factors involved in THR have been extensively studied and newer and better prosthesis have become available every day. There are many indications for THR but the primary one remains osteoarthritis, which may be primary or secondary—to any number of causes including rheumatoid arthritis, developmental hip dysphasia, and slipped capital femoral epiphysis (SCFE) to name the most common.

All of the complications mentioned in the introduction occur in THR. Loosening was a common complication in the old prostheses, particularly in the femoral component, and it was not uncommon to see a lucent line appearing between the cement and native bone. It was more unusual to see a line between the metal prostheses and the cement. Once again the patient did not have to be symptomatic even with extensive loosening. Remember, "Treat the patient and not the film." Loosening will lead to other

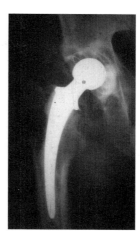

Figure 22 Loosening. A lucent line can be seen between the cement and the underlying femoral component. The acetabular component is also loose.

complications including fractures and particle disease, which will be dealt with later in the chapter. Loosening can be progressive or not, symptomatic or not, and is biomechanically related to one of three forces: (*i*) a pistoning effect, (*ii*) a pivoting effect, equivalent to a windshield wiper, or (*iii*) a bending or cantilever effect. The diagnosis is usually made on plain films (Fig. 22), but if there is any doubt, a combined indium 111 white cell and technetium bone scan can be performed (Fig. 23).

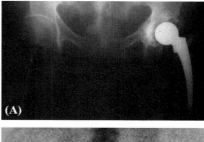
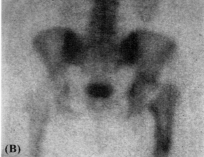

Figure 23 (**A**) Loosening. Plain film appears relatively normal. (**B**) Bone scan showing uptake around both the femoral and acetabular components, typical of loosening. Infection would have a higher signal as well as be more focal.

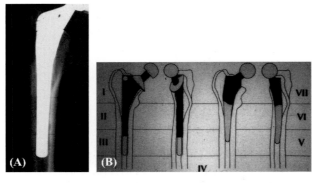

Figure 24 (**A**) Gruen zones. Film of femoral component with the zones marked. There is loosening in three zones. (**B**) Diagram to show the seven zones.

The overall incidence of loosening used to be about 10% but nowadays it is between 2% and 4% and more frequently affects the femoral component.

To better identify significant degrees of loosening in the more recent porous coated femoral prostheses, Gruen divided the length of the prosthesis into seven zones. If any three of these show evidence of loosening, then the prosthesis can be considered to be loose (Fig. 24).

They also commented on migration of the prosthesis, the presence or absence of a bony pedestal at the distal end of the femoral component, as well as calcar hypertrophy or atrophy. Particle shedding can also occur if there is deterioration of the interface and small metal beads can be seen scattered around the joint as a result of continued loosening (Fig. 25) (7).

Migration of the prosthesis is also quite common—the acetabular component will migrate in a cranial direction and if the patient is young and active may actually protrude into the pelvis (Fig. 26).

Infection can be a problem following any orthopedic procedure and about 2% of THRs get infected. This is bimodal with about half occurring in the immediate post-

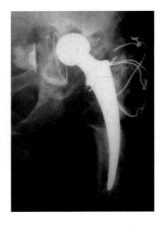

Figure 26 Loosening with protusion of the acetabular component through the medial acetabular wall into the pelvis. This was an extremely active younger patient who felt something give while playing golf.

operative period and half occurring four to six years later. The agent is usually one of the staphylococcal organisms such as the *S. aureus*. Infection is usually difficult to diagnose radiologically, although a joint aspiration will often provide the diagnosis. If a "dry tap" is achieved, then a radionuclide study is usually diagnostic—often using a combination of a technetium bone scan and either a gallium or indium white cell scan (Fig. 27).

One method of separating loosening from infection in bone scanning is that infection is hot on all three phases of the bone scan whereas loosening is usually only hot on the delayed images and not during the vascular phase or blood pool phase. In a recent paper, Aliabadi et al. (8) compared the sensitivity and specificity of combining radiography and bone scanning in the differentiation of loosening versus infection. Bone scanning alone was 73% sensitive and 96% specific in the diagnosis of loosening but combined with the radiographs bone scanning achieved a 84% sensitivity and 92% specificity.

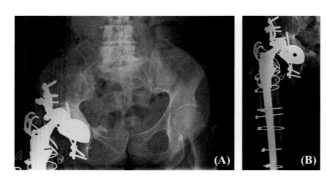

Figure 25 (**A**) Loosening with stray beads. (**B**) Loosening with stray beads.

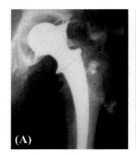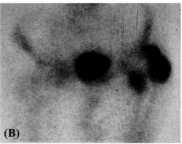

Figure 27 (**A**) Infection. A film taken from an aspiration arthrogram showing multiple sinus tracks. (**B**) A bone scan showing focal uptake mostly around the femoral head and neck. This is typical of infection.

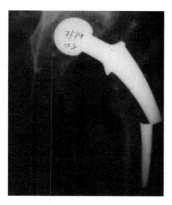

Figure 28 Fractured component.

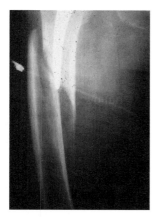

Figure 29 Fractured femur. This is the classical oblique fracture running across the distal end of the femoral component.

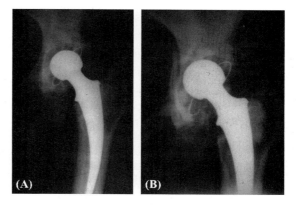

Figure 30 (**A**) Fractured acetabular component. Film taken three years after THR, which was normal. (**B**) Film taken a year later with a fracture of the bony acetabulum as well as of the acetabular component itself. *Abbreviation*: THR, total hip replacement.

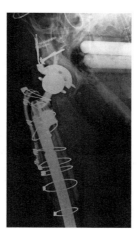

Figure 31 Postoperative fixation with a plate and screw placed following a fracture, which occurred after a THR. *Abbreviation*: THR, total hip replacement.

Fractures were also common in the early days, particularly fractures of the prosthesis but as the manufacturing process became more stringent, these became less common. The majority of fractures seen following THR are oblique fractures running across the proximal femoral shaft adjacent to the distal end of the stem of the femoral prosthesis (Figs. 28 and 29).

Fractures across the acetabular component are much rarer but do occur (Fig. 30) and fractures or separation of the greater trochanter can still be seen today. Factors involved in postoperative fracturing of the femur include weight (over 90 kg), height (over 1.8 m), and bilateral hip disease. Thus, they occur usually in men with a high level of activity (Fig. 26). In 1989, Roffman et al. (9) introduced the classification of upper femoral fractures following THR and suggested that the majority of patients can be treated conservatively. However, nowadays, as patients get larger and heavier, most of them have interoperative reduction with a long lateral plate and cerclage wires (Fig. 31).

Stress and insufficiency fractures also occur following THR and the characteristic ones (and a typical radiology boards case) is a vertical fracture of the ischial ramus adjacent to and on the same side as the THR (Fig. 32).

Dislocation and subluxation occurs in up to 2% of patients and is also bimodal with half occurring within the immediate postoperative period and the rest occurring five to six years later. The majority occurs as a result of improper placing of the components, particularly of the acetabular cup, which may be too vertical (Fig. 33).

However, dislocations also occur in patients who have a confused mental status or neuromuscular disorder. Treatment is usually by closed reduction, although a revision arthroplasty is in order if the dislocation keeps reoccurring (Fig. 34).

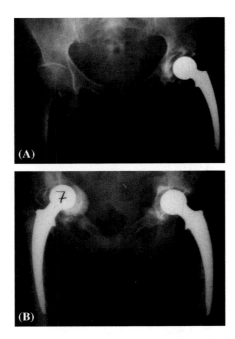

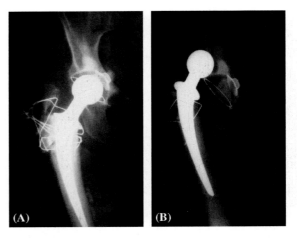

Figure 33 (**A**) Dislocated THR. In place. (**B**) Dislocated superiorly and dorsally. *Abbreviation*: THR, total hip replacement.

Figure 32 (**A**) Stress fracture of the ischial ramus. A 64-year-old female who has had the hip replacement for three years and is now complaining of left hip pain. (**B**) Stress fracture of the ischial ramus in a different patient.

We recently had a case of recurrent subluxation because a loose fragment of cement became interposed between the acetabular component and the femoral head (Fig. 35).

Heterotopic bone formation used to be a major problem with the use of methyl methacrylate and in fact a

classification evolved ranging from class I (very minor which was common) to class IV (which was fused) (Figs. 36–38).

But it became obvious that there were certain groups of patients who were susceptible to form bone and these are known as the bone formers. Patients with excessively large osteophytes, patients with DISH, patients with ankylosing spondylitis, and patients with acromegaly all form excess bone. Thus, the answer was to find ways to stop osteoblasts laying down extra bone. Various methods were tried but the most reliable seem to be the use of NSAIDS such as ibuprofen and low-dose radiation. The radiation used to be given in 300 millisievert

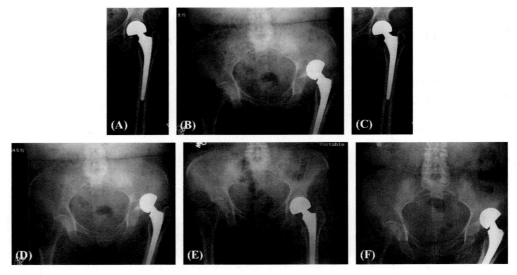

Figure 34 (**A**) Dislocating endoprosthesis. In position. (**B**) Dislocating endoprothesis. Twelve months later, showing the dislocation. (**C**) Dislocating endoprosthesis. Reduced. (**D**) Dislocating endoprosthesis. Nine months later, endoprosthesis is out again. (**E**) Dislocating endoprosthesis. Reduced. (**F**) Dislocating endoprosthesis. Now replaced with a THR. *Abbreviation*: THR, total hip replacement.

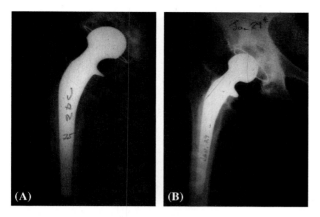

Figure 35 (A) Cement interposed between cup and femoral head. Initial postoperative film with loose cement lying below joint. (B) Film taken four days later with cement in the joint causing subluxation of the femoral head.

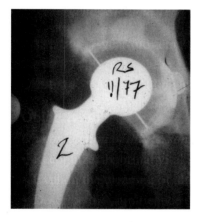

Figure 36 Grade I heterotopic bone formation with discrete areas of myositis ossificans seen laterally to the femoral head.

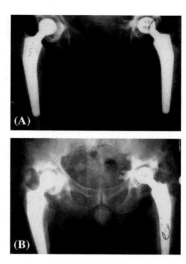

Figure 37 (A) Progressive heterotopic bone formation. Film taken six months after a THR. There is Grade II heterotopic bone formation on the left. The right side appears clear. (B) Film taken one year later. There is a grade III heterotopic bone formation on the right and Grade IV on the left. *Abbreviation*: THR, total hip replacement.

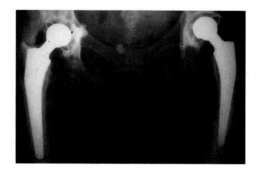

Figure 38 Grade IV heterotopic bone formation on the right with complete fusion of the joint. The left side is clean because the patient was given 1000 millisieverts of radiation.

increments—the day before the operation, three days and 10 days after the operation, although some people advocated a single dose of 700 millisievert given within 72 hours of operation. Lo et al. (10) used this regimen on 24 hips in 23 patients and only one patient developed grade II heterotopic bone formation.

Other complications of THR include deep vein thrombosis and pulmonary embolism, pulmonary embolism from the use of cement, intraoperative hemorrhage, and finally, granulomatous foreign body reaction, which will be discussed separately below.

One final comment about hip prostheses, about 30 years ago, because of the then high failure rate with conventional two-component THR, resurfacing procedures of the femoral hip were introduced. These consisted of a traditional acetabular cup but with a metal prosthesis resurfacing the femoral head without a metal neck or stem. Although the short-term results were good, these uniformly failed about three to five years after implant (Fig. 39).

Howie et al. (11) reviewed 100 Wagner hip arthoplasties in 93 patients at 10 years. Seventy percent had failed because of loosening at five years and a further 50% of the remainder by eight years.

Total Knee Replacement

Total knee replacements (TKR) were introduced in the 1960s and similar to THRs were initially not very successful. In 1990, the Mayo clinic (12) reviewed over 9000

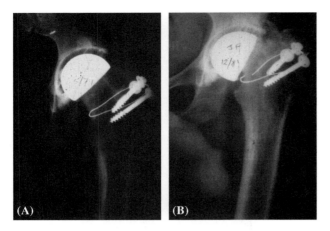

Figure 39 (**A**) Femoral resurfacing procedure. Film taken one year postoperatively. (**B**) Film taken six months later, where the femoral cup has slipped and the femoral head is fragmenting.

TKRs performed between 1971 and 1987. They found a 10-year survival rate of 82% in patients older than 60 and an 80% survival right in patients with rheumatoid arthritis. However, if the patients were younger, this rate dropped to 74%, and if the underlying etiology was posttraumatic arthritis, the survivorship dropped to 60%. These authors found that good prognostic factors were older age, primary operation, rheumatoid arthritis, and the use of a femoral condylar prosthesis with a metal-backed tibial component. TKRs suffer from all the same complications that are seen following THR. Dislocations have now become quite rare (Fig. 40) because of the introduction of constrained knee prostheses and fractures are also not

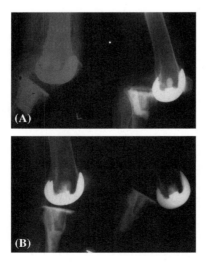

Figure 40 (**A**) Left side. TKR dislocation. (**B**) Right side. Note the normal alignment on the left side of each image and the dislocated prosthesis on the right. This patient could dislocate both his knees at will. *Abbreviation*: THR, total knee replacement.

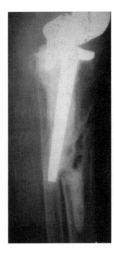

Figure 41 Fractured tibia. A typical oblique fracture across the base of the tibial prosthesis occurred with only minor stress.

as common since the length of the stem of the tibial prosthesis has been reduced considerably. Fractures occur characteristically across the distal end of the tibial component and run obliquely across the bone (Fig. 41).

Insufficiency fractures can be seen in elderly patients anywhere but in the knee following TKR, they usually run across the distal femur just above the femoral component (Fig. 42).

Loosening will occur in 2% to 4% of TKRs and if the femoral component loosens, it usually does so in the sagittal plane with the femoral component "rocking" on the distal femur (Fig. 43).

Loosening initially presents as a lucent line between the cement and underlying bone or between the cement and the metal of the prosthesis (Fig. 44).

Loosening of the tibial component may also show lucent lines but more often the tibial component gets impacted

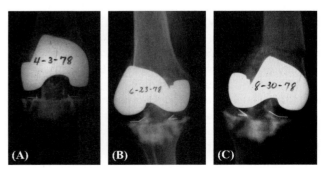

Figure 42 (**A**) Insufficiency fracture in an 80-year-old lady. Initial film without a fracture. (**B**) Film taken two months later following a fall in the bath and read as normal. (**C**) Film taken two months after the fall, showing a displaced insufficiency fracture running across the distal femur. Note the fragmentation of the cement in the proximal tibia.)

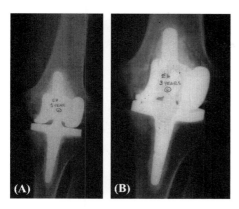

Figure 43 (A) Loosening. Initial film. Shows no abnormality. (B) Film taken two years later shows a clear cut lucent zone between the cement and femur.

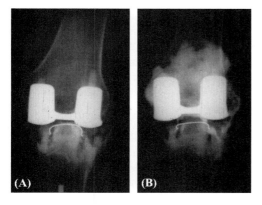

Figure 44 (A) Loosening. Initial film showing loosening and fragmentation of the tibial component. (B) An arthrogram shows the contrast running between the cement and the tibia and extending out through the region of fragmentation.

down into the tibia and so loosening is more difficult to diagnose. However, it is important to realize that many of the modern prostheses have plastic inserts (spacers) to make them fit and these can appear loose on an X-ray if you are not aware of this type of new prosthesis (Fig. 45).

Infections occur in approximately 2% of TKRs also, in a bimodal fashion, either in the first six months following operation or four to six years postoperatively. The diagnosis usually cannot be made on radiological grounds alone, but either an aspiration or an arthrogram will often make the diagnosis correctly. Once again the radionuclide study can be diagnostic (Fig. 46).

Heterotopic bone formation is less common following TKR than THR probably because of the restricted range of motion of the knee. However, it can still be seen occasionally in the quadriceps tendon mechanism (Fig. 47).

The most interesting and the most frequent complication of TKR involves the patellofemoral joint. It has been

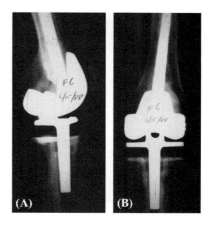

Figure 45 (A) New type of prothesis with variable-sized spacer, which is radiolucent, and thus making it appear that the prothesis is loose or malpositioned. (B) New type of prothesis with variable-sized spacer, which is radiolucent, and thus making it appear that the prothesis is loose.

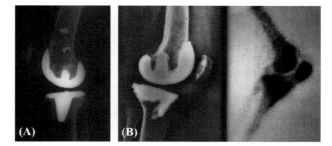

Figure 46 (A) Infection. There is a large effusion present. At aspiration, frank pus was removed. (B) Infection in a different patient. On the left, a lateral film shows a large joint effusion. On the right, a radionuclide scan shows the characteristic focal areas of high uptake characteristic of an infection.

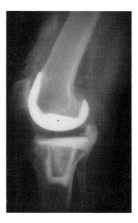

Figure 47 Heterotopic bone formation in the quadriceps tendon following TKR. *Abbreviation*: THR, total knee replacement.

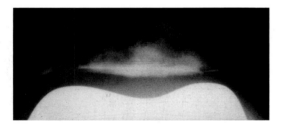

Figure 48 Fractured patellar component. Note the fracture of the metal plate on the left.

estimated that approximately 50% of complications seen following TKR are related in some way to the extensor mechanism. Apart from the more general complications discussed above, such as fractures and infections, there are two subgroups of complications involving the patella. The first group can be considered to be tracking complications. About 10% of patients develop the patellofemoral syndrome following TKR. This is due to an imbalance in the extensor muscles often favoring the lateral side of the knee. Simple exercises showed correct this. However, any patellofemoral imbalance will lead to wear and tear of the polyethylene surface of the patella component. This is caused by the patellar tracking abnormally in the trochlear groove of the femoral component. Modern prostheses are carefully machined so that the patella component articulates smoothly with the femoral component. Thus, any degree of angulation of one surface to the other will lead to wear and tear and to the formation of debris, which will fall into the joint (Fig. 48).

In time, this can lead to a chronic foreign body synovitis, which can occur as a reaction to particles of polyethylene, cement, or metal in the synovial fluid. Although this rarely leads to any major clinical problems,

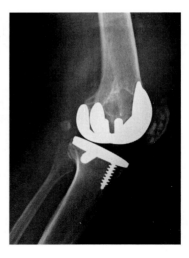

Figure 50 Patella femoral joint complications. Fragmentation and collapse of the patellar component.

it can cause marked synovial hypertrophy and swelling with decreased range of motion (Fig. 49).

The second group of complications can be considered under the general heading of component failure. Probably the most common patellar complication is loosening and this can be seen in up to 2% of knees following TKR. The plane of loosening is usually between the prosthesis (with the pegs intact) and the patella. The grinding action of this motion will lead to the patella fragmenting (Figs. 50 and 51) and ultimately to complete separation of the prosthesis from the underlying bone with the dislocated prosthesis often moving elsewhere in the joint (Fig 52).

Obviously, a number of other complications can be seen with this scenario, such as fracture and failure of the pins, failure of the prosthesis, and ultimately fracture of the patella. Keating et al. (13) found an incidence of 3.8

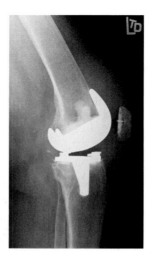

Figure 49 Patella femoral joint complications. Synovial hypertrophy seen in the region of the suprapatella pouch and Hoffa's fat pad.

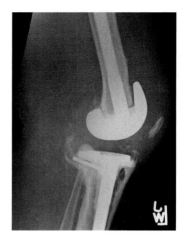

Figure 51 Patella femoral joint complications. This lateral film shows both marked synovial hypertrophy and wearing down of the patient's native patella.

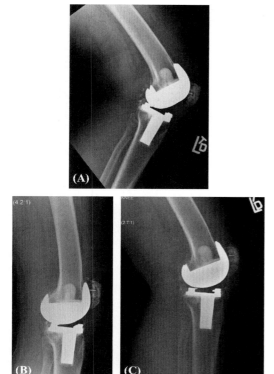

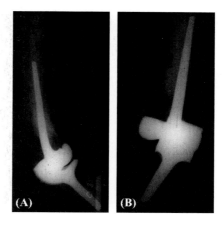

Figure 53 (**A**) Loosening of a total elbow replacement. Initial film). (**B**) Film taken two years later showing subluxation and loosening.

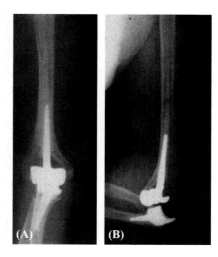

Figure 52 (**A**) Patella femoral joint complications. Initial film is normal. (**B**) Patella femoral joint complications. Film taken one year later shows loosening of the patella component. (**C**) Patella femoral joint complications. Film taken six months after the previous one shows further fragmentation and collapse of the patella component.

patellar fractures in 4583 patients following TKR. They found that 114 of their patients had an intact extensor mechanism with a loose patellar component.

Total Elbow Replacement

Unfortunately, the elbow joint is not a simple hinge joint otherwise there could be a simple hinged prosthesis. Most total elbow joint replacements require the excision of the radial head as well as placing a hinged prosthesis between the distal humerus and the proximal ulna. Obviously, this leads to inherent instability. In a recent report by Schneeberger et al. (14), following up 41 patients with posttraumatic osteoarthritis of the elbow who received total joint replacements, only 40% reported excellent results over an average follow-up of five years. Seventeen percent rated their results fair to poor. On the other hand, 78% of the patients experienced either no pain or only mild discomfort. However, 11 patients had major complications including three patients with infections, three patients with failure of the prosthesis, and five

Figure 54 (**A**) Dislocation. Initial film shows normal alignment. (**B**) Film taken two years later shows posterior dislocation.

patients whose ulnar component fractured. We have seen loosening, dislocation, and fractures associated with total elbow replacement (Figs. 53 and 54).

Infections are also quite common and occur in up to 10% of patients following total elbow replacement (Fig. 55).

The best results appear to be in patients with severe rheumatoid arthritis who are not very mobile. In primary total elbow replacement, the capitellocondylar prosthesis produces excellent results. In secondary replacements, radial head resection and synovectomy should precede the placement of a simple hinged prosthesis.

Total Ankle Replacement

Total ankle replacements are rare because there is little underlying bone stock and the normal human ankle

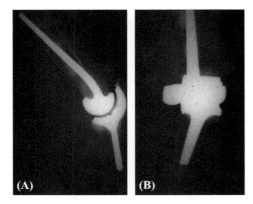

Figure 55 (**A**) Lateral film. Loosening and infection. (**B**) AP film shows marked loosening of the humeral component secondary to a windshield wiper effect. At operation, infection was also found. *Abbreviation*: AP, anteroposterior.

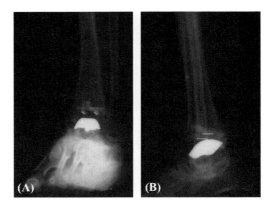

Figure 57 (**A**) Total ankle replacement with loosening of the talar component. (**B**) Total ankle replacement with loosening of the talar component.

mortise is carefully designed to take a lot of weight on a relatively small surface area. Although the normal ankle joint is a hinged joint and thus theoretically should be easy to replace, most of the complications of total ankle replacement are mechanical with loosening, dislocation, and disintegration being the most common (Figs. 56 and 57).

Obviously, infection can also occur. Nowadays most surgeons prefer to perform an ankle fusion, i.e., a fusion of the tibiotalar joint usually accompanied by fusion of the subtalar joints or with a triple arthrodesis. This procedure also has many complications such as nonunion and disintegration as well as infection (Fig. 58).

Total ankle replacements are rarely performed today but I am sure that a new generation of ankle joint

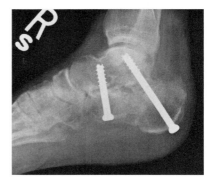

Figure 58 Subtalar fusion using two long cannulated screws running between the calcaneus and talus.

replacements is being developed while this book is being written.

Total Shoulder Replacement

There are probably as many types of total shoulder prosthesis on the market as there are shoulder surgeons. In fact, the latest is called a "reverse" prosthesis with a "ball" replacing the glenoid and a "cup" replacing the humeral head. However the true history of total shoulder replacement has been fraught with complications of which loosening and disintegration are the most common. In the early days, the pioneers proclaimed great results but only in patients with a short-term follow-up. For instance Barrett et al. (15) followed 50 total shoulder replacements (TSR) on 44 patients and at three years, 88% were pain free and there were only four cases of loosening. Radiologically, a lucent line could be seen between the humeral prosthesis and the underlying bone in 10% and in 74% of the glenoid prostheses. There was frank loosening of the prosthesis in

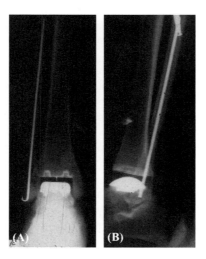

Figure 56 (**A**) Total ankle replacement in good alignment but with collapse and fragmentation of the talar bone. (**B**) Total ankle replacement in good alignment but with collapse and fragmentation of the talar bone.

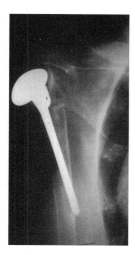

Figure 59 Loose humeral prosthesis. Note that the humeral prosthesis is loose, markedly rotated, and protrudes through the medial cortex of the humerus.

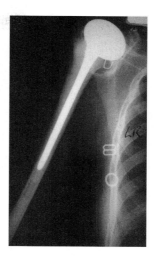

Figure 61 Upward subluxation of the humeral prosthesis through the rotator cuff, causing marked impingment on the undersurface of the acromion.

8% of the outpatients. However, in a longer-term follow-up, the same authors (16) reported on a 60%-failure rate.

In my own experience, loosening appears to be the commonest complication of total shoulder replacement, and this can involve the humeral prosthesis (Fig. 59) as well as the glenoid (Fig. 60).

Dislocations can also occur and in time the humeral prosthesis can wear through the supraspinatus tendon to cause marked impingement (Fig. 61).

Heterotopic new bone can also rarely be seen following a total shoulder replacement (Fig. 62).

One of the problems with assessing total shoulder replacements radiologically is that on many of the radiographs, the prosthetic humeral head appears to lie too superiorly (Fig. 63).

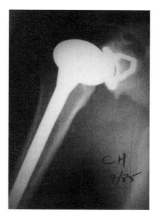

Figure 62 Heterotopic bone following total shoulder replacement. Note the discrete ossification lying below the glenohumeral joint.

A template can be drawn to assess the relative position of the prosthetic humeral head to the glenoid (Fig. 64) to see if it is well placed.

1. Draw a vertical line bisecting the shaft of the humerus.
2. Draw a horizontal line through the equator of the glenoid.
3. Draw a 1-cm^2 box above and inside these two lines where they intersect. This is usually rhomboidal in shape rather than square.
4. Assume that the humeral head is round like a tennis ball and find its center of circumference. This should lie within the box if the prosthesis has been correctly placed (Fig. 64).

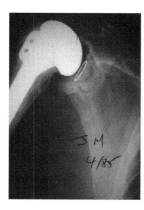

Figure 60 Loose total shoulder replacement—glenoid component. Note the lucent line between the cement and the underlying bone.

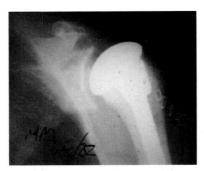

Figure 63 TSR with humeral head apparently subluxed upwards but is actually in a normal position.

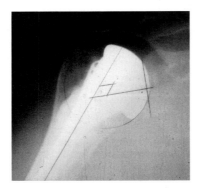

Figure 64 Template for assessing to see if the humeral head is correctly placed. See text.

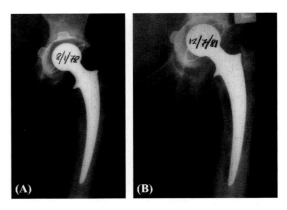

Figure 65 (**A**) Foreign body granulomatous disease. Early films taken one year after THR. *Abbreviation*: THR, total hip replacement. (**B**) Film taken three years later, showing marked loosening as well as rounded or ovoid bony defects typical of foreign body granulomatous disease.

In 1988, Aliabadi et al. (17) reviewed their results of 98 shoulders in 76 patients with an average follow-up time of three years. Thirty-eight percent of the shoulders had complications: upward migration in 24%, loosening of the glenoid component in 15%, loosening of the humeral component in 5%, and subsidence of the humeral component in 7%. However, they found no correlation between the radiological findings and the patient's symptoms or clinical findings.

FOREIGN BODY GRANULOMATOUS DISEASE OR "PARTICLE" DISEASE

Foreign body granulomatous disease has several other names including "aggressive giant-cell foreign body reaction" and, more recently, "Particle disease." It occurs in approximately 2% to 4% of patients following THR, 15% patients following TKR, and in about 40% of patients with silicone implants who do not have rheumatoid arthritis. The underlying pathogenesis starts with microloosening, which proceeds onto more marked loosening. In turn, this will lead to fragmentation of cement at the bone/cement interface and possibly even of metal as well as of the surrounding bone. Macrophages move into remove the debris and giant cells become abundant to help in the healing process. This in turn will lead to localized destruction of bone, cement, and anything else that is in the way, usually producing ovoid or rounded destructive areas adjacent to the prosthesis itself. In the case of the acetabulum, these will often extend into the soft tissues of the pelvis as large soft-tissue masses. If the process involves the joint as is frequently seen secondary to silicone implants, then generalized synovial hypertrophy can occur, causing multiple subchondral synovial cysts scattered throughout the joint.

Foreign body granulomatous disease occurs in three main situations, following either THR or TKR and adjacent to silicone implants. In the hip, often the loosening is observed to be increasing over several years and then rounded or ovoid areas of primary bony destruction can be seen adjacent to the prosthesis mainly around the stem of the femoral component (Fig. 65).

These areas of destruction can encompass trabecular bone, cortical bone, and even methylmethacrylate, all of which become progressively engulfed and destroyed. Obviously, this will lead to instability of the prosthesis, although only rarely to fractures (Fig. 66).

In the knee, the foreign body granulomatous reaction seems to mainly involve the synovium probably because there is a large amount of synovium within the knee joint, which is retained after a TKR. Thus, swelling of the synovium in the suprapatellar pouch as well as in the region of Hoffa's fat pad can be clearly seen (Fig. 49).

Weissman et al. (18) described 18 patients with metal-induced synovitis in the knee where an actual dense "metal" line of deposition can be seen in the synovium

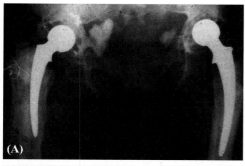

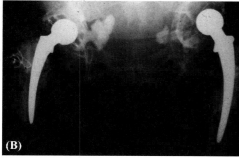

Figure 66 (A) Foreign body granulomatous disease. Film taken two years post–op, showing an apparently normal left THR but a right one that is obviously loose and has a foreign body granulomatous disease with many rounded bony defects. (B) Film taken two years later, showing marked destruction of both the left acetabular and proximal femur with multiple rounded lucencies typical of particle disease. The right side is basically unchanged. *Abbreviations*: THR, total hip replacement.

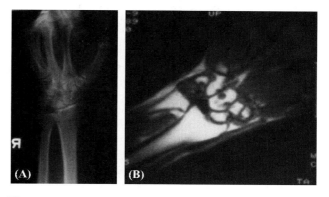

Figure 67 Image (**A**) is an oblique view of the right wrist showing a silicone prosthesis replacing the lunate. Image (**B**) is a proton density MRI. The lunate can be seen as the black square in the middle of the proximal carpal row. The synovial reaction can be seen as gray synovially based overgrowth at the level of the distal ulna and throughout the carpus. *Abbreviation*: MRI, magnetic resonance imaging.

along with marked soft tissue changes. The soft-tissue swelling is characteristically seen on the lateral radiograph and appears to affect between 5% to 10% of knees following TKR. The "metal line" is much rarer in our own experience.

The third situation in which foreign body granulomatous disease is seen is in association with silicone implants. These have been used for over 50 years to replace the interphalangeal joints of patients with rheumatoid arthritis generally without complication. However, if a silicone implant is placed into an otherwise fit patient who is not immunocompromised, foreign body reactions routinely occur. I have seen them in association with a number of silicone implants in the hand, particularly of the scaphoid and the lunate, and also in the foot with interphalangeal implants in the first metatarsophalangeal joint (Fig. 67).

The etiology is the same: motion leads to an invasion of macrophages, which in turn attracts osteoclastic activity and giant cells into the surrounding synovium. Obviously, this can involve the whole joint even away from the implant. Foreign body granulomatous disease also has a characteristic MR appearance.

REFERENCES

1. D'Ambrosia RD. Orthopaedics in the new millennium. A new patient-physician partnership. JBJS 1999; 81(4): 447–451.
2. Drez D Jr., Finney TP, Roberts TS. Sepsis in orthopedic surgery. Orthopedics 1991; 14(2):157–162.
3. Maurer DJ, Merkow RL, Gustilo RB. Infection after intramedullary nailing of severe open tibial fractures initially treated with external fixation. JBJS Am 1989; 71(6): 835–838.
4. Mahan J, Seligson D, Henry SL. Factors in pin tract infection. Orthopedics 1991; 14(3):305–308.
5. Griffiths HJ, Bullis. Complications of Spinal surgery (unpublished data).
6. Boachie-Adjei O, Lonstein JE, Winter RB. Management of neuromuscular spinal deformities with Luque segmental instrumentation. JBJS Am 1989; 71(4):548–562.
7. Gruen TA, McNeice GM, Amstutz HC. "Modes of failure" of cemented stem-type femoral components: a radiologic analysis of loosening. Clin Orthop Relat Res 1979; (141): 17–27.
8. Alibadi P, Tumeh SS, Weissman BN. Cemented total hip prosthesis: radiologic and scintigraphic evaluation. Radiology 1989; 173(1):203–206.
9. Roffman M, Mendes DG. Fracture of the femur after total hip arthroplasty. Orthopedics 1989; 12(8):1067–1070.
10. Lo TC, Healy WL. Re-irradiation for prophylaxis of heterotopic ossification after hip surgery. Br J Radiology 2001; 74(882):503–506.
11. Howie DW, Campbell D, McGee M. Wagner resurfacing hip arthroplasty. The results of one hundred consecutive arthroplasties after eight to ten years. JBJS Am 1990; 72 (5):708–714.

12. Rand JA, Ilstrup DM. Survivorship analysis of total knee arthroplasty. Cumulative rates of survival of 9200 total knee arthroplasties. JBJS Am 1991; 73(3):397–409.

13. Keating EM, Haas G, Meding JB. Patella fracture after post total knee replacements. Clin Orthop Relat Res 2003; (416):93–97.

14. Schneeberger AG, Adams R, Morrey BF. Semiconstrained total elbow replacement for the treatment of post-traumatic osteoarthrosis. JBJS Am 1997; 79(8):1211–1222.

15. Barrett WP, Franklin JL, Jackins SE. Total shoulder arthroplasty. JBJS Am 1987; 69(6):865–872.

16. Barrett WP, Thornhill TS, Thomas WH. Nonconstrained total shoulder arthroplasty in patients with polyarticular rheumatoid arthritis. J Arhtroplasty 1989; 4(1):91–96.

17. Aliabadi P, Weissman BN, Thornhill T. Evaluation of a nonconstrained total shoulder prosthesis. AJR Am J Roentgenol 1988; 151(6):1169–1172.

18. Weissman BN, Scott RD, Brick GW. Radiographic detection of metal-induced synovitis as a complication of arthroplasty of the knee. JBJS Am 1991; 73(7):1002–1007.

8

MRI and Ultrasound

MRI OF THE KNEE

The standard knee protocol should include three sagittal sequences—T1, proton density, and delayed T2. There should be two coronal sequences—proton density and a fat saturation T1. Although one fat saturation T1 axial sequence may be sufficient, I personally like to add a proton density axial.

Like assessing a chest X-ray, one needs to be systematic for looking at knee MRIs. I begin with the sagittal sequences moving from lateral to medial, then onto the coronal sequences going from posterior to anterior, and finally going to the axial sequences and moving from the top to the bottom.

The Menisci

The menisci present as black triangles. Normally, there should be two slices in which they both appear like a bow tie and then appear as black triangles anteriorly and posteriorly. The medial meniscus is usually larger than the lateral meniscus (Fig. 1).

In normal adults, there should be no internal signal. However, there is a grading system for internal signals in the menisci, and this is as follows:

Grade I: horizontal line: normal up to age 15, in middle (equivalent to vascular channel), and occasionally in adults.

Grade II: "degenerative" myxoid changes common in over 40s should not touch any surface but may be widespread (Fig. 2).

Grade III: actual tear: signal touches any surface—top, bottom, meniscocapsular junction (Fig. 3).

Helpful hint:
Approximately 80% of tears are in the posterior horn of the medial meniscus.

There are different types of tears including horizontal, vertical, undersurface, and complex. Most intersubstance tears are considered to be grade 2 tears if they occur in a young person, although grade 2 high signal in older patients is usually secondary to myxoid degeneration. A bucket handle tear is a long vertical tear, and the meniscus flips over, often into the intercondylar notch and may occur anteriorly or posteriorly. Signs associated with bucket handle tears: double cruciate sign, clipped meniscus sign (Figs. 4 and 5).

Parrot beak tear: It is a combination of a horizontal and vertical tear so that looking down on the meniscus, it looks like a parrots beak (Fig. 6).

Recurrent tear: After attempted surgical repair of meniscal tear, I think all (most) bets are off. However,

1. if you can see fluid running through the repair, then retear.
2. if the meniscus is uniformly black, then it is successfully repaired.

Anything else is useless.

Discoid menisci are usually lateral and occur in 2% of the population. On the sagittal cuts, the bow ties appear in at least four cuts (and not in the normal 2), since the meniscus is a disc and not a half moon. Discoid menisci

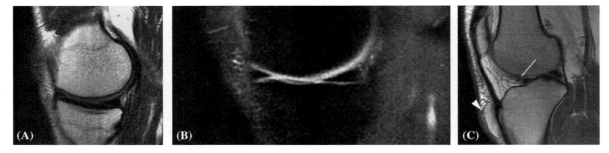

Figure 1 Normal medial meniscus. (**A**) Proton density. (**B**) T1 fat sat sequence. (**C**) Normal lateral meniscus—medial proton density slice. A patient with a transverse ligament (*arrow*). Note that he also has bursitis in his pretibial bursae. *Abbreviation*: fat sat, fat saturation.

are much more prone to tears with approximately 50% torn at age 50 (Fig. 7).

Helpful hints:

1. *Remember the association between a tear of the posterior horn of the medial meniscus and a tear of the anterior cruciate ligament (ACL) and one of the medial collateral ligament (McDonough's terrible triad).*
2. *Remember that there is an intermeniscal ligament, which occurs in 20% of the population. This runs from the anterior aspect of the anterior horn of the lateral meniscus (where it can look like a tear!) across the intercondylar notch to the anterior horn*

of the medial meniscus. This finding can be confirmed on the axial sequences (Fig. 8).

Cruciate Ligaments

The ACL has some fat separating the fibrous tissue bands, particularly at its insertion into the tibia, so it is never as dark as the posterior cruciate ligament (PCL). If a suspected tear is seen on sagittal slices, check with the coronal slices (Fig. 9).

The origin of the ACL is from the posterior roof of the femur in the intercondylar notch, and it inserts into the anterior part of the tibial plateau, anterior to the tibial spine.

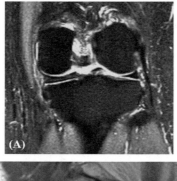

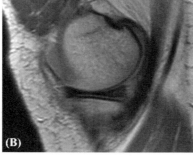

Figure 2 Myxoid degeneration of the posterior horn of the medial meniscus. (**A**) Coronal T1 fat sat sequence. (**B**) Proton density. *Abbreviation*: fat sat, fat saturation.

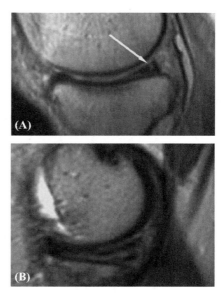

Figure 3 Actual tears. (**A**) Posterior horn of the medial meniscus has a vertical tear (*arrow*). (**B**) Undersurface tear in the posterior horn of the medial menicus extending both to the undersurface of the meniscus as well as to its capsular insertion.

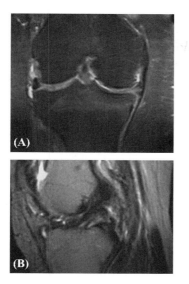

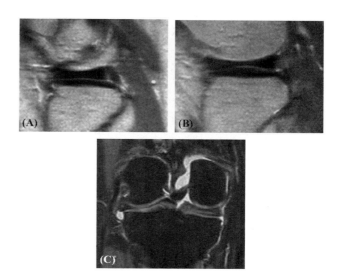

Figure 4 Bucket handle tear. (**A**) Coronal T1 fat sat slice. There are tears of both the medial meniscus and lateral meniscus. (**B**) Sagittal view. Note the "double" ACL sign (arrow) for a bucket handle tear of the lateral meniscus. *Abbreviation*: fat sat, fat saturation.

Figure 7 Discoid meniscus. (**A**) Two proton density slices taken at different places in a discoid meniscus, which is intact. (**B**) Two proton density slices taken at different places in a discoid meniscus, which is intact. (**C**) Discoid Meniscus in a different patient with central tears of both menisci.

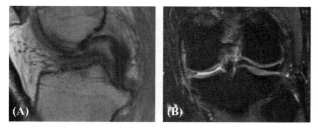

Figure 5 Bucket handle medial meniscus tear. (**A**) Sagittal proton density with double PCL sign. (**B**) Coronal fat sat showing a missing medial meniscus and something lying horizontally in the intercondylar notch (the medial meniscus!). *Abbreviations*: fat sat, fat saturation; PCL, posterior cruciate ligament.

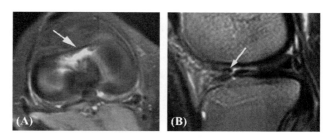

Figure 8 Transverse ligament. (**A**) Axial (*arrow*). (**B**) Sagittal delayed T2 (*arrow*).

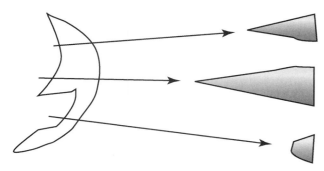

Figure 6 "Parrot Beak" tear of a medial meniscus.

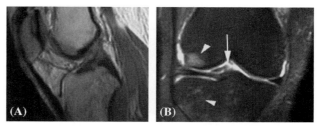

Figure 9 Complete tear of the ACL (*arrows*): Note that the origin of the ACL has been separated from the roof of the intercondylar notch. (**A**) Sagittal. (**B**) Coronal: Note the accompanying and classical bone bruising (arrowheads). *Abbreviation*: ACL, anterior cruciate ligament.

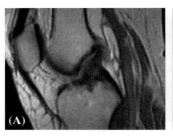

Figure 10 Partial tear of the ACL. (**A**) Proton density sagittal view. (**B**) Coronal T1 fat sat sequence (*arrows*). Note that the patient also has a grade II MCL tear (*arrowheads*). *Abbreviations*: fat sat, fat saturation; ACL, anterior cruciate ligament; MCL, medial collateral ligament.

The ACL splays out at its insertion and should be shown to be contiguous with the anterior horn of the lateral meniscus.

A tear can be *partial* in which case the ligament is swollen and of high signal. If only one fiber can be seen going from the femur to the tibia, this is still considered to be a partial tear (Fig. 10).

A *complete* tear is when the ACL is avulsed off its origin, and it may end up lying flat on the floor of the intercondylar notch. It can also be avulsed off its insertion going posteriorly and curled up adjacent to PCL. ACL tears are usually associated with large effusions as well as a classical bone bruise pattern—lateral aspect of the lateral femoral condyle and posterior tibia.

An old, healed ACL tear usually has a fibrosis tissue reaction, so it is dense and often adheres to the PCL, and thus appears L shaped (Fig. 11).

A surgical rule of thumb is a complete ACL tear should be fixed within 72 hours—after that, it is too late. So a magnetic resonance imaging (MRI) should be done immediately because this is a genuine emergency in an elite athlete with a suspected ACL tear.

Important note: The cruciate ligaments are extraarticular and covered by a synovial tent. It is thus possible to

have a partial and/or complete tear of either cruciate ligament *without* an effusion. In fact, partial tears of the ACL are only associated with effusions in about 40% of patients.

Posterior Cruciate Ligament

This ligament is not as important a stabilizer as the ACL, and in fact, if it is torn as a solitary injury, the orthopedists rarely do anything about it. The origin of the PCL is from the lower aspect of the roof of the intercondylar notch. It runs horizontally, then obliquely, and finally vertically to insert into the far posterior aspect of the central tibial plateau.

It has an oblique supporting ligament running low laterally to high medially, known as Humphrey's ligament in the front and Wrisberg's ligament at the back. These are embryologically the same ligament.

The PCL has very low intensity on all sequences because of its tight fibrous tissue construction. Tears of the PCL are rarely complete and are usually only associated with a knee dislocation (Fig. 12).

Partial tears are not uncommon, usually running along the line of the ligament and usually in its oblique central portion.

The PCL may also show central high signal with obvious disruption as well as swelling and enlargement, thus acting more like grade I tendonitis in a tendon elsewhere.

Helpful hint:

Tears of the PCL are rarely solitary so look especially hard for meniscal tears PHMM (posterior horn medial meniscus) and collateral ligament tears [medial collateral ligament (MCL)].

Medial Collateral Ligament

The MCL originates from the upper surface of the medial femoral condyle. It extends down to the undersurface of the medial tibial plateau. It is approximately 5 cm wide from front to back. It is closely adherent to both bones and

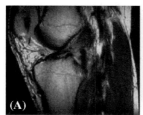
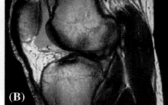

Figure 11 Posterior knee dislocation. (**A**) Complete tears of both the ACL and PCL. (**B**) Note the radiological drawer sign. The patient had also torn his MCL and posterior horn of the medial meniscus.

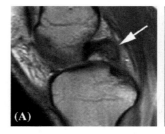
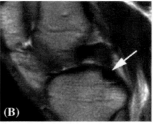

Figure 12 Partial tear of the PCL on two sagittal slices. (**A**) Note the high intensity in the region of its insertion into the posterior aspect of the tibia (*arrow*). (**B**) On this image it looks as though this is a near complete tear. *Abbreviation*: PCL, posterior cruciate ligament.

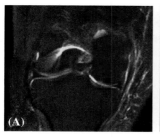 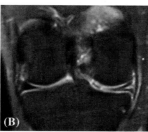

Figure 13 MCL tears. (**A**) There is fluid on both sides of the ligament (grade II) with some menisculocapsular separation. (**B**) Grade II MCL tear in a different patient with an accompanying tear of the medial meniscus. *Abbreviation*: MCL, medial collateral ligament.

to the medial meniscus; in fact in normal knees, the meniscocapsular separation should be no greater than 1 or 2 mm between the medial meniscus and the MCL seen on coronal views. If it is greater, then meniscocapsular separation has occurred (Fig. 13).

Tears of the MCL are classified into three clinical types orthopedically. The deeper fibers of the MCL are relatively weaker and are thus more frequently torn and are often associated with meniscocapsular separation and tears of the lateral meniscus. Tears of the deeper fibers may be partial or complete. The grading of MCL tears is as follows:

Grade I—fluid running inside and adjacent to the tendon.
Grade II—fluid running on both sides of the tendon with or without fraying of the tendon itself.
Grade III—complete tear with either an avulsion off its origin, a transverse midtendon tear, or an avulsion off its insertion into the tibia (Fig. 14).

Helpful hint:
For MCL tears, use the fat-suppressed coronal sequence.
The superficial layer is what really constitutes the MCL, and complete tears render the knee unstable. They

are usually "avulsion"-type injuries with the tear involving the ligament's origin or insertion. But if a major valgus injury occurs to the knee, complete tears of the central part of the MCL can occur not infrequently.

Lateral Collateral Ligament

The *anterior part of the lateral collateral ligament (LCL)* is in reality part of the patella retinaculum and will get dealt with in that section.

The *central part of the lateral collateral ligament* is really the iliotibial band or the tensor fascia lata and is made up of various tendons and ligaments running down from the hip. It inserts into the lateral part of the lateral tibial plateau. It is about 2 cm wide. Avulsion injuries of the iliotibial band from the outermost part of the lateral tibial plateau are known as *segond* fractures.

What the orthopedists now call the LCL is what I was taught was the femoral fibular ligament, which lies posteriorly and runs obliquely from the distal femur to insert on the head of the fibula adjacent to the insertion of the biceps femoris (Fig. 15).

Helpful hint:
Start on the most posterior slices of the T1 coronal sequence and identify the biceps femoris tendon and move anteriorly from there: biceps femoris, popliteus muscle and tendon, and LCL.

Under the femoral fibular ligament, but difficult to see on MRI, is a Y-shaped arcuate ligament, extending from the tip of the fibula proximally with one arm going obliquely and vertically across the back of the joint and the other arm going anteriorly and horizontally. This ligament holds the posterior horn of the lateral meniscus in place and forms the tunnel for the popliteus tendon. It is important to identify the various muscles and tendons on an MRI because damage to the posterolateral corner of the knee leads to profound instability of the knee joint. The popliteus muscle is important because it locks the knee so that we can stand (Figs. 16 and 17).

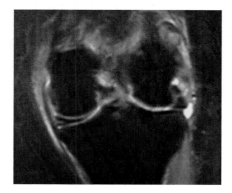

Figure 14 Complete grade III MCL tear. Note that the ligament has been pulled off its origin from the femoral condyle. *Abbreviation*: MCL, medial collateral ligament.

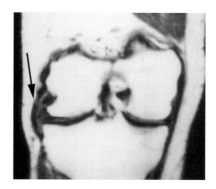

Figure 15 Normal femorofibular ligament (*arrow*).

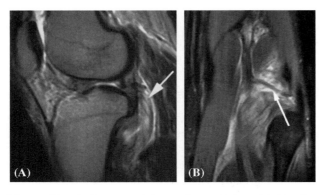

Figure 16 (**A, B**) Tear of the popliteus tendon with bleeding into its muscle belly (*arrows*).

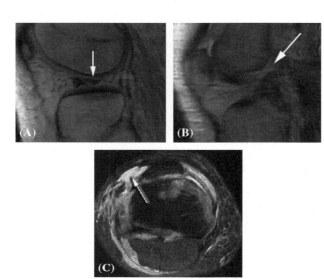

Figure 17 (**A**) Dislocation of the knee. Sagittal slice showing a bucket handle tear of the lateral meniscus (*arrow*). (**B**) Sagittal slice at another level showing complete avulsion of the ACL from its origin. (**C**) An axial cut shows extensive bleeding into the lateral aspect of the knee with tears of the lateral retinaculum (*arrow*) and blood surrounding the popliteus muscle. *Abbreviation*: ACL, anterior cruciate ligament.

Helpful hint:
Starting posteriorly, identify the (oblique) popliteus muscle running from the posterior medial aspect of the tibia to the lateral aspect of the knee joint itself. It is the only oblique muscle in this region. Then identify the LCL, which is usually seen on three consecutive cuts. If it appears on one single cut, then an ACL tear has occurred.

Patellofemoral Mechanism

This consists of the quadriceps tendon, which covers the superior surface of the patella and spreads out medially

and laterally to become the patellar retinaculum. It then reforms below the patella to become the patellar tendon inserting on the tibial tuberosity.

Remember Osgood-Schlatter's disease, which is an avulsion-type injury to the tibial tubercle in tall athletic adolescents and is best seen on sagittal slices.

Chondromalacia Patellae

Represents degenerative osteoarthritis of the patellar cartilage.

There are five grades of chondromalacia. Grades I and II cannot be seen radiographically. Grade III has some high signal within the cartilage itself and early irregularity of its surface. Grade IV shows increasing degenerative changes. Grade V is severe degenerative arthritis with marked loss of cartilage (Fig. 18).

Helpful hint:
Best sequence for patellar cartilage is a fat-saturated early T1 short-TE 3D spoiled gradient echo axial sequence.

Patellar Tendonitis (Jumper's Knee)

This presents as swelling and high signal just below the origin of the patellar tendon. It is due to chronic impingement of the lower pole of the patella on the tendon. It is best seen on sagittal sequences in patients with pointed lower patellae. Patellar tendonitis can occur elsewhere, for example, at the insertion of the tendon into the

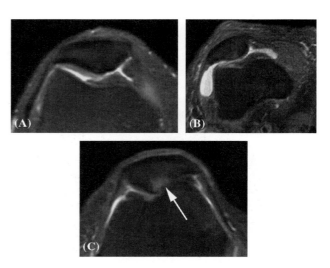

Figure 18 Chondromalacia patella—different stages. (**A**) Grade III. (**B**) Grade IV where most of the cartilage is missing. (**C**) Grade V with subchondral changes in the underlying patella (*arrow*) and complete loss of the articular cartilage.

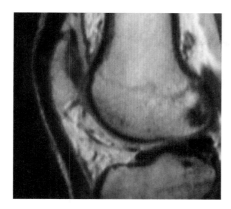

Figure 19 Jumper's knee: Note the high signal and thickening of the patellar tendon as it inserts into the tibial tubercle.

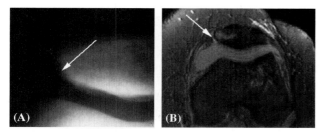

Figure 20 Dislocation of the patella. (**A**) Plain film. On the plain film, a small bony fragment can be seen lying laterally (*arrow*). (**B**) Axial T1 fat sat. In a different patient, on the MRI a tear of the retinaculum is obvious (*arrow*), but note the typical bone bruising on the lateral femoral condyle and medial side of the patella itself. *Abbreviation*: fat sat, fat saturation.

tibia with swelling of the tendon and increased signal (Fig. 19).

Patellar Dislocations

Look for bone bruising on the medial pole of the patella and the lateral aspect of the lateral femoral condyle. Look also for tears (usually avulsion injuries) of the medial retinaculum pulled off the patella (Fig. 20).

Tears of both the patellar tendon and quadriceps tendons can be seen in elderly patients with diabetes or who are receiving steroids or who are being treated with dialysis (Figs. 21 and 22).

Bursae and Cysts

Baker's cysts are well known to occur posteromedially and are associated with tears of the posterior horn of the medial meniscus and in patients with rheumatoid arthritis. Anatomically, we all have a bursa lying between the

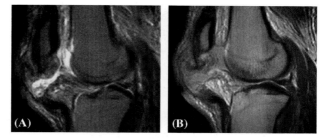

Figure 21 Complete tear of the patella tendon. (**A**) Sagittal delayed T2 view. (**B**) Sagittal proton density view.

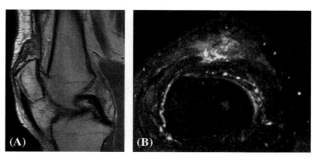

Figure 22 Almost complete tear of the quadriceps tendon. (**A**) On the sagittal proton density view, note the disruption of the vastus intermedius and rectus femorus tendons as they enter the patella. (**B**) This is confirmed by the disruption of the fibers and the high signal centrally. The vastus lateralis and vastus medialis are intact on the axial fat sat view. *Abbreviation*: fat sat, fat saturation.

insertion of the semimembranosis tendon and the origin of the medial head of the gastrocnemius. In fact, it remains connected to the knee joint until the age of two, it then closes off only to reopen if the patient develops a rapid onset effusion (Fig. 23).

Helpful hint:
If you find a Baker's cyst, look for a tear of the posterior horn of the medial meniscus.

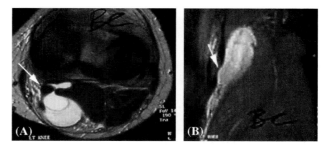

Figure 23 Typical Baker's cyst lying posteriorly between the semimembranosus tendon (*arrow*) and the medial head of the gastrocnemius. (**A**) Axial slice. (**B**) Four coronal slices.

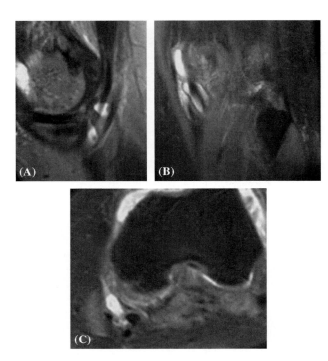

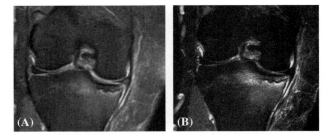

Figure 25 Osteochondral fracture in an elderly female patient. (**A**) Delayed T2 coronal. The fracture line is of low intensity on both sequences and parallels the medial tibial condyle. It is surrounded by high-signal bone bruising. Note that the patient has grade II changes in the medial meniscus and a grade II tear of the adjacent MCL. (**B**) T1 fat sat coronal. *Abbreviations*: fat sat, fat saturation; MCL, medial collateral ligament.

Figure 24 Pes anserinus bursitis. (**A**) Proton density sagittal slice. All of the images in this sequence show the semitendonous tendon surrounded by fluid in the posterior, medial side of the knee. (**B**) Delayed T2 coronal slice. (**C**) Axial T1 fat sat. *Abbreviation*: fat sat, fat saturation.

However, it is said that we have 19 potential bursae around the knee joint of which the most common are:

1. posteromedially on the femur adjacent to the insertion of the adductor magnus;
2. posterolaterally adjacent and below the proximal tibiofibular joint;
3. adjacent to the insertion of the semitendinosis muscle, anteromedially in an area known as the "pes anserinus" where the tendons of the gracilis, sartorius, and semitendinosis combine (Fig. 24); and
4. ganglion cysts that can occur adjacent to and deforming either the ACL or the PCL.

Any of these bursae can fill with fluid and become a ganglion cyst, which may be of unknown etiology, posttraumatic, or post-inflammation. Subchondral cysts also can occur in the bone, usually the tibia, following direct trauma or partial avulsion at the insertion of either the PCL or the ACL.

Meniscal cysts can occasionally be seen in association with tears of the menisci associated with meniscocapsular separation, thus allowing joint fluid through the meniscal tear into the soft tissues. These classically occur medially and anteriorly where the retinaculum is relatively thin (Fig. 15).

Bone Bruises and Osteochondral Fractures

Bone bruises signify direct trauma to the bone, appear within 48 hours of the blow, and may persist up to six months. A bone bruise represents bleeding into the trabecular bone with microfractures. Classically, bone bruises of the lateral aspect of the lateral femoral condyle and of the posterior aspect of the tibia accompany acute ACL tears (Fig. 9).

Osteochondral fractures occur because a greater force has been applied to the bone, and these represent a true fracture through both the bone and the articular cartilage and can result in damage to the cartilage with a step-off, flattening of its contour or, more importantly, a loose body, and ultimately premature degenerative arthritis (Fig. 25).

Helpful hint:
If you see a bone bruise, look locally for damage to surrounding structures, i.e., meniscus tear or collateral ligament damage. However, the commonest situation with bone bruising is in association with degenerative arthritis (Fig. 26).

Osteochondritis Dissecans

This condition is of unknown etiology and occurs probably as either a developmental or posttraumatic event. It classically involves the lateral aspect of the medial femoral condyle (LAME) but may be seen anywhere in the knee.

The articular cartilage may be intact in which case the underlying bone heals. Or it may be fractured, and then the bone does not heal and remains as fragments, leading to loose body formation.

Helpful hint:
If you find either osteochondritis dissecans or an osteochondral fracture, look at the articular cartilage to see if it is intact or not. If not, look for loose bodies.

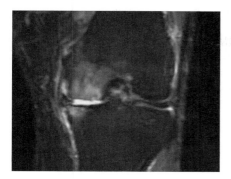

Figure 26 Bone bruising in a patient with severe DJD in the medial compartment of his left knee with complete loss of the articular cartilage, a degenerative tear in the medial meniscus, and bone bruises in both the femoral condyle and the proximal medial tibia secondary to eburnation. *Abbreviation*: DJD, degenerative joint disease.

MRI OF THE SHOULDER

I believe that the shoulder is the most difficult joint to interpret on MRI, and this is mainly due to the anatomy of the rotator cuff. There are four muscles and tendons–three of which are major movers of the shoulder. The *subscapularis* is in front of the scapula under the coracoid process and is basically vertically oriented. It inserts into the lesser tuberosity. The *supraspinatus* lies over the spine of the scapula and is horizontal. The *infraspinatus* starts vertically but moves up and over the humeral head to insert horizontally and obliquely. Both of these tendons insert into the greater tuberosity. The *teres minor* runs vertically and inserts into the proximal humeral metaphysis below the greater tuberosity posteriorly. Where the first three of these insert into the humeral head, there is a virtually continuous "rotator cuff", but there are three spaces: (*i*) The *rotator interval* for the biceps tendon lies in the intertuberous notch between the subscapularis "in front" and the supraspinatus above and behind. (*ii*) The quadrilateral space (which is not square!) lies between the coracoid process, the subscapularis tendon, the supraspinatus tendon, and the combined insertion of these two tendons into the humeral head. (*iii*). The *bare area* lies between the insertion of the supraspinatus and infraspinatus as the tendons come together to merge onto the greater tuberosity of the humerus and is variable in size and may in fact be absent.

Because the scapular is oriented roughly 45° to the coronal (or sagittal) plane, sequences for shoulder MRI are axial, 45° coronal, and 45 degrees sagittal, which are usually called paracoronal and parasagittal but may be known as oblique coronal and oblique sagittal. The technician should orient the sequences on the basis of the alignment of the scapula on an axial scout film with the understanding that the paracoronal and parasagittal sequences should be 90° apart in orientation (Fig. 27).

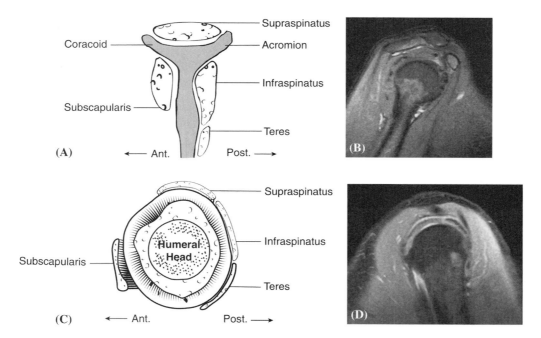

Figure 27 Parasagittal slices showing the configuration of the four components of the rotator cuff. (**A**) Drawing. (**B**) MRI of a central parasagittal slice. (**C**) Drawing of a peripheral parasagittal slice. (**D**) MRI of a peripheral parasagittal slice. *Abbreviation*: MRI, magnetic resonance imaging.

Helpful hint:

If you are not able to orient yourself on the sagittals, the blade of the scapula lies obliquely running from the coracoid process superiorly down to the blade posteriorly at approximate an angle of 50° tilted forward because of the rib cage.

Suggestion sequences are as follows:

1. Axial proton density
2. Axial fat saturation (or special sequence for articular cartilage)
3. Coronal proton density
4. Coronal delayed T2
5. Coronal fat saturation T2 (or inversion recovery)
6. Sagittal proton density
7. Sagittal delayed T2 (or inversion recovery sequence for fluid)

Many people have different methods of looking at shoulder MRIs, but certainly a sensible approach would be to peruse a sagittal sequence to look at the four individual muscles and to follow their tendons onto their insertion into the humeral head. However, with respect to rotator cuff pathology, the money shots are paracoronal sequences: start at the front and move back: subscapularis, supraspinatus, infraspinatus, and teres minor.

Subscapularis Muscle and Tendon

This runs continuously from its origin into its insertion into the lesser tuberosity. The muscle usually ends in four to six separate tendons before becoming part of the rotator cuff. The biceps tendon can be seen running vertically in the intertuberous notch just lateral to the insertion of the subscapularis and below the insertion of the supraspinatus. Question to be asked: Is there any high signal on the fat saturation sequences either in the muscle or in the tendon? If there is high signal in the tendon itself, it probably represents "tendonosis" (chronic) or tendonitis (acute) (Fig. 28).

Is the tendon closely adherent to the undersurface of the coracoid process and scapula? If not, is there fluid between the two (check the sagittal sequences)? If there is fluid between the subscapularis and the scapula, it probably represents a joint effusion. However, if the fluid runs up over and in front of the tendon, this almost certainly represents a grade I tear (or worst). Note that there is a separate subcoracoid bursa, which does not connect to the shoulder joint in normal circumstances and may contain fluid (i.e., bursitis). If it does connect to the joint, then this represents at least a grade I tear.

Grading system of tears of the subscapularis muscle and tendon is as follows:

Grade I: upper fibers only, involving no more than one-third of vertical height of the entire tendon/muscle.

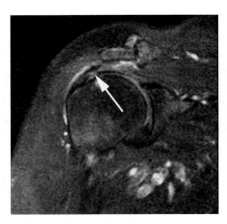

Figure 28 Paracoronal slice showing tendonosis in the supraspinatus tendon with a small undersurface tear (*arrow*).

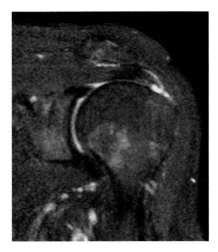

Figure 29 Discrete tear at the insertion of the supraspinatus tendon into the humeral head.

Grade II: involving upper and mid but no more than two-thirds of the tendon (Fig. 29).
Grade III: Complete tears, which are mainly at the musculotendinous junction or of the tendon itself at its insertion (avulsion injury) (Fig. 30).

The Supraspinatus Muscle and Tendon

On the parasagittal sequences, this muscle belly lies in between the coracoid process anteriorly and the "spine" of the acromion posteriorly and under the distal clavicle and acromioclavicular joint. It runs horizontally paralleling the line of the blade of the scapula. Before turning into the anterior superior part of the rotator cuff, the supraspinatus forms into two main tendon complexes. The most vulnerable parts of the supraspinatus are (*i*) at the musculotendinous

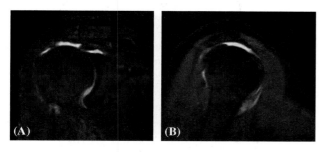

Figure 30 Complete tears of both the supraspinatus and infraspinatus tendons with marked retraction of the tendons and atrophy of the muscle bundles. (**A**) Paracoronal T2 fat sat. (**B**) Parasagittal peripheral slice to see the narrowing of the space between the undersurface of the acromion and the humeral head signifying a complete tear of both the supraspinatus and the infraspinatus tendons. *Abbreviation*: fat sat, fat saturation.

junction, which lies below the distal clavicle and somewhat medial to the acromioclaviclar joint and (*ii*) its insertion into the greater tuberosity where most of the full thickness tears occur.

The Infraspinatus Muscle and Tendon

This is probably the most difficult part of the rotator cuff to follow since it starts as a vertical muscle under the spine of the acromion, hence "infraspinatus." As it emerges laterally, it starts turning anteriorly and finally inserts into the superior posterior part of the greater tuberosity with the final anterior part of the tendon running horizontally conjoined to the supraspinatus tendon. The posterior aspect of the tendon inserts obliquely into the posterior aspect of the greater tuberosity. Tears of the infraspinatus tendon are similar to those of the supraspinatus (Fig. 31).

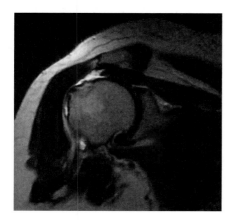

Figure 31 Complete tear of the infraspinatus tendon with retraction.

The Teres Minor Muscle and Tendon

This is a minor part of the rotator cuff (as the name implies) and starts medially as the inferior component of the combined intraspinatus muscle belly to separate from the latter when it starts shifting course. The teres minor continues to run horizontally and inserts into the proximal humeral metaphysis posteriorly where it becomes the lower posterior part of the rotator cuff.

The Glenoid Labrum

This should be easy, but is not. First, the labrum is triangular in shape and surrounds as well as is attached to the glenoid articular cartilage. Second, its superior and anterior aspects are larger than the inferior ones that are more inclined to be either globular (in its inferior and posterior aspects) or smaller. The labrum is fibrocartilage (dark signal on all sequences) and inserts onto the hyaline articular cartilage (which is high signal on all sequences), and so it often appears that there is a separation of the labrum from the underlying bone when it is not there (Fig. 32).

To make matters worst, 75% of us have a normal rounded defect in our superior labrum (called the sublabral foramen or sulcus), which can also look like a tear. However, most tears are either linear or oblique, or degenerative with fragmentation, so it is usually relatively easy to tell them apart from various congenital anomalies of which there are many. I will only mention one more: In the Buford complex, the anterior superior one-quarter of the labrum is missing completely. This occurs in 2% of the population and is always associated with thickening of the middle glenoid ligament. Tears can either be easy or impossible to see (Figs. 33–35).

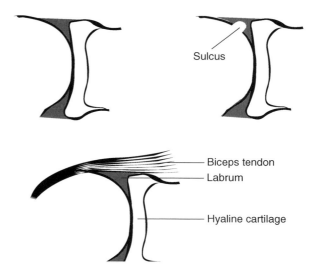

Figure 32 Line drawing of labral insertions.

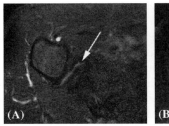
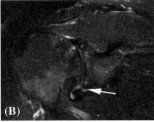

Figure 33 Labral tears. (**A**) Axial slice showing an inferior labral tear in a patient with severe DJD (*arrow*). (**B**) Paracoronal slice in the same patient showing the tear (*arrow*). *Abbreviation*: DJD, degenerative joint disease.

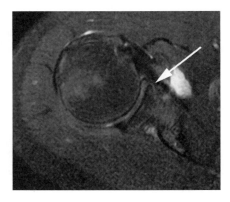

Figure 34 Discrete tear in the anterior labrium (*arrow*).

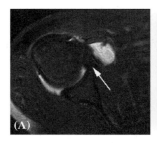
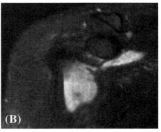

Figure 35 Large tear with a fluid collection anteriorly. (**A**) Axial slice (*arrow*). (**B**) Anterior paracornal slice showing a large fluid collection.

The Biceps Tendon

This originates from the upper surface of the glenoid just above the labrum and runs horizontally and obliquely through the joint until it turns vertically to exit via the intertuberous notch between the lesser tuberosity and greater tuberosity. The tendon should be black on all sequences.

The Glenohumeral Ligaments

Everyone makes a big deal about these. Don't! (*i*). The superior glenohumeral ligament (GHL) represents a thickening of the superior capsule of the joint running under the supraspinatus tendon and merging into it at its insertion. It originates above and behind the biceps tendon, which, in turn, runs above the superior glenoid labrum. (*ii*) The middle GHL runs anteriorly and horizontally from in front of the glenoid labrum starting just above the equator of the joint (i.e., the middle part of the glenohumeral joint) and runs horizontally into the humeral head. It is usually separate from the labrum but sometimes appears to merge with it. This is the only one of the glenohumeral ligaments, which is easy to find on an MRI. (*iii*) The inferior GHL is simply a thickening of the inferior capsule of the joint.

S.L.A.P. Lesions

Articles have been written about these, and over nine different types have been described, but the simplest and most useful classification has only four types. S.L.A.P (superior labral anterior posterior) injuries occur when the humeral head is driven upward and obliquely into the shoulder socket. The significant S.L.A.P. lesions mainly occur in young people (younger than 40 years) and are often associated with bone bruises in the humeral head, superior aspect of the glenoid, distal clavicle, and acromion (type II).

Type I: fraying of the superior labrum and occurs commonly in older people (74%).

Type II: the most common and consists of separation of the biceps labral complex from the glenoid rim from nine o'clock (posteriorly) to three o'clock (anteriorly) (21%).

Type III: A bucket handle tear of the superior glenoid labrum. This has only been seen in a very few patients (1%).

Type IV: An extension of this tear into the long head of the biceps tendon. This is also very rare (4%).

Alphabet soup: There are a lot of other acronyms related to the shoulder—basically forget them all. You can look them up in a textbook. Oh, all right!

ALPSA—anterior ligamentous periosteal sleeve avulsions—seem best on sagittal views with separation of the subscapularis from the scapula.

GLAD—glenoid labral articular disruption—often seen in association with a bony Bankart lesion.

HAGL—humeral avulsion of glenohumeral ligament.

Other eponyms of importance:

Hill-sachs deformity—is an impacted fracture of the posterior lateral aspect of the humeral head usually following a (recurrent) anterior shoulder dislocation.

Bankart lesion—is a tear of the anterior-inferior glenoid labrum usually as a result of an anterior shoulder dislocation. This may or may not be seen with a fracture on plain films and is then known as a bony Bankart lesion.

Other things to look for are as follows:

Osteochondritis dissecans—occurs in either the glenoid or in the humeral head and looks like osteochondritis dissecans in the knee.

Acromioclavicular joint changes—someone named Griffiths wrote the definitive article! The *only* significant MR changes of acromioclavicular joint disease are high signal in the acromion, fluid in the joint, and/or high signal in the distal clavicle. But remember that we have trouble differentiating degenerative joint disease, posttraumatic osteolysis and rheumatoid arthritis without plain films.

Ganglion cysts—occur anywhere around the shoulder but more especially look in the suprascapular notch where a ganglion cyst may compress the suprascapular nerve, causing atrophy of either the deltoid or the infraspinatus muscle.

For the rest of this chapter, the reader is referred to other sections of the book to see examples of all the conditions that are mentioned.

MRI OF THE PELVIS AND HIPS

Coronal and axial, proton density, T2 , and fat saturation sequences are all you will need unless you are assessing the soft tissues of the pelvis when sagittal slices can be useful. The majority of pelvic and hip MRIs are done to look for either a fracture or avascular necrosis although soft tissue injury such as muscle tears and hematomas are also fairly common indications.

For the pelvis, I start with the coronal slices and go through from the symphysis pubis to the sacrum. Look for signal abnormalities in the bone marrow, soft tissue abnormalities, and for avascular necrosis in the femoral heads. Also look at the acetabular labrum, which, like the glenoid labrum, may be torn or subluxed. On the axial slices, look for the same things although much of the musculature is easier to see on the axial slices than on the coronal slices. Also look at the sacrum and coccyx and lower abdominal musculature such as the psoas muscles. These are easier to evaluate on the coronal and sagittal slices. Remember that both soft tissue and bony tumors occur in the lower abdomen and pelvis. Sacral tumors also occur, and the two commonest of these include chordoma and chondrosarcomas.

MRI OF THE ANKLE

MRI of the ankle is fairly straightforward. Start from the lateral aspect where the first thing one sees is the fibula. Note that this lies behind the plane of the medial malleolus.

Behind the fibula, lie the two peroneal tendons. They often begin as a conjoined tendon in the lower leg and then split into two distinct tendons as they turn around the tip of the fibular and run into the foot. The peroneus brevis tendon inserts into the base of the fifth metatarsal where an avulsion injury leads to a Jones fracture. The peroneus longus tendon inserts into the metatarsal heads. Note that 20% of the population has an accessory peroneus muscle, and this can be seen lying between the two normally occurring peroneal muscles just anterior to the Achilles tendon.

Next we come to the calcaneus. Assess for bone marrow signal as well as the general shape of the bone. The Achilles tendon is inserted into the superior posterior aspect. Look at its width and see if there is any high signal within the tendon itself to suggest either a tear or tendinosis. Look at the plantar fascia and make sure that it is neither thickened nor disrupted. The next bone is the talus—again look at the bone marrow signal and the bones overall shape. Remember to look for osteochondritis dissecans of the talar domes. The talus has a posterior process, which may become detached in adolescence when it becomes known as the os trigonum—more of which will be discussed later. Directly behind this runs the tendon of the Hallucis longus ("Harry" of Tom, Dick, and Harry fame). Obviously, this tendon may become involved in any trauma that occurs in this region.

Anterior to the calcaneus lies the cuboid and anterior to the talus lies the navicula and then the cuneiforms. Once again, assess the bone marrow signal as well as the alignment of the bones and their relationship with each other. Remember that early neuropathic changes in a diabetic foot are often signaled by a collapse of the midfoot with relationship to the hind foot and forefoot. Anatomically, there is a small groove on the undersurface of the talus, which is known as the tarsal tunnel and contains an artery, a vein, and a nerve. Note should also be made of the distal tibia and the subtalar joints at this point in your overall survey.

On the medial side of the foot is the medial malleolus with the two other major tendons running behind it and around it. These are the posterior tibial tendon in front with the digitorum longus tendon running behind ("Tom" and "Dick" of Tom, Dick, and Harry fame).

Now we will turn to the coronal slices starting posteriorly. But remember what is axial in the foot is coronal in the ankle and vice versa. The coronal ankle slices show the Achilles tendon posteriorly: Look at its insertion into the calcaneus. The ankle mortise consists of the distal fibula, distal tibial plafond, and medial malleolus with the talus, lying inside like a carpenter's mortise joint. Look at the talar domes to make sure the patient does not have osteochondritis dissecans. The medial and lateral collateral ligaments of the ankle are complex. Laterally, there are individual fibulotalar and fibulocalcaneal ligaments as well as a generalized ankle retinaculum. Medially, we have the deltoid ligament, which consists of three main parts: The posterior part is oblique and difficult to see on an MRI: The middle part is the classical "deltoid ligament" as we know it with deep and superficial portions. The deep portion goes from the medial malleolus to the medial aspect of the talus, and the superficial portion, which is much the stronger of the two goes to the calcaneus and mainly to the sustentaculum tali. This is by far the strongest medial ligament. The anterior portion of the deltoid ligament is also oblique, running round from the medial malleolus to the anterior aspect of the talus primarily. Continue going through the coronal slices moving anteriorly. Remember that navicular stress fractures are nearly all in the sagittal plane and thus not easy to see on the sagittal views.

On the axial slices (of the ankle), start above the joint. Follow the Achilles tendon into its insertion: It should be basically curved with its convex surface posteriorly. Then follows the two peroneal tendons from behind the fibular and around into the foot. Usually, the peroneus brevis is easy to follow to its insertion into the base of the fifth metatarsal, but the peroneus longus gets lost under the metatarsal heads. Then follow the hallucis longus tendon around the posterior aspect of the talus and into the foot. Similarly, follow the tendons of the posterior tibialis and digitorum longus into the foot. The tendons should be black and contain no high signal, and they should not be surrounded by any fluid. These five tendons, like most tendons in the body, are surrounded by tenosynovium, and when inflammation occurs, this gets filled with fluid, leading to tenosynovitis. Remember the one major tendon in the body, which does not have a tenosynovium is the Achilles tendon.

Finally on the axial views, there are small anterior and posterior tibiofibular ligaments supporting the distal tibia—fibular syndesmosis. These should be easy to see on an MRI. Also look at the tarsal bones and confirm that there are no stress fractures, particularly of the navicular and the metatarsal necks.

Diseases and conditions to be looked for and which are discussed elsewhere in this book include osteochondritis dissecans, fractures of the calcaneus, talus, and navicular, ligamentous tears, tenosynovitis, infections, os trigonum syndrome, and various bony and soft tissue tumors.

MRI OF THE FOOT

Similar to the ankle, use sagittal, coronal, and axial slices. Take proton density and T1 fat saturation sequences and run through the anatomy. In the *foot,* we are mostly

looking for infection or tenosynovitis and so sagittal fat saturation sequences are the best. It is easiest to have the sagittal images on one monitor and axial images on the other so that the identification of the correct toe and metatarsal may be made. Remember that most of us only have sesamoid bones under our first metatarsophangeal joint, which makes this easy to identify.

Diseases and conditions to look for include infection (both cellulitis and osteomyelitis), tenosynovitis, sesamoiditis, discrete fractures, and tumors such as Morton's neuroma (usually lying between and below the third and fourth metatarsal heads).

MRI OF THE ELBOW, WRIST, AND HAND

Once again you need coronal, sagittal, and axial sequences for all of these joints. Proton density and fat saturation T1 sequences are useful in all the three plains. In the *elbow,*

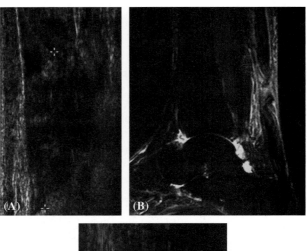
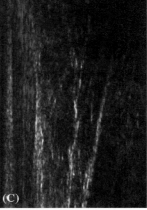

Figure 36 Achilles tendon tear. (**A**) Gap delineated by crosshairs. (**B**) MRI demonstrates tendon gap with irregular contour and abnormal signal of torn and retracted tendon margins. (**C**) Normal contralateral Achilles tendon for comparison.

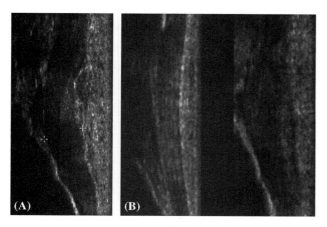

Figure 37 (A) Torn patellar tendon. (B) Normal right versus torn left patellar tendon. The left side is on the left.

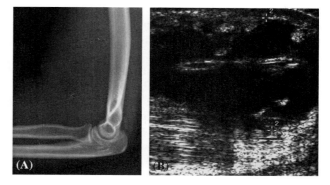

Figure 39 (A) Radiograph of the anticubital fossa in a patient with an abscess demonstrated on ultrasound. (B) Complex hypoechoic mass in antecubital fossa representing an abscess.

an additional delayed T2 sagittal sequence is useful to look for loose bodies and Panner's disease. The radial collateral ligament (RCL) is easy to see since it runs vertically down from the humerus to the radius, but the ulnar collateral ligament (UCL) is Y shaped and so it often looks as though there is a tear off its origin. One should just page through the coronal slices to follow its normal course. In the elbow, diseases to look for include Panner's disease of the capitellum with or without loose bodies, tears of either the RCL or UCL, various forms of arthritis, and tears of the insertion of the biceps tendon, which can be partial or complete when there is retraction of the muscle and tendon itself.

In the wrist, an additional very early T1 sequence can be useful for looking for tears of the triangular fibrocartilage (TFC). The TFC runs between the ulnar styloid process where it has two main points of origin and the distal radius. It is attached to the hyaline cartilage of the ulnar aspect of the distal radioulnar joint. The TFC is fibrous tissue and is of low signal on all sequences. The hyaline cartilage is of high or medium signal, and hence to the unwary, it appears that everyone has a tear of the insertion of the TFC into the radius. So be warned.

In the wrist and hand, look for tears of the TFC, avascular necrosis of the lunate (Kienbock's disease), ganglion cysts, evidence of early erosive arthritis (particularly early rheumatoid arthritis), conditions involving the carpal tunnel, tenosynovitis and such rarities as amyloidosis of the carpal tunnel, which can be seen in long-term dialysis patients.

MUSCULOSKELETAL ULTRASOUND

Lori Deitte M.D.

Musculoskeletal ultrasound imaging has been increasing in frequency and popularity over the past decade. Because of their superficial location, tendons of extremities are particularly amenable to sonographic assessment with a linear array high frequency (7–15 MHz) transducer. Normal tendons are echogenic in appearance and display a fibrillar echotexture with longitudinally oriented parallel lines corresponding to interfaces between collagen bundles and endotendineum septa (1). Tendon pathology such as a tear often results in the demonstration of discontinuity of fibers with an adjacent hematoma on ultrasound imaging. When evaluating tendon disorders, it is helpful to

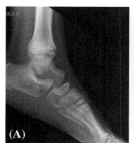
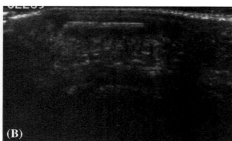
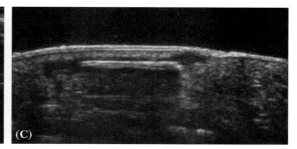

Figure 38 (A) Normal foot radiograph. (B) Echogenic splinter on ultrasound. (C) Echogenic splinter demonstrated on scanning with a standoff pad.

perform comparative imaging of the normal contralateral tendon. Examples of tendon pathology include an Achilles tendon tear with MRI correlation and a patellar tendon tear (Figs. 36 and 37).

Ultrasound is also a useful imaging modality for assessing extremity soft tissue abnormalities in the emergency room patient, including retained foreign bodies and abscesses. Although nonradiopaque foreign bodies such as splinters cannot be detected on plain radiographs, they are often visible on ultrasound imaging, typically appearing hyperechoic with varying degrees of shadowing and adjacent inflammatory changes (Fig. 38).

Soft tissue abscesses demonstrate a similar sonographic appearance to abscesses elsewhere, hypoechoic and complex (Fig. 39).

REFERENCE

1. Martinoloi C, Derchi LE, Pastorino C, et al. Analysis of echotexture of tendons with US. Radiology 1993; 186: 839–843.

9

Lumbar Spine

INTRODUCTION

It may be unusual to have a specific chapter on the lumbar spine in a musculoskeletal textbook, particularly since infections, arthritis, tumors, and trauma to the spine are covered in their respective chapters. However, there are some unique conditions that involve the lumbosacral spine, which do not fit under the normal chapter headings. These conditions include spondylolysis, spondylolisthesis, Schmorl's nodes, anterior disc herniation, and Scheuermann's disease. I also thought that I would include a brief discussion on degenerative disc disease, disc herniation, and spinal stenosis as well.

SPONDYLOLYSIS

The importance of spondylolysis and its relationship to low back pain is still improperly understood. The word "spondylolysis" comes from the Greek "spondylo" (vertebra) and "lysis" (coming apart, referring to a break in the pars interarticularis), and since it occurs in about 5% of the normal white male population, spondylolysis is not an uncommon finding. As far as we know, it was first described in 1743 by Andry, but it was Neugebaur, in 1895, who could be described as the father of clinical spondylolysis.

Etiology

The reported incidence of spondylolysis in the adult population varies considerably. Roche and Rowe (1) looked at 4200 skeletons and found spondylolysis in 6.4% of white men, 2.3% of white women, 2.8% of black men, and 1.1% of black women.

An overall incidence rate of 5% to 6% in the adult male white population is a reasonably accepted number. On the other hand, there are specific subgroups of patients with a much higher incidence of spondylolysis, such as gymnasts, active athletes, and certain Eskimo populations. Some of the original work on gymnasts was done in Edinburgh in 1953. A group of active gymnasts was followed for over 30 years. There was a 5% incidence of spondylolysis at age six; however, by the age of 30 the incidence of pars defects in this same group had increased to 17%, and of those people who continued their gymnastics until the age of 40, no less than 34% had spondylolysis. These authors postulated that it was the repetitive hyperextension and hyperflexion as well as the increased vertical stress loading that led to the increased incidence of spondylolysis. They also noted that although spina bifida occurs in approximately 5% of normal people, it was present in over 30% of the gymnasts.

Rossi (2) reported a 50% incidence of spondylolysis in the Italian Olympic gymnastic team, as well as an increased incidence of spondylolysis in many members of other Olympic athletic teams and found that apart from gymnastics, skiing, hurdling, and the combination of multiple sports seem to lead to a higher incidence of spondylolysis.

The increased incidence of spondylolysis in the Eskimo population has been discussed in detail by Wiltse and others (3). Apparently, some of the isolated Eskimo communities have a nearly 60% incidence of spondy-lolysis, but even the more civilized tribes have an incidence of 20% or over. The reasons for this finding are not fully understood but probably a combination of hereditary factors and forced hyperextension due to squatting over ice fishing holes are both responsible.

Of equal interest is the fact that there are almost no reports of spondylolysis occurring in utero or under the age of four. In fact, in reviewing the world literature over the years, there have been fewer than 10 reported cases of children under the age of five with isolated spondylolysis. However, by the first grade, Wiltse (3) found a 5% incidence of spondylolysis and by the second grade a 6% incidence.

Thus, although there are undoubtedly hereditary factors involved in the etiology of spondylolysis, no true congenital cases have been described. The hereditary factors involved include a hypoplastic pars, often associated with other anatomic variations that will be discussed later.

The main etiologic factor involved in the formation of spondylolysis is a fatigue or stress fracture presumably due to repetitive minor trauma, although of course a single incident of real trauma can also produce a true fracture of the pars interarticularis (Fig. 1).

It is very rare to see any callus, although occasionally cases of spontaneous healing of spondylolysis have been described (Fig. 2).

Spondylolysis tends to persist rather than to heal. The nature of the chronic stress that occurs in gymnasts and

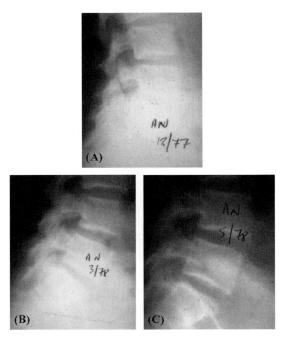

Figure 2 Healing of spondylolysis. (**A**) Lateral film taken in December 1977, showing a typical spondylolysis posteriorly at L3. (**B**) Film taken in March 1978, showing healing. (**C**) Film taken in May 1978, showing that the spondylolysis has completely healed.

other athletes, in heavy workers, and possibly in certain Eskimo populations is mechanical hyperextension, which when associated with a rotational force, produces a maximum shear stress at the L5 level. If this occurs in a patient with an already congenitally hypoplastic pars, then spondylolysis will probably be inevitable.

Finally, a number of interrelationships between other spinal anomalies and spondylolysis have been described, particularly between spondylolysis and spondylolisthesis. Various authors have found a 25% incidence of spondylolysis in patients with spondylolisthesis. Similarly, an incidence of 35% of both spondylolysis and spondylolisthesis has been described in patients with scoliosis. More recently, Ogilvie and Sherman (4) found a 50% incidence of asymptomatic spondylolysis in a group of 18 patients with Scheuermann's disease with increased lumbar lordosis. These authors proposed that the shear forces on the pars interarticularis increase as the lordosis increases, and hence hyperlordosis is associated with an increased incidence of spondylolysis.

Thus, it can be seen that a number of interesting facts have emerged about spondylolysis: It appears that it is not congenital in origin but rather is associated with an inherited predisposition to a hypoplastic pars through which a fatigue fracture occurs either due to minor repetitive stress or more forceful stresses, such as are encountered by athletes, which leads to spondylolysis.

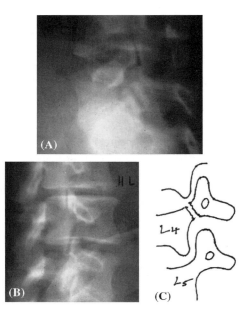

Figure 1 Two examples of spondylolysis. (**A**) Classical break in the Scotty dogs neck at L4 on the left with clear-cut sclerotic margins. (**B**) Wide spondylolysis at L4 on the left in a different patient. (**C**) Scotty dog with spondylolysis L4 and intact L5.

Symptoms Associated with Spondylolysis

Approximately 5% of the population experience significant back pain at some stage in their lives and 5% of the population have either spondylolysis or spondylolisthesis. However, only about 2% to 3% of patients with spondylolysis experience lower back pain. The most common causes of lower back pain are associated with degenerative disc disease and facet joint arthrosis.

Radiographic Diagnosis of Spondylolysis

Classically, the diagnosis of a pars defect depends on good oblique views of the lumbar spine. These are normally angled at 45° and should show virtually 100% of pars defects at L4, but often defects at the L5/S1 junction are more difficult to see even on adequate oblique views (Fig. 3).

In a recent Australian review article, Pierce (5) reported on the sensitivity of the various radiographic projections. As can be expected, the anteroposterior (AP) view was worst with a 32% sensitivity, the lateral view had a 75% sensitivity, and the oblique view had a 77% sensitivity, but a coned-down L5/S1 lateral view had an 84% sensitivity. I agree with these results and often find that the coned-down lateral view will confirm my suspicions of a true spondylolysis at L5/S1 if the oblique views are equivocal (Fig. 4).

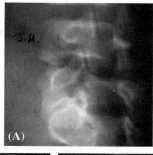
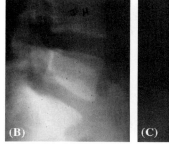
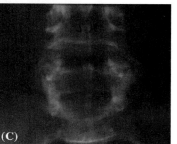

Figure 4 An example of spondylolysis at L4. (**A**) An oblique view. (**B**) A lateral view. (**C**) An AP view. Note that the spondylolysis is easy to see on Figures A and B but much more difficult on Figure C. *Abbreviation*: AP, anteroposterior.

Single photon emission computed tomography (SPECT) produces better and more focused images than ordinary bone scanning. Collier et al. (6) performed SPECT bone scans of the lower lumbar region of 19 patients. Six patients were normal with no low back pain but had a spondylolysis radiographically. In the rest of the group, SPECT was positive, implying that the spondylolysis was recent and presumably due to either a stress fracture or a true fracture through the pars and thus suggesting that the patient should be treated (Fig. 5).

Finally, the use of magnetic resonance imaging (MRI) has been advocated by a number of authors. The pars defect is best seen using sagittal views on the proton density T2 sequences or with a gradient-echo protocol. A defect is shown as an intermediate signal running perpendicularly to the facet joint (Fig. 6).

However, MRI only poorly showed bone fragments but was helpful in diagnosing other things, such as disc herniation, nerve root encroachment, and spondylolisthesis.

Spondylolysis at Other Levels

Although it is not infrequent to find spondylolysis in association with various congenital anomalies, such as a block vertebra, meningomyelocele, and spinal dysraphism, isolated spondylolysis has also been described throughout the length of the spine at all levels. Fewer

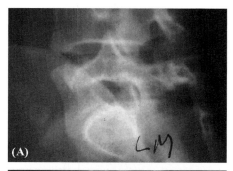
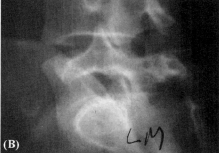

Figure 3 Patient with dysplastic pars bilaterally at L4. (**A**) A lysis on the left probably post-traumatic in origin. (**B**) A healing fracture on the right with callus formation.

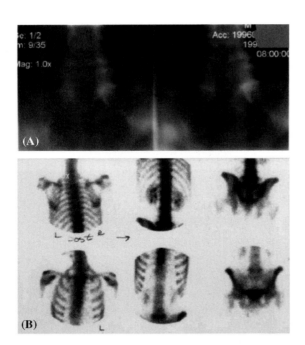

Figure 5 The use of a bone scan in spondylolysis. (**A**) On a tomogram, sclerosis is noted of the pars at L5 bilaterally. (**B**) A bone scan shows bilateral increase uptake of radionucleotide at L5.

than 30 cases of lower cervical pars defects have been described in the literature. I have recently seen two cases in the cervical region.

One of these patients (a 16-year-old adolescent) was incidentally found to have a C7 pars defect following an automobile accident, and the other was a 32-year-old man with no history of trauma who had a spina bifida, a hypoplastic lamina, and a pars defect at C6 that was thought to be congenital in origin (Fig. 7).

SPONDYLOLISTHESIS

The word "spondylolisthesis" comes from the Greek "spond" (spine) and "olisthesis" (to slip) and refers to the slippage of one vertebral body anteriorly on the one below. The term "retrolisthesis" has been used for the reverse situation, with the vertebral body above slipping posteriorly on the one below, but I do not like this term and use spondylolisthesis for all types of vertebral slips. Spondylolisthesis was first described by Herbiniaux in Belgium in 1782, but it was not until 1854 that Kilian discussed spondylolisthesis in any detail. It only occurs in humans and is presumably related in some way to our upright posture. The incidence of spondylolisthesis in the

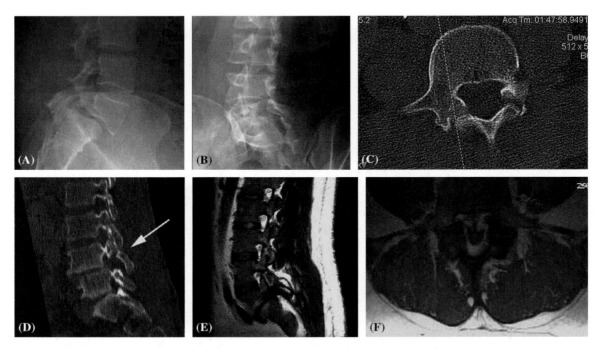

Figure 6 Spondylolysis (**A**) Shown in two different patients. First patient: lateral lumbar spine showing bilateral spondylolysis at L5-S1 with grade 2 spondylolisthesis. (**B**) Oblique view showing the spondylolysis on the right. (**C**) CT scan: axial cut showing spondylolysis bilaterally. (**D**) CT scan: sagittal reconstruction showing the spondylolysis on the left (*arrow*) at L4. (**E**) Second patient: Sagittal MR showing spondylolysis at both L4 and L5 with grade 2 spondylolisthesis. (**F**) Axial MR scan: showing how difficult the diagnosis can be. *Abbreviations*: CT, computed tomography; MR, magnetic resonance.

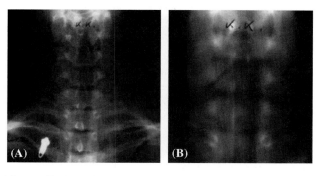

Figure 7 Spondylolysis at C7. (**A**) This was an incidental finding in a young patient following a motor vehicle accident. Plain film. (**B**) This was an incidental finding in a young patient following a motor vehicle accident. Tomogram.

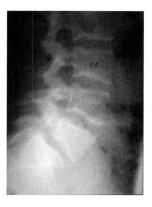

Figure 8 Spondylolysis and spondylolisthesis. Note the horizontal sacrum and acute lumbosacral angle. The body of L5 is wedged, and a spondylolysis is apparent at L5.

general population varies according to various authors; 4% to 5% is a reasonable figure (Fig. 8).

It occurs three times as often in men as in women. Only three cases have been described in infancy, and no intra-uterine cases have been described. The majority of cases of spondylolisthesis seem to appear between ages 5 and 15, with 5% of the adolescent population over the age of 15 having the condition. It does not appear to occur de novo after the age of 20, although obviously posttraumatic, postsurgical, and degenerative spondylolisthesis all occur in older adults. Spondylolisthesis is familial and occurs in 20% to 40% of probands of patients with the condition. The etiology is unknown, but since it is not congenital, it must be "developmental" or associated with either acute or chronic trauma. Spondylolisthesis occurs in association with a number of other spinal anomalies, including spondylolysis, which occurs in at least one-third of cases of spondylolisthesis. Similarly, spina bifida is seen in 50% to 75% of patients with spondylolisthesis, and scoliosis with a range of 14% to 60% spinal curvature

(mean, 27°) has been described in association with spondylolisthesis in up to 50% of patients. Most of the curves seen in association with spondylolisthesis are small and postural and will correct themselves once the spondylolisthesis has been corrected.

Classification

Wiltse (3) was the first person to attempt to classify spondylolisthesis. He suggested five categories:

1. Dysplastic
2. Isthmic
3. Degenerative
4. Traumatic
5. Pathologic

However, more recently a number of authors have postulated that the dysplastic type of spondylolisthesis, which is due to elongated posterior elements of the spine, will progress and become the isthmic variety associated with spondylolysis and spondylolisthesis. An alternative classification that I prefer is as follows:

1. Spondylolytic spondylolisthesis, which is associated with bilateral spondylolysis.
2. Congenital spondylolisthesis, which is associated with a number of anomalies including spina bifida, agenesis of the facets, and a long pars intra-articularis and is rare.
3. Degenerative spondylolisthesis, which occurs almost exclusively in association with degenerative disc disease and is most frequently seen in women 50 years or older and mostly either as L4-L5 or L3-L4. It is rare at L5/S1. It also occurs more frequently in black patients than white patients and obesity seems to predispose to it (Fig. 9).

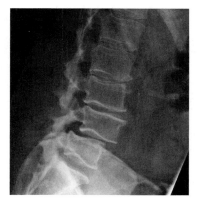

Figure 9 Lateral lumbar spine showing grade I spondylolisthesis with loss of disc height at L4-L5, typical of degenerative spondylolisthesis.

4. Traumatic spondylolisthesis, following a fracture or dislocation, which is invariably associated with fractures of the posterior elements. In 75%, the fractures will heal leaving the radiographic appearance to be apparently that of spondylolisthesis alone.
5. Postspinal fusion and instrumentation, in which spondylolisthesis occurs due to the abnormal stresses exerted above and below the fused segment. It is more usually seen at the level below the level of the fusion.
6. Spondylolisthesis secondary to some pathologic process, such as infection, metastasis, and Charcot joints.

Clinical Manifestations

The majority of patients with spondylolisthesis have no symptoms. However, some patients develop low back pain, and the age of onset of the symptoms will vary between 7 and 23 years, with a mean between 13 and 15 years. Some of the classic signs are a characteristic crouched posture, contracted hamstrings, and low back pain, which characteristically can have a sciatic radiation. If this situation progresses, scoliosis will occur, and this is known as "sciatic scoliosis."

The majority of people with a minor slip (grades I and II) will remain asymptomatic throughout their lives. Many patients with grade III and grade IV slips will have symptoms, including low back pain and tight hamstrings as well as a disturbance of gait. Unfortunately, some of these patients will go on to develop neurologic complications later in life as well as degenerative disc disease.

Radiology

Spondylolisthesis is graded into four stages, with grade I being minimal and grade V being maximal Wiltse (3) describes a grade V slip where the vertebral body above has slipped completely off the body below and he terms this "spondyloptosis" (Fig. 10).

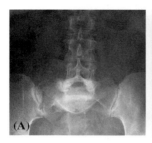
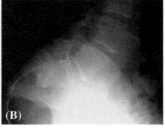

Figure 10 Spondyloptosis. (**A**) AP view of lumbosacral junction showing the "Napolean's hat" appearance. This results from seeing the sacrum directly end on. (**B**) Lateral view confirming that L5 lies completely in front of the sacrum. *Abbreviation*: AP, anteroposterior.

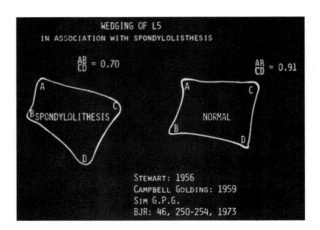

Figure 11 Measurement of spinal index.

There are a number of radiologic measurements that are of importance in this condition. Probably, the measurement that is used most is known as the lumbar index (Fig. 11), which refers to the degree of wedging of the body of L5. In the general population the body of L5 is normally wedged, with the posterior end plate having only 90% of the height of the anterior end plate. However, in spondylolisthesis, the body of L5 becomes increasingly wedged, often with the posterior end plate being only 70% of the height of the anterior one (Figs. 6 and 9).

This index was first described in the 1930s, but more recently, it has been reevaluated for use in the assessment of spondylolisthesis.

Various authors have described special views for the diagnosis of spondylolisthesis, including lateral flexion and extension views. Penning and Blickman (7) used standing flexion and extension lateral views in 24 patients who had spondylolytic spondylolisthesis. A parallel shift of the end plates was not seen, but hypermobility at the level of the spondylolisthesis was seen through the disc space. Similarly, other authors used standing rather than supine films and found an overall 5% increase in the degree of spondylolisthesis (range +31% to −10%) in these patients.

Recently, a number of complications of long-standing spondylolisthesis have been described, including the presence of intraspinal synovial cysts. These are often associated with secondary facet joint arthritis and particularly occur in patients with degenerative spondylolisthesis.

Elster and Jensen (8) described the use of computed tomography (CT) in the diagnosis of 165 patients who had spondylolisthesis out of a total of 2500 patients whose lumbosacral spines they examined.

Seventy percent of the patients with spondylolisthesis had other findings that were apparent on the CT scan; these included spondylolysis, facet joint arthritis, disc disease, and disc protrusion, as well as spinal stenosis.

These authors emphasized that while the primary diagnosis of spondylolisthesis may be based on the plain films, CT scanning is very useful for analyzing the various complications that may be associated with the condition.

Various orthopedic surgeons have stated how they think spondylolisthesis should be managed. I basically agree with their thoughts that are as follows:

1. Patients with grade I and grade II spondylolisthesis who have no symptoms should be left alone.
2. Patients with grade I and grade II spondylolisthesis who have symptoms, but without radicular extremity pain or radiculopathy, should be treated conservatively, preferably with a Milwaukee brace.
3. Patients who have radiculopathy and nerve root compression should be decompressed and fused.
4. Patients who have spondylolisthesis with low back pain and/or radicular extremity pain should be fused.

SCHEUERMANN'S DISEASE AND SCHMORL'S NODES

Scheuermann's disease was first described in 1920, and at that time the cause was thought to be due to avascular necrosis in the apophyseal growth centers on the end plates of the vertebral bodies, particularly in the midthoracic region. Thus, in many of the older texts, Scheuermann's disease remains classified as one of the group of conditions under the term "osteochondritis." However, it is now realized that it is due to a defect in the cartilage formation in the vertebral end plates.

The typical findings of Scheuermann's disease are radiographic and include at least three of the following (Fig. 12):

1. Irregular end plates
2. Anterior wedging of a vertebral body
3. Schmorl's nodes
4. Loss of disc height
5. Separated apophysis

Scheuermann's disease is restricted to humans, presumably because of our erect posture and is aggravated by continued weight bearing, continued heavy lifting, or strenuous athletic activity that produced the changes in the first place. Clinically, many minor cases of Scheuermann's disease are asymptomatic, but there is a subgroup, usually of boys who are often tall and frequently heavy and who also develop back pain in association with the classic radiographic changes; this clinical condition is referred to as "painful juvenile kyphosis." The pain is relieved by ceasing the activity that produces it; however, some of these patients need to be actively treated so that the kyphosis does not progress. Incidentally, the differential diagnosis between Scheuermann's disease and postural round back syndrome

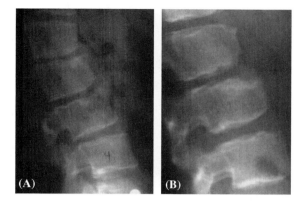

Figure 12 (**A**) Classical Scheuermann's disease. Marked irregularity and wedging of the vertebral end plates and bodies are noted throughout the lumbar spine. L1 and L2 are notably wedged. The end plates of L1, L2, L3, and L4 are all irregular, and there is an appearance of Schmorl's nodes at the upper surfaces of L2 and L3. (**B**) Typical Scheuermann's disease. There is loss of the vertebral edges, irregularity of many of the end plates, wedging of many vertebral bodies, and even wedging of one disc associated with a large anterior "erosion," presumably secondary to anterior disc herniation.

depends on the fact that there are no structural abnormalities in the round back syndrome and that the kyphosis corrects itself when the patient lies flat. On the other hand, Scheuermann's disease has specific radiographic abnormalities and does not naturally correct itself at rest.

History

Scheuermann's disease was first described by Scheuermann (9) in 1920 in a group of adolescent boys who were agricultural workers or sons of farmers living in the southern part of the Netherlands and northern Germany. Scheuermann noticed that their symptoms were seasonal, occurring in the boys during times of strenuous activity such as at harvest time and in the spring when they were tilling the fields. Because of the many farming fatalities, he was able to acquire some histologic material, which he thought showed that the vertebral end plate changes were due to avascular necrosis. However, a few years later, Schmorl (10), on reviewing Scheuermann's material, could find no evidence of avascular necrosis and was really unable to find a specific etiologic factor. Since then our interest in the condition has waxed and waned, but at the moment there seems to be more interest in Scheuermann's disease.

Anatomy

Each vertebral body has a number of growth centers, and there are two apophyseal rings that run around and are adjacent to the upper and lower end plates (Fig. 13).

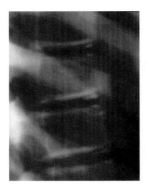

Figure 13 Normal spinal apophyses in a child of 11 years.

These rings appear at age 5 and fuse somewhere between ages 15 and 18, usually at a younger age in girls and an older age in boys. Incidentally, the ring is thinner in its middle than at its periphery.

The overall incidence of Scheuermann's disease appears to be about 5% of the population of whom 2% have minimal changes, 2% moderate changes, and 1% severe changes. The age range is mainly between 20 and 50, although once acquired, the findings of Scheuermann's disease persist. Seventy percent of the patients are male.

Etiology

Scheuermann's disease was first thought to be due to avascular necrosis of the apophysis and thus similar to Kienbock's disease of the lunate, Kohler's disease of the tarsal navicular, and Kummel's disease of the vertebral body. However, no one has been able to substantiate the presence of avascular necrosis, and more recently Scheuermann's disease has been found to be due to abnormalities in both the cartilaginous and bony end plates, as well as in the apophysis itself.

Most cases of Scheuermann's disease are associated with some form of strenuous activity, either agricultural or other work, or associated with sports activities. This activity, which is often repetitive, causes herniation of disc material into the end plate of the vertebral body or actually through the end plate, causing disruption of the apophyseal growth plate itself. This condition was well described by Schmorl (10) in 1930, and of course a single herniation is known as a Schmorl's node. Multiple areas are known as Scheuermann's disease and are related to heavy work, vibration (woodsmen using chainsaws), strenuous physical efforts, and athletics such as rowing, gymnastics, weight lifting, and waterskiing.

It has been found that the incidence of Scheuermann's type changes increased with the length of time spent waterskiing. Less than five years of activity was associated with a 26% incidence of changes, five years with a 50% incidence, and greater than nine years with a 100% incidence.

Pathologic Findings

Ippolito and Ponseti (11) from the Mayo Clinic were able to examine the spine of a 16-year-old male adolescent with known Scheuermann's disease who was killed in a traffic accident and whom they had been following clinically for four years. They also examined the spine of a similar 16-year-old boy without Scheuermann's disease. They found no evidence of either avascular necrosis or osetoporosis, but they did find

1. abnormal cartilage in the end plate and apophysis
2. a loose cartilaginous matrix, with numerous chondrocytes but containing few glycoproteins
3. abnormal collagen
4. stunted ossification
5. disc material extruded into the vertebral body

Thus, it appears that Schmorl was correct: There is an abnormality of the cartilaginous end plate that predisposes to herniation of disc material either up into the cartilage or through it into the apophyseal ring, or actually into the vertebral body itself. This situation is exaggerated by repetitive strenuous activity, either manual labor or athletics, during which, as the stress loading on the spine increases, there is increasing risk of herniation of the disc up into the end plate, particularly during adolescence.

Clinical Manifestations

Few patients with the radiologic findings of Scheuermann's disease ever present to the clinician; however, there is a subgroup of patients with increasingly painful juvenile kyphosis who presents in the late teens. They are often tall, heavy, male children with some history of strenuous activity, a single traumatic episode, or a continuous stooped posture (i.e., nowadays, bent over a computer keyboard). But on the whole Scheuermann's disease is found unexpectedly on routine spine radiographs frequently in asymptomatic patients. Even on cross-questioning the majority of patients will say they had never had any back pain during adolescence or young adulthood.

Radiology

The radiographic features of Scheuermann's disease include some or all of the following. First, anterior wedging of vertebral bodies should be present in 100% of cases and should involve at least two (usually adjacent) vertebral bodies. This is usually seen in the mid-thoracic region in patients with painful juvenile kyphosis but in the thoracolumbar region in the majority of patients with asymptomatic Scheuermann's disease (Fig. 14).

Second, irregular end plates should be present in 100% of cases. The whole end plate is usually involved, with marked irregularity and fragmentation. However, in early cases of Scheuermann's disease (i.e., in younger patients) there is often only "vertebral edge separation," with separation of the apophysis and little evidence of other changes (Fig. 15).

Third, apophyseal separation should be present in the majority of cases; however, in younger patients, vertebral edge separation is a characteristic finding of early Scheuermann's disease. It appears to be an almost "inflammatory" reaction, with an "erosion" of the anterior margin of the vertebral body and loss of the normal triangular apophysis. In due time, this will mature into simple anterior wedging of the vertebral body and irregular end plates (Figs. 16 and 17).

Fourth, since disc herniation into the vertebral body and end plate is what we are talking about, then Schmorl's nodes should occur, at least histologically, in 100% of patients. In fact, they do occur elsewhere in the spine

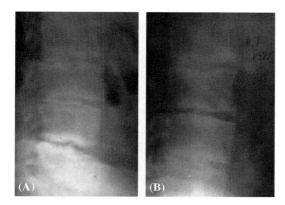

Figure 14 (**A** and **B**) Scheuermann's disease. This is another young patient with almost total loss of disc height throughout the lumbar spine as well as irregularities of many of the end plates. This could represent either Scheuermann's disease or idiopathic chondrolysis.

Figure 16 Scheuermann's disease/vertebral edge separation. Loss of the corner of the end plate is noted at L2 in this 14-year-old boy. This is associated with some sclerosis, and irregularities are equivalent to "erosions." Similar changes are apparent adjacent to the inferior end plate above, and there is loss of anterior disc height.

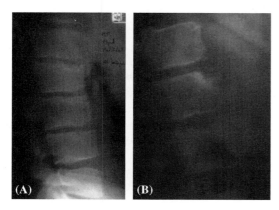

Figure 15 Scheuermann's disease. (**A**) Loss of disc height and irregular end plates are associated with long, thin vertebral bodies, which typify Scheuermann's disease in this young 23-year-old medical student who has no back pain. (**B**) Classical vertebral edge seperation and irregularity can be seen at the anterior margins of a number of vertebral end plates. Characteristically, there is a large defect on the anterior margin of L1, with slight loss of anterior disc height.

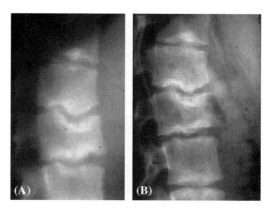

Figure 17 This 40-year-old lawyer had never experienced back pain but came in for an intravenous pyelogram. On nephrotomography, this unusual appearance was found in his lumbar spine and so formal films of the spine were taken. (**A**) The end plates are irregular and apparently dovetail into each other; presumably this represents a form of Scheuermann's disease. (**B**) Tomograms confirm this appearance; note the curious irregularity of the vertebral bodies and end plates.

away from the area of Scheuermann's disease in about 75% of patients; however, Schmorl's nodes also occur in at least 10% of the normal population. Certainly there appear to be more Schmorl's nodes present in patients who have evidence of Scheuermann's diathesis.

Finally, there should be loss of disc height, an inevitable accompaniment of the pathologic process that leads to the radiographic appearance of Scheuermann's disease. Thus, loss of disc height, particularly anteriorly, should be present in 100% of cases of Scheuermann's disease.

Complications

Few true complications of Scheuermann's disease have been reported, although there are some complex interrelationships between various other types of spinal disease and Scheuermann's disease, which will be discussed later.

SCHMORL'S NODES

In 1927, Schmorl (10) described herniation of disc material up into the vertebral body through the cartilaginous end plate (Fig. 18).

This finding was subsequently confirmed by various other authors. The etiology of this finding is similar to that of Scheuermann's disease, although since Schmorl's nodes occur frequently in the normal population and are localized, I assume that the herniation occurs on the whole as a result of a single traumatic episode. The reported incidence of Schmorl's nodes in the general population varies from 25% to 40% of all spines but can be as high as 75%.

The characteristic radiographic appearance of a Schmorl's node is a curvilinear indentation of the vertebral end plate, often on the inferior surface of the vertebral body and in the anterior or posterior third rather than in

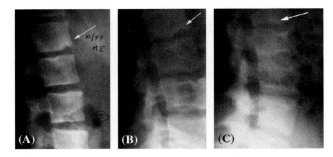

Figure 19 (A) In 1977, this lateral film of the L5 spine shows what appears to be atypical anterior disc hernation (*arrow*). (B) Eight months later, this is beginning to look like a Schmorl's node (*arrow*). (C) By 1979, this is a typical Schmorl's node (*arrow*).

the center. Usually, there is a clear-cut narrow sclerotic margin surrounding the indentation (Fig. 19).

Occasionally, one can follow the progression and formation of a Schmorl's node from a vertebral edge defect (or anterior disc herniation) to a classic Schmorl/s node.

ANTERIOR DISC HERNATION

Anterior disc herniation has a characteristic appearance: A small triangular piece separates slightly from off the corner of a vertebral body and the underlying bone (Fig. 20).

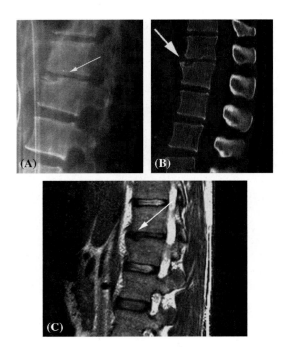

Figure 20 Lateral projections of a young male patient involved in an MVA, showing typical anterior disc herniation (*arrow*). (A) Plain film. (B) CT scan. (C) Sagittal MRI. He was treated as though this was a fracture. *Abbreviation*: MVA, motor vehicle accident.

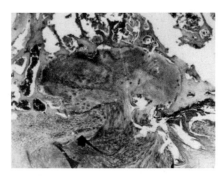

Figure 18 Histology of Schmorl's node. There is an obvious herniation of disc material up into the vertebral body through a hole in the cartilaginous end plate.

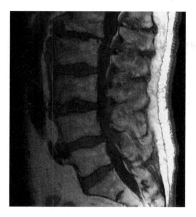

Figure 21 Anterior disc herniation: sagittal MR showing a large asymptomatic anterior disc herniation at L4/L5 (*arrow*). *Abbreviation*: MR, magnetic resonance.

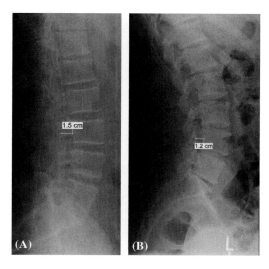

Figure 22 (**A**) Lateral L5 spine showing narrow AP diameter of the lower lumbar spine. (**B**) Lateral L5 spine showing narrow AP diameter of the lower lumbar spine in a different patient. *Abbreviation*: AP, anteroposterior.

Usually, there are sclerotic margins on both sides and anterior disc space narrowing. In an exhaustive review, Hilton et al. (12) autopsied 50 spines of people aged 13 to 96. They found evidence of anterior disc herniation in no less than 76%; it was more common in men and in the lower vertebral end plate and usually associated with anterior disc space narrowing and degenerative disc disease. They found that anterior disc herniation was more common between T10 and L1 than between L2 and L5 (Fig. 21).

Similarly, Kozlowski (13), in a review article, found that anterior disc herniation was due to rupture of the annulus fibrosus, with extrusion of the nucleus pulposus beneath the annulus and through the epiphyseal ring in the adolescent spine, and hence it really represents an anterior Schmorl's node. In his group of patients, anterior disc herniation appeared to occur in association with excessive sports activity or repetitive minor trauma. He found that anterior disc herniation can be seen in 1% of the normal population and in patients with sickle cell anemia, epilepsy (with or without anticonvulsant therapy), patients on steroid therapy, and patients with renal disease.

SPINAL STENOSIS

Radiologically, spinal stenosis can occasionally be diagnosed on a lateral view of the lumbar spine if it is primarily bony in origin. The normal sagittal diameter of the lumbar spinal canal is greater than 20 mm although this is variable. One measures the distance from the posterior end plate of a vertebral body to the front of the lamina (Fig. 22).

However, the lamina is often difficult to identify on plain films in large patients or in those with severe facet joint arthrosis. Moreover, in the vast majority of patients with significant spinal stenosis, the narrowing is caused by a combination of hypertrophy of the ligmentum flavum and hypertrophy and arthrosis of the facet joints with large osteophytes encroaching on the spinal canal from the lateral direction. Thus, both CT and MRI are far more accurate in diagnosing and assessing the degree of narrowing seen in spinal stenosis.

On the other hand, a patient with a wide spinal canal will probably never develop spinal stenosis, however large the osteophytes associated with facet joint arthrosis become.

Spinal stenosis has been described as being of two principal types: central or lateral. The central type is most typically seen in association with a centrally herniated disc but has also been described in association with hypertrophy and buckling of the ligamentum flavum, as well as in association with various congenital conditions associated with spinal stenosis (Fig. 23).

The lateral type can be associated with a lateral herniated disc but is more frequently seen associated with the degenerative process and hypertrophic osteophyte formation seen as a result of degenerative arthritis of the facet joints. In facet joint hypertrophy associated with facet joint degenerative disease, there is narrowing of the lateral recess where the dural sac and root sleeves emerge (Fig. 23).

Spinal stenosis has been seen in association with many different diseases and conditions and is probably best classified as being of either congenital or acquired origin.

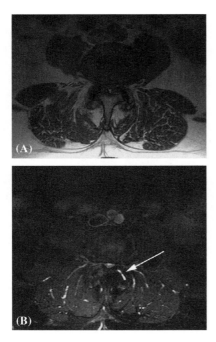

Figure 23 Similar axial MR slices of the lower lumbar region to show spinal stenosis. (**A**) Proton density image showing hypertrophy of the ligamentum flavum and severe facet joint arthrosis. (**B**) Fat Sat T1 image confirms these findings. Note the facet joint hypertrophy and fluid on the left (*arrow*). *Abbreviations*: MR, magnetic resonance, Fat Sat T1, fat saturated T1-weighted image.

THE LUMBAR INTERVERTEBRAL DISCS

The discs act as buffers between one vertebral body and the next. Obviously, those in the lumbar spine take more weight than those higher up in the spine and hence degenerative disc disease largely occurs in the cervical region where there is more motion and in the lumbar region where there is more weight. Each disc consists of a central hydrated core known as the nucleus pulposus and an outer primarily fibrous tissue rim called the annulus fibrosis (Fig. 24).

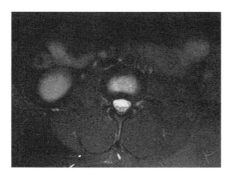

Figure 24 Normal disc. Note the high signal in the nucleus pulposis surrounded by the lower signal in the fibrous tissue annulus fibrosis.

There are many causes of degenerative disc disease, although a significant percentage follows trauma to the spine; however, there is also a hereditary association. At the age of 40, most discs remain well-hydrated but there is a gradual decline as one ages. This becomes readily apparent

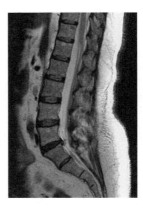

Figure 25 Disc dessication in a 50-year-old female patient. The discs are normal down to L4/L5, which is somewhat darker, and L5/S1, which is herniated posteriorly and is black due to dessication of the disc.

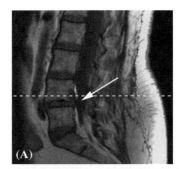

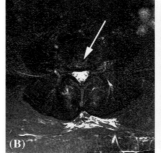
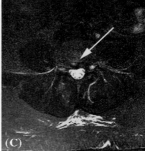

Figure 26 Herniated L4/L5 disc, which remains contiguous with the disc space but lies mainly behind the L4 body compressing the cauda equina. (**A**) Sagittal MRI showing the disc herniation. (**B**) Axial T1 Fat Sat at the level of L5 disc showing same high signal suggested a cleft in the annulus fibrosis (*arrow*). (**C**) Axial T1 Fat Sat at a higher level showing the actual disc (*arrow*). *Abbreviations*: Fat Sat T1, fat saturated T1-weighted image; MRI, magnetic resonance imaging.

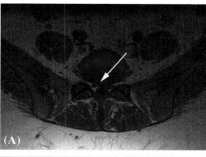

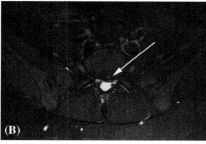

Figure 27 Disc herniation in a different patient. (**A**) Axial PD image shows a definite paracentral disc bulge (*arrow*). (**B**) Axial Fat Sat T1 image shows the herniated disc as high signal (*arrow*). *Abbreviations*: PD, proton density; Fat Sat T1, fat saturated T1-weighted image.

on sagittal T2 lumbosacral spine MRIs where, instead of the disc being of high signal, it starts to lose its normal signal intensity and becomes desiccated. This can be seen as a normal aging process but will occur earlier if there is recurrent trauma, or if the patient is on various drugs of which the corticosteroids are the best example, and if degenerative disc disease runs in the family (Fig. 25).

If a more acute event occurs in a younger patient and the disc prolapses, then the nucleus pulposus usually does so by bursting through the annulus fibrosis. The nucleus pulposus can herniate (slip) in any direction, although they usually tend to slip anteriorly, which usually produces few symptoms, or posteriorly, where they usually become symptomatic. In younger patients, a cleft can be seen running through the annulus fibrosis through which the nucleus pulposus has become extruded (Figs. 26 and 27).

In most patients, this cleft heals and the slipped disc becomes separated and sequestered. It can migrate up or down in the spinal canal, often causing radicular symptoms.

In older patients, it is more usual to see the annulus fibrosis bulge in one direction or another or all around. Central posterior bulges may or may not cause symptoms but paracentral bulges often encroach on the intervertebral foramen and displace or actually compress the nerve root as it exits obviously leading to reticular symptoms usually of acute onset. Finally, a disc may collapse completely and the fragments become resorbed when all one sees is a collapsed disc space without either a herniated disc or a bulge. On a plain film, this situation will usually present as discogenic vertebral sclerosis.

REFERENCES

1. Roche MB, Rowe CG. Incidence of separate neural arch and coincident bone variations. Anat Rec 1951; 109: 233–235.
2. Rossi F. Spondylolysis, spondylolisthesis and sports. J Sports Med Phys Fitness 1978; 18:317–340.
3. Wiltse LL. Etiology of spondylolisthesis. Clin Orthop 1957; 10:48–58.
4. Ogilvie JW, Sherman J. Spondylolysis in Scheuermann's disease. Spine 1987; 12:251–253.
5. Pierce ME. Spondylolysis: what does it mean? Australas Radiol 1987; 31:391–394.
6. Collier DB, Johnson RP, Carrera GF. Painful spondylolysis or spondylolisthesis studied by radiography and single proton emission computed tomography. Radiology 1985; 154:207–211.
7. Penning L, Blickman JR. Instability in lumbar spondylolisthesis: a radiologic study of several concepts. AJR Am J Roentgenol 1980; 134(2):293–301.
8. Elster AD, Jensen KM. Computed Tomography of spondylolisthesis: patterns of associated pathology. J Comput Assist Tomogr 1985; 9:867–874.
9. Scheuermann HW. Dorsalis juvenilis. Ugesk Laeger 1920; 82:385–393.
10. Schmorl G. Die pathogenese the juvenilen kyphose. Fortshr Geb Rontgenstr Nuklearmed Erganzungsband 1930; 41:359.
11. Ippolito E, Ponseti IV. Juvenile kyphosis. JBJS 1981; 63A:175–182.
12. Hilton RC, Ball J, Been RT. Vertebral end-plate lesions (Schmorl's nodes) in the dorsolumbar spine. Ann Rheum Dis 1976; 35:127–132.
13. Kozlowski K. Anterior intervertebral disc herniations. Fortschr Geb Rontgenstr Nuclearmed Erganzungsband 1978; 129:47–49.

Index